ALLE ZEIT WACH
SJ
1842

Therapy of Feto-Placental Insufficiency

I. International Symposium
Parma, May 19th and 20th 1973

Edited by B. Salvadori

With 263 Figures

Springer-Verlag
Berlin Heidelberg New York 1975

Professor Dr. BRUNO SALVADORI
Istituto di Clinica Ostetrica e Ginecologica, Parma, Italy

ISBN-13: 978-3-642-66010-8 e-ISBN-13: 978-3-642-66008-5
DOI: 10.1007/978-3-642-66008-5

Softcover reprint of the hardcover 1st edition 1975
Library of Congress Cataloging in Publication Data. Main entry under title: Therapy of feto-placental insufficiency. 1. Pregnancy, Complications of - Congress. 2. Fetus - Diseases - Congresses. 3. Maternal - fetal exchange - Congresses. 4. Obstetrical pharmacology - Congresses. 1. Salvadori, Bruno, ed [DNLM: 1. Fetal deseases - Therapy - Congresses. 2. Placenta disorders - Therapy - Congresses. WQ212T398.1974]. RG627.T48. 618.3. 74-22028.

Preface

The progess in biological sciences and its applications in obstetrics in the last twenty years have formed the base for feto-placental semeiotics. In this way, it has been possible to diagnose placental insufficiency even in patients whose clinical conditions gave all the indications of a perfectly normal feto-placental condition. On the other hand, observations have shown that in certain conditions some deficiencies can improve until normality is reached again. On the basis of the above one feels justified to talk about the therapy of feto-placental insufficiency. Until now this therapy has been aimed at the obstetrical pathology of the mother. Our aim is to illustrate the various steps which should be taken to execute an efficient therapy of the conditions relating to the pathology of the fetus, realizing full well that fetal pharmacology is only now being taken into consideration. The various steps to be taken, the length of therapy, and all the other correlated factors are still the object of individual experiences, and we are fortunate to have amongst us researchers in this field who have accepted our invitation and can supply us with their personal experiences which can also be compared.

The first international symposium on the therapy of feto-placental insufficiency has been organized in conjunction with the Samil-Pabyrn Foundation whom I would lik to thank, and especially so its president, Mrs. INGE SAXON-MILLS.

The aim stated may seem too ambitious, but we are amongst those who believe that, ambition if well used, can be a very useful stimulous.

Parma, February 1975

B. SALVADORI

Table of Contents

1st Session
Chairman Prof. B. Salvadori

2nd Session
Chairman Prof. P. Quinto

3rd Session
Chairman Prof. BERTACCINI

Participants

Agostoni, G., Ospedale Civile Fornaroli Magenta (Milano) Italy
Ambrosini, L., Department of Clinical Chemistry Istituto Gaslini, Genova, Italy
Andrew, J. D., Red Hill General Hospital Surrey, England
Arnò, E., Clinica Ostetrica e Ginecologica Università Cattolica Sacro Cuore, Roma, Italy
Athanassiades, N. S., State and University Maternity Hospital "Alexandra" Athene, Grecia

Badini-Confalonieri, F., Clinica Ostetrica e Ginecologica Università di Torino, Italy
Baumgarten, K., II. Universitäts-Frauenklinik Wien, Austria
Beaconsfield, P., Royal Free Hospital Liverpool Road, Branch London N1 England
Bellati, U., Università Cattolica Sacro Cuore Roma, Italy
Benassi, L., Clinica Ostetrica e Ginecologica Università di Parma, Italy
Benbassa, A., Clinic of Obstetrics and Gynaecology of Grenoble, France
Benito, J., Department of Obstetrics and Gynaecology University of Barcelona, Spain
Berle, P., Universitäts-Frauenklinik, Hamburg, Germany
Bevilacqua, G., Institute for Child – Welfare and Neonatal Medicine, University of Parma, Italy
Bieling, C., Universitäts-Frauenklinik, Tübingen, Germany
Bieniarz, J., Department of Obstetrics and Gynaecology, Michael Reese Medical Center and the Pritker School of Medicine of the University of Chicago, Illinois, U.S.A.
Bocci, A., Clinica Ostetrica e Ginecologica Università di Torino, Italy
Bompiani, A., Università Cattolica S. Cuore. Clinica Ostetrica e Ginecologica, Roma, Italy
Boog, G., Centre Medico – Chirurgical et Obstetricale de la Caisse Primaire de Securite sociale, Clinique Gynecologique et Obstetricale I°, Institut de Chimie Biologique Faculte de Medicine, Strasbourg, France
Brettes, J. P., Clinique Gynecologyque et Obstetricale Hopital Civil Strasbourg, France
Brigato, G., Ospedale Civile Este (Padova) Italy
Brosens, I. A., Department of Obstetrics and Gynaecology Catholic University of Leuven, Belgium
Brunel, G., 59 Avenue Foch Nancy, France

Cabero, L., Department of Obstetrics and Gynaecology University of Barcelona, Spain
Calaf, G., Department of Obstetrics and Gynaecology, University of Barcelona, Spain
Campbell, S., Upton Hospital, Slough Bucks, England
Carli, F., Pediatric Hospital, Trieste, Italy
Carlomagno, G., Pediatric Hospital, Trieste, Italy
Cavatorta, E., Clinica Ostetrica e Ginecologica Università di Parma, Italy
Cekanski, A., Institut of Obstetrics and Gynaecology of Silesian Medical School, Katowice, Poland
Celasco, G., Laboratori Ricerche e Sviluppo Vister, Casatenovo, (Como) Italy
Ceruti, M., Clinica Ostetrica e Ginecologica Università di Parma, Italy
Cevasco, L., Department of Pathology, Istituto Gaslini, Genova, Italy
Chavas, A., Clinique Gynecologique et Obstetricale, Hôpital Civil, Strasbourg, France
Chef, R., 2e Avenue N° 7, Marcinelle, Belgium
Codaccioni, X., 293 Rue Nationale, Lille, France

COLUCCI, G., School of Obstetrics, General Hospital of Udine, Udine, Italy
COSTANTINESCO, A., Clinique Gynecologique et Obstetricale, Hôpital, Civil, Strasbourg, France
COPPOLA, F., Clinica Ostetrica e Ginecologica Università di Parma, Italy
CROSIGNANI, P. G., Section of Endocrinology, Department of Obstetrics and Gynaecology, University of Milan, Italy

DEBIASI, D., Clinica Ostetrica e Ginecologica, Università di Parma, Parma, Italy
DEGOY, J., Clinique Gynecologique et Obstetricale, Toulouse, France
DELL'ACQUA, S., Clinica Ostetrica e Ginecologica, Università Cattolica del S. Cuore, Roma, Italy
DELECOUR, P., 293 Rue Nationale, Lille, France
DEMEY-PONSSART, L., Service de Pathologie Medicale, Universite de Liege, Belgium
DENZER, E., Krankenhaus Bethesda, Duisburg, Germany
DESOLE, E., School of Obstetrics, General Hospital of Udine, Udine, Italy
DE VITO, L., Ospedale Civile Fornaroli, Magenta (Milano) Italy
DI CHIARA, F.: School of Obstetrics, Ospedale Civile di Udine, Udine, Italy
DITTMAR, F. W., Universitäts-Frauenklinik, Kiel, Germany
DIXON, H. G., Department of Obstetrics and Gynaecology, University of Bristol, England
DIVERSI, F., Pediatric Hospital, Trieste, Italy
DMOWSKI, W. P., Department of Obstetrics and Gynaecology, Michael Reese Medical Center and the Pritker School of Medicine of the University of Chicago, Chicago, Illinois, U.S.A.
DONALDSON, D., Redhill general Hospital, Surrey, England
DRAŽANČIĆ, A., Department of Obstetrics and Gynaecology, University Medical School, Zagreb, Jugoslavia
DUBLER, O., Department of Obstetrics and Gynaecology, Kantonspital Munsterlingen, Switzerland

ENGLARO, G. C., Institute of Nuclear Medicine and Radiotherapy General Hospital of Udine, Udine, Italy

FAVRETTO, R., Clinique Gynecologique et Obstetricale, Toulouse, France
FLYNN, M. J.: Department of Clinical Research, Philips-Duphar, Weesp, Holland
FOX, H., Department of Pathology, University of Manchester, England
FRANZOLINI, L., School of Obstetrics, General Hospital of Udine, Udine, Italy
FREYSZ, H., 8 Rue d'Oslo, Strasbourg, France
FRIEDMAN, S., Department of Obstetrics and Gynaecology, Beilinson Medical Center and Tel Aviv University Medical School, Tel Aviv, Israel
FRÖHLICH, H., II. Universitäts-Frauenklinik, Spitalgasse 13, Wien, Austria

GAMISSANS, O., Department of Obstetrics and Gynaecology, University of Barcelona, Spain
GANDAR, R., Clinique Gynecologique et Obstetricale, Hopital Civil, Strasbourg, France
GARDEY, G., Clinique Obstetricale, Faculte de Medicine, Montpellier, France
GASPARD, U., Service de Gynecologie Obstetrique, Universite de Liege, Belgium
GASPARRI, F., Clinica Ostetrica e Ginecologica Università di Firenze, Policlinico Careggi, Firenze, Italy
GERNER, R., Universitäts-Frauenklinik, Frankfurt a. M., Germany
GINSBURG, J., Royal Free Hospital, Liverpool Road, Branch London N 1, England
GIRAUD, J. R., Service de Gynecologie-Obstetrique, Hotel Dieu, Poitiers, France
GOLDMAN, J. A., Department of Obstetrics and Gynaecology, Beilinson Medical Centre, and Tel Aviv University, Medical School, Israel

Gombert, J., Service de Gynecologie-Obstetrique, Hotel Dieu, Poitiers, France
Grandjean, H., Clinique Gynecologique et Obstetricale, Toulouse, France
Grella, P., Clinica Ostetrica e Ginecologica, Università di Verona, Verona, Italy
Gruber, W., II. Universitäts-Frauenklinik, Spitalgasse 13, Wien, Austria
Guiraud, R., Clinique Gynecologique et Obstetricale, Toulouse, France

Halberstadt, E., Universitäts-Frauenklinik, Frankfurt a. M., Germany
Heller, S., Universitäts-Frauenklinik, Tübingen, Germany
Hochuli, E., Department of Obstetrics and Gynaecology, Kantonsspital, Münsterlingen, Switzerland
Hutchinson, D. L., Department of Obstetrics and Gynaecology, Academisch Ziekenhuis, Rotterdam-Dijkzigt, Holland

Ionaşcu, D. R., Faculty of Medicine of Bucharest, Romania
Irrmann, M., Clinique Gynecologique et Obstetricale, Hôpital Civil, Strasbourg, France

Jakowicki, J., Institut of Obstetrics and Gynaecology, Medical Academy, Lublin, Poland
Janisch, H., I. Universitäts-Frauenklinik, Spitalgasse 13, Wien, Austria
Jasna, I., Department of Obstetrics and Gynnaecology, University Medical School, Zagreb, Jugoslavia

Kides, E., Universitäts-Frauenklinik, Tübingen, Germany
Kieszkiewicz, J., Institute of Gynaecology and Obstetrics, Medical Academy, Lodz, Poland
Kirstetter, L., Centre Medico Chirurgical et Obstetrical de la Caisse Primaire, de Sécurité sociale, Strasbourg, France
Klopper, A., Department of Obstetrics and Gynaecology, University of Aberdeen; U.K.
Koehl, C., Centre Medico Chirurgical et Obstetrical de la Caisse Primaire de Securite Sociale, Strasbourg, France
Koliopoulos, C., State and University Maternity Hospital "Alexandra", Athene, Grecia
Kolodie, F., Clinic of Obstetrics and Gynaecology of Grenoble, Grenoble, France
Krauze, M., Institut of Obstetrics and Gynaecology, Medical Academy, Lublin, Poland
Kunz, S.: Universität-Frauenklinik, Tübingen, Germany
Künzig, H. J., Universität-Frauenklinik, Köln, Germany
Kuvacic, I., Department of Obstetrics and Gynaecology, University Medical School, Zagreb, Jugoslavia

Lamedica, G. M., Department of Clinical Chemistry, Istituto Gaslini, Genova, Italy
Lauritzen, Ch., Department of Obstetrics and Gynaecology, University of Ulm, Germany
Leodolter, S., Universitäts-Frauenklinik, Spitalgasse 13, Wien, Austria
Longatti, A., Ospedale Civile Fornaroli, Magenta (Milano), Italy
Lucisano, A., Clinica Ostetrica e Ginecologica, Università Cattolica S. Cuore, Roma, Italy
Macchia, M., Obstetrical and Gynaecological Clinic of the University of Trieste, Trieste, Italy
Mac Rae, D. J., The Mother's Hospital, London, England
Mandruzzato, G. P., Obstetrical and Gynaecological Clinic of the University of Trieste, Trieste, Italy
Mannherz, K. H., Krankenhaus Bethesda, Duisburg, Germany
Mansani, F. E., Clinica Ostetrica e Ginecologica, Università di Parma, Parma, Italy
Margaria, E., Clinica Ostetrica e Ginecologica, Università di Torino, Torino, Italy
Marzetti, L., I° Clinica Ostetrica e Ginecologica, Università di Roma, Roma, Italy
Mas, M., Clinic of Obstetrics and Gynaecology of Grenoble, Grenoble, France

MASSOBRIO, M., Clinica Ostetrica e Ginecologica, Università di Torino, Torino, Italy
MAZER, J., Department of Obstetrics and Gynaecology, Academisch Ziekenhuis, Rotterdam-Dijkzigt, Holland
MELCHIOR, J., Service de Gynecologie Obstetrique, Hôpital Foch, Suresnes, France
MENINI, E., Clinica Ostetrica e Ginecologica, Università Cattolica S. Cuore, Roma, Italy
MERIALDI, A., Clinica Ostetrica e Ginecologica, Università di Parma, Parma, Italy
MESCOLI, G., Ospedale Civile, Este (Padova), Italy
MOHAMEDALLY, S. M., The Mother's Hospital, London, England
MOLINAS, Y., Clinic of Obstetrics and Gynecology of Grenoble, Grenoble, France
MONETA, E., Clinica Ostetrica e Ginecologica, Università Cattolica S. Cuore, Roma, Italy
MORETTI, M., Institute for Child-welfare and neonatal Medicine, University of Parma, Parma, Italy
MORICI, A., Clinica Ostetrica e Ginecologica, Università Cattolica S. Cuore, Roma, Italy

NAGL, F., Department of Obstetrics and Gynaecology, Munsterlingen, Switzerland
NISI, F., Obstetrical and Gynaecological Clinic of the University of Trieste, Trieste, Italy

PAJSZCZYK-KIESZKIEWICZ, T., Institute of Gynaecology and Obstetrics Medical Academy, Lodz, Poland
PALAZZI, C., Ospedale Civile, Este (Padova) Italy
PANAYOTOU, P. P., State and University Maternity Hospital "Alexandra" Athene, Grecia
PANAITESCU-MIRESCU, A., Institute "Filantropia" of Obstetrics and Gynaecology, University of Bucarest, Romania
PARINI, A., Ospedale Civile Fornaroli, Magenta (Milano) Italy
PARLATI, E., Clinica Ostetrica e Ginecologica, Università Cattolica S. Cuore, Roma, Italy
PEREZ-LOPEZ, F. P., Department of Obstetrics and Gynaecology, University of Barcelona, Spain
PERSELLO, C., Obstetrical and Gynaecological Clinic of the University of Trieste, Trieste, Italy
PIANETTI, F., Ospedale Civile Fornaroli, Magenta (Milano) Italy
PISANO, G., Ospedale Civile, Este (Padova) Italy
PLOTTI, G., Università Cattolica S. Cuore, Clinica Ostetrica e Ginecologica, Roma, Italy
PONTONNIER, G., Clinique Gynecologique et Obstetricale, Toulouse, France
PORRO, E., Department of Obstetrics, Genetics and prenatal care, Istituto Gaslini, Genova, Italy
PUJOL-AMAT, P., Department of Obstetrics and Gynaecology, University of Barcelona, Spain

RACINET, C., Clinic of Obstetrics and Gynaecology of Grenoble, Grenoble, France
REINOLD, E., I. Universitäts-Frauenklinik, Spitalgasse 13, Wien, Austria
REISS, D., Service de Gynecologie Obstetrique, Hotel Dieu, Poitiers, France
RENAUD, R., Centre Medico-Chirurgical et Obstetrical de la Caisse Primaire de securite sociale, Strasbourg, France
ROBERTSON, W. B., St. George's Hospital, Medical School, London, England
ROBYN, C., Department of Obstetrics and Gynaecology, University of Barcelona, Spain
ROMANINI, C., Clinica Ostetrica e Ginecologica, Università Cattolica S. Cuore, Roma, Italy
RÖMER, E., Universitäts-Frauenklinik, Frankfurt a. M., Germany
RONDINELLI, M., Clinica Ostetrica e Ginecologica, Università di Padova, Padova, Italy
ROSSI, G., Department of Clinical Chemistry, Istituto Gaslini, Genova, Italy

SABBATI, M. C., Obstetrical and Gynaecological Clinic of the University of Trieste, Trieste, Italy

Salmaggi, L., I° Clinica Ostetrica e Ginecologica, Università di Roma, Roma, Italy
Salvadori, B., Clinica Ostetrica e Ginecologica, Università di Parma, Parma, Italy
Santi, F., Department of Obstetrics, Genetics and prenatal care, Istituto Gaslini, Genova, Italy
Sarramon, M. F.: Clinique Gynecologique et Obstetricale, Toulouse, France
Scafidi, M., Department of Clinical Chemistry, Istituto Gaslini, Genova, Italy
Scapin, F., Ospedale Civile Fornaroli, Magenta (Milano), Italy
Schafer, L., Universitäts-Frauenklinik, Hebammenlehranstalt, Kiel, Germany
Schmid, J., Universitäts-Frauenklinik, Zurich, Switzerland
Schmidt, W., Universitäts-Frauenklinik, Kiel, Germany
Schumacher, J. C., Clinique Gynecologique et Obstetricale I, Strasbourg, France
Scommegna, A., Department of Obstetrics and Gynaecology, Michael Reese Medical Center and the Pritker School of Medicine of the University of Chicago, Chicago, Illinois, U.S.A.
Serrano, J. J., Clinique Obstetricale, Faculte de Medicine, Montpellier, France
Sieroszewski, J., Institute of Gynaecology and Obstetrics, Medical Academy, Lodz, Poland
Skalba, P., Institut of Obstetrics and Gynaecology, of Silesian Medical School, Katowice, Poland
Spanio, P., Obstetrical and Gynaecological Clinic of the University of Trieste, Trieste, Italy
Springolo, E., School of Obstetrics, General Hospital of Udine, Udine, Italy
Sulon, J., Service de Pathologie Medicale, Universite de Liege, Liege, Belgium
Szymanski, W., Institut of Obstetrics and Gynaecology, Medical Academy, Lublin, Poland

Thoulon, J. M., Clinique Obstetricale du 2. Dumont Hôpital de la Croix Rousse, Lyon, France
Thoumsin, H., Service de Gynecologie Obstetrique, Universite de Liege, Liege, Belgium
Tosolini, G. C., School of Obstetrics, General Hospital of Udine, Udine, Italy
Tykal, P., Universitäts-Frauenklinik, Kiel, Germany

Vadora, E., Clinica Ostetrica e Ginecologica, Università di Parma, Parma, Italy
Vangelista, R., Clinica Ostetrica e Ginecologica, Università di Padova, Padova, Italy
Van Kessel, H., Laboratory of the Department of Obstetrics and Gynaecology, Academic Hospital, Free University, Amsterdam, Holland
Viala, J. L., Clinique Obstetricale, Faculte de Medicine, Montpellier, France
Villemin, D., Clinic of Obstetrics and Gynaecology of Grenoble, Grenoble, France
Vincedon, G., Clinique Gynecologique et Obstetricale I, Strasbourg, France
Vrettos, A. S., State and University Maternity Hospital "Alexandra", Athene, Grecia

Wallenburg, H. C. S., Department of Obstetrics and Gynaecology, Academisch Ziekenhuis, Rotterdam-Dijkzigt, Holland
Weber, H., Universitäts-Frauenklinik, Tübingen, Germany
Wernicke, K., Universitäts-Frauenklinik, Frankfurt a.M., Germany
Willard, D., Clinique Gynecologique et Obstetricale I, Strasbourg, France

Zardini, E., Clinica Ostetrica e Ginecologica, Università di Verona, Verona, Italy
Zichella, L., Clinica Ostetrica e Ginecologica I, Università di Roma, Roma, Italy
Zinelli, G., Clinica Ostetrica e Ginecologica, Università di Parma, Parma, Italy

Plasma Oestriol in Obstetric Disease

A. Klopper and G. Masson

The advent of radioimmunoassay has made it possible to measure steroid hormones in plasma under clinical circumstances. It is the purpose of this paper critically to examine the role which measurements of one such steroid - oestriol - might be expected to play in obstetric practice. Before, however, considering the changes in plasma oestriol concentration which might occur in obstetric disease it is well to examine briefly the implications of a plasma concentration measurement and the factors which might be supposed to have an effect on it.

Plasma concentration measurements are quite a different entity from the urinary assays to which clinicians are accustomed. The latter bear some relevance to the total amount of oestriol produced over the preceding 24 hours while a plasma measurement is only a moment in time, - that second when the blood was drawn. Also urinary measurements are at the end of a series of physiological processes while blood measurements are in the middle. Plasma concentration is a complex entity; a point of balance between many diverse elements. Essentially it is a balance between inflow into the plasma and outflow from it, but each of these is in turn constituted by several different components. Inflow into maternal plasma may be from the foeto-placental unit or from adjacent maternal compartments such as interstitial fluid, which also contain oestriol. Outflow again may be into such adjacent compartments or may be by further metabolism by the liver or by renal excretion. All of these need to be examined critically before it can be assumed that maternal plasma oestriol levels necessarily reflect the steroid production of the feto-placental unit.

Even the chemical entity, oestriol, itself needs to be looked at more closely. We speak as though there were one single molecular species in the circulation. This is not the case. There is unconjugated oestriol which may or may not be bound to protein. There is also a great variety of conjugated forms of oestriol, chiefly oestriol-3 sulphate, oestriol-16 glucosiduronate and oestriol-3 sulphate-16 glucosiduronate. Each of these may, in turn, be protein bound or free. Each steroid moiety enters and leaves the maternal plasma compartment by different processes and at different rates. Should one measure just one of these entities or all? Unconjugated oestriol is easiest to measure for technical reasons and one is tempted to suppose that it might represent foetal activity most directly and perhaps have some functional significance. I propose to examine the choice between measurements of unconjugated oestriol and of total oestriol, that is the sum of unconjugated oestriol and all the conjugated forms taken together, with some care. In the course of this examination it may be possible to glance briefly at the measurement of other oestrogens such as oestradiol-17β or 15α-hydroxyoestriol (oestetrol) but the main choice to be explored is that between unconjugated and total oestriol.

Two criteria are most pertinent to the choice between unconjugated oestriol and total oestriol. The first is how variable the levels are from time to time in the same subject and the second concerns the spread of the universe from one subject to another. Mention has already been made of the snapshot quality of plasma measurements. Unless the value at one moment is representative of what will obtain in an hour or a day, there can be no clinical purpose in plasma measurements. The first consideration was therefore to determine the variability of oestriol concentration levels at short intervals. The data on 5 patients measured at 1/2 hour intervals is shown in Table 1.

Table 1. Variability of total oestriol concentration in plasma at 38 weeks gestation

Thirty minute intervals (12 samples)

Patient	Mean Value (μg/100 ml)	Standard Deviation (μg/100 ml)
A	10.94	1.16
B	14.08	2.56
C	17.93	2.30
D	13.40	2.19
E	23.14	3.70

Average coefficient of variation = 14.8 %

Clearly the total oestriol in plasma, i. e. the sum of the conjugated and the unconjugated oestriol, is stable from time to time over short periods and, in a normal subject, the assay result at one moment can be expected to be representative of the value which will obtain over the next few hours. Whether this concentration changes in keeping with the clinical state in obstetric disease, and how rapidly, remains to be demonstrated.

A second consideration was to determine whether there was any diurnal variation in total plasma oestriol in order to ascertain whether it would be necessary always to take blood samples at a fixed time of day. The experiments examining the possibility of diurnal variations were combined with those designed to find out whether plasma oestriol was altered by activity. Four patients, all at 38 weeks gestation, were used in this trial. On the first day they stayed at rest and blood was withdrawn at 3 hourly intervals for 15 hours. The mean plasma oestriol of the six observations was calculated for each subject and the individual observations expressed as a percentage of that mean. The results of the experiment under resting conditions are shown in Fig. 1.

On the next day a similar experiment was repeated on the same subjects but on this occasion the patients were exercised by walking up and down 3 flights of stairs before each blood sample was taken. The results of assays under conditions of exercise are shown in Fig. 2.

It is evident from Fig. 1 and Fig. 2 that there is no diurnal variation in plasma oestriol and that rest or exercise do not influence the plasma concentration of the steroid.

Of course to the obstetrician the definitive value is that of variability from day-to-day as this is the measurement that is likely to obtain under clinical circumstances. The day-to-day variation in total plasma oestriol was determined in 10 patients measured daily for 6 days. All patients were primigravidae at the same stage of gestation (38 weeks) and blood was drawn from each subject at the same time of day. The results of experiment are summarized in Table 2.

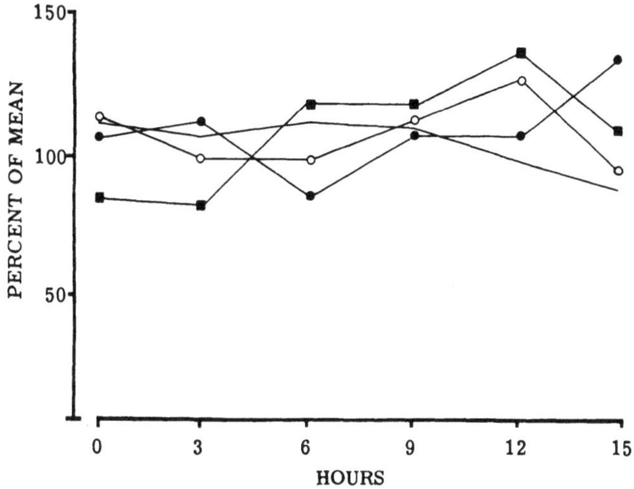

Fig. 1. Diurnal variation of plasma oestriol under resting condit

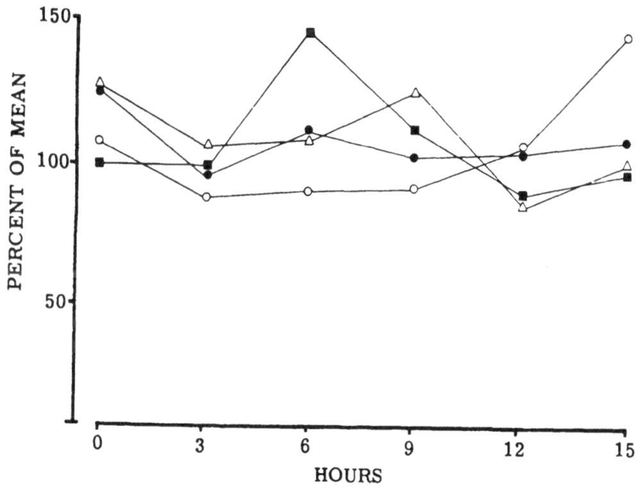

Fig. 2. Diurnal variation of plasma oestriol under conditions of exercise

Table 2. Day-to-day variation of plasma oestriol concentration in pregnancy (6 days; 10 patients)

Group mean value	= 16.3 μg per 100 ml plasma
Average standard deviation	= 1.8 μg per 100 ml plasma
Average coefficient of variation	= 13.2 %

Clearly the day-to-day variability of plasma oestriol concentration in the same patient is of the same order as the variability over 3 hour intervals in one day. There is no diurnal variation and diet or exercise do not affect the levels.

In short, plasma oestriol concentration may be expected to stay reasonably stable from time to time in the same healthy subject and in serial estimations a sustained rise or fall is likely to be indicative of a real change in the conditions determining the plasma level.

Of course serial measurements in which each patient acts as her own control are not always possible under clinical circumstances. The value of one or two estimations can be expected to be proportionate to the spread of the universe, that is by how much one normal woman may differ from another at the same stage of gestation.

In order to eliminate the effect of non-significant day-to-day variations in the same individual we have compared the mean value over 6 days in one patient with that found in 10 similar women over 6 days. The results are shown in Table 3. By way of contrast the variation in urinary oestriol excretion and the unconjugated plasma oestriol is also shown.

Table 3. Subject-to-subject variation in total plasma oestriol concentration (10 subjects over 6 days)

Assay	Mean Value	Standard deviation	Coefficient of variation (%)
24 h urinary oestriol excretion	33.34 mg	9.3	28.0 %
Total plasma oestriol concentration	16.8 μg/ 100 ml	5.7 μg	33.9 %
Unconjugated plasma oestriol concentration	3.3 μg/ 100 ml	1.1	31.9 %

The conclusions to be drawn from this examination of the normal subject are that if total oestriol is measured day by day in the same subject reasonably steady results are obtained but that the variation from one normal subject to another is so large that single estimations can do very little to locate an individual in a category of risk.

The encouraging findings anent serial plasma oestriol assays do little to establish their clinical value. To be of use in obstetric practice such values must not only be steady in normal subjects but must change in keeping with the severity of disease in obstetric pathology. It is inherently improbable that all forms of obstetric disease will affect the process of oestriol biogenesis, or indeed affect it equally. It is therefore of the essence that each form of obstetric pathology should be strictly categorised and examined separately. In the time available it will not be possible to consider many obstetric diseases and we propose to choose a few almost at random.

The first obstetric disease to be examined is pre-eclamptic toxaemia. We have endeavoured to get a picture of the genesis of this condition by doing assays week by week on a group of high risk subjects (defined in terms of parity and weight gain). The average weekly value of those patients who developed a mild pre-eclamptic toxaemia is shown in Fig.3.

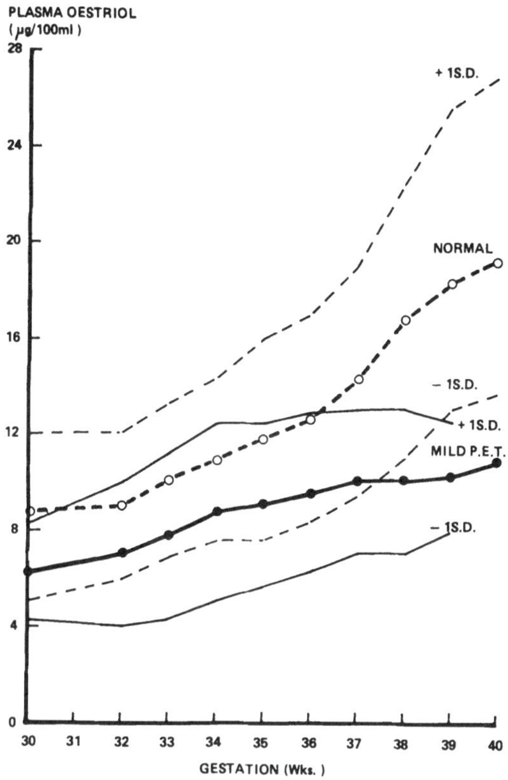

Fig. 3. Plasma oestriol in mild pre-eclamptic toxaemia: mean values and standard deviation contrasted with the values obtaining in normal pregnancy

It can be seen that, although originally the universe of plasma oestriol in pre-eclampsia is very similar to that of the normal, as pregnancy advances the values in mild toxaemia deviate more and more from the normal. The findings in the case of those patients who developed a severe toxaemia is shown in Fig. 4.

In severe pre-eclampsia the changes are more marked and in this condition the mean values of plasma oestriol concentration are significantly less than in normal pregnancy.

The pertinent question in any analysis of pre-eclampsia is whether the oestriol values are dependent on the blood pressure level or whether other factors such as the degree of placental infarction or of foetal growth retardation have a bearing. In a quicksilver disease like toxaemia, changing from moment to moment, often in response to therapy, it is not possible to isolate such factors. We have therefore examined the situation which obtains in essential hypertension where the high

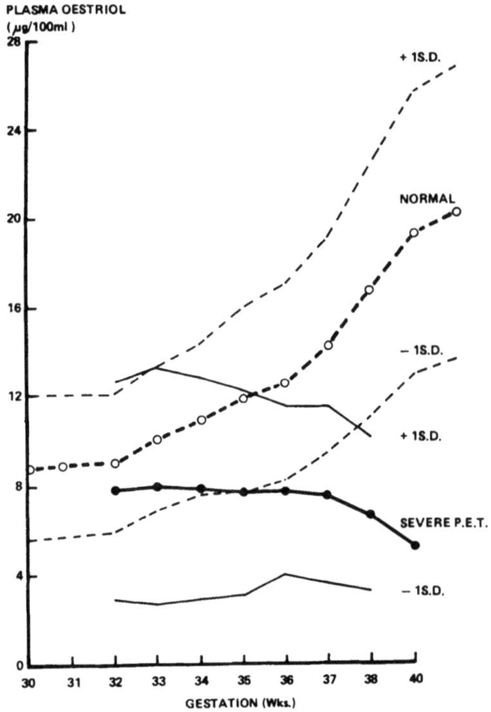

Fig. 4. Plasma oestriol in severe pre-eclamptic toxaemia: mean values and standard deviation contrasted with the values obtaining in normal pregnancy

blood pressure was present from an early stage of pregnancy without the development later of other signs of pre-eclampsia. Statistical examination here shows that the day-to-day changes in blood pressure are mirrored by similar changes in plasma oestriol. The findings are summarized in Fig. 5.

Indeed this correlation is so close that it can be seen from time to time in an individual patient as in Fig. 6.

Of course retarded foetal growth is a frequent concomitant of hypertension in pregnancy and it is therefore proper to enquire how much influence foetal size has on oestriol levels. We have examined the plasma oestriol concentration in a group of women who gave birth to growth retarded babies. Some of these women had a pre-existing hypertension. Others did not. As can be seen in Fig. 7 the presence or absence of hypertension did not affect the oestriol level in women carrying a growth retarded foetus.

Foetal growth retardation is one of the most nettlesome problems with which obstetricians are faced and it has become almost traditional to rely on urinary oestriol assays in this condition. It remains to be determined how valuable plasma assays are in this context. It is easy enough to show that in general the plasma oestriol in women carrying a growth retarded foetus tends to level off in late pregnancy when it should be rising. But before coming to any final verdict about plasma

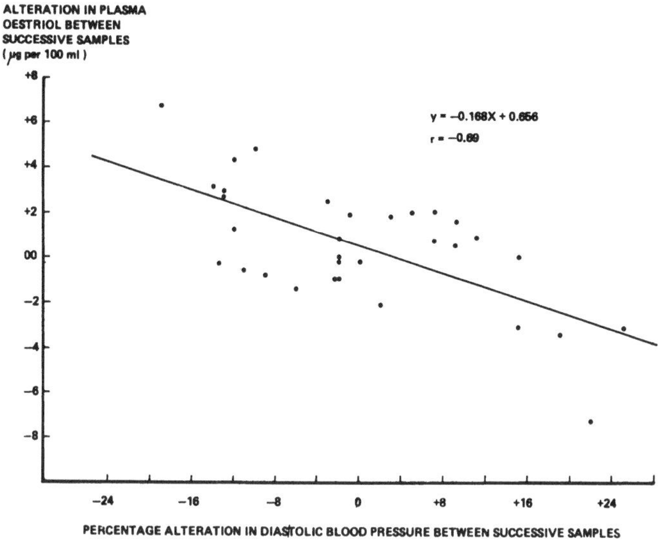

Fig. 5. Relationship between changes in plasma oestriol and changes in diastolic blood pressure

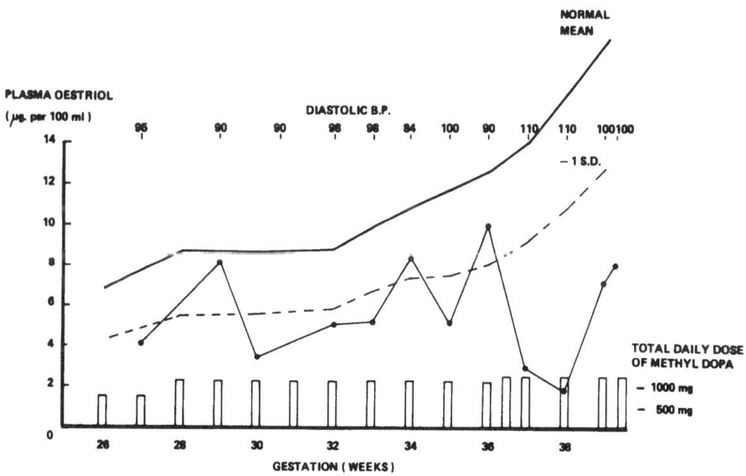

Fig. 6. Relationship between plasma oestriol and diastolic blood pressure in an individual patient

assays in growth retardation it would be well to take thought. Growth retardation is a general expression of many possible causes operating through different mechanisms. It is unlikely that they will all affect plasma oestriol levels equally. It is necessary to split such large grouping into more homogenous fractions; eg with or without hypertensiona, with or without low maternal weight gain, by parity and previous history and whether or not a foetal abnormality is present. When such categorisation

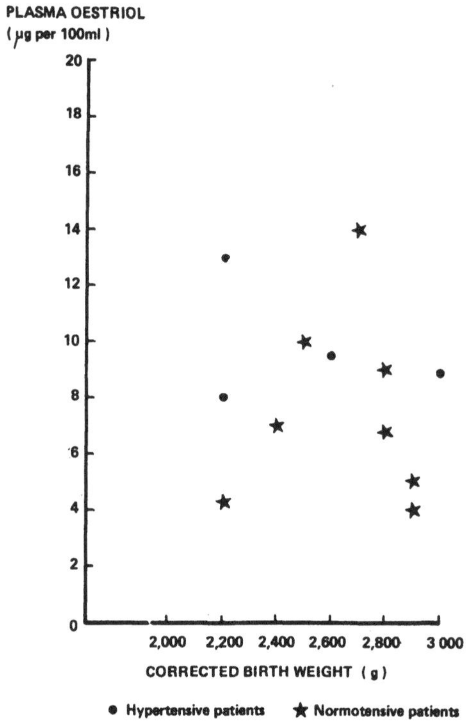

Fig. 7. Plasma oestriol levels in normotensive and hypertensive patients correlated with birth weight

is done the pattern of plasma oestriol becomes easier to reconcile with the clinical findings. Some findings bearing on this generalisation are shown in Fig. 8.

Retarded foetal growth shades into the further problem of intrauterine death. Here too, the findings on plasma oestriol should be assessed in relation to the cause which leads to foetal death. The last figure summarizes some findings on the oestriol levels obtaining before and after foetal death.

Conclusions

It is too early yet to fell a final verdict on the clinical value of plasma oestriol measurements. They have so many advantages over urinary assays that if the order of change is at least as extensive and as consistent with the foetal state as is the case with urinary levels, then plasma determinations will inevitably displace the urinary measurements. One ghost at least has been laid: Provided total plasma oestriol and not just the unconjugated fraction is measured, plasma levels do not have a snapshot quality but reflect a steady state. It may well be that when the foeto-placental unit is adversely affected they change more quickly and dramatically than does the urinary excretion.

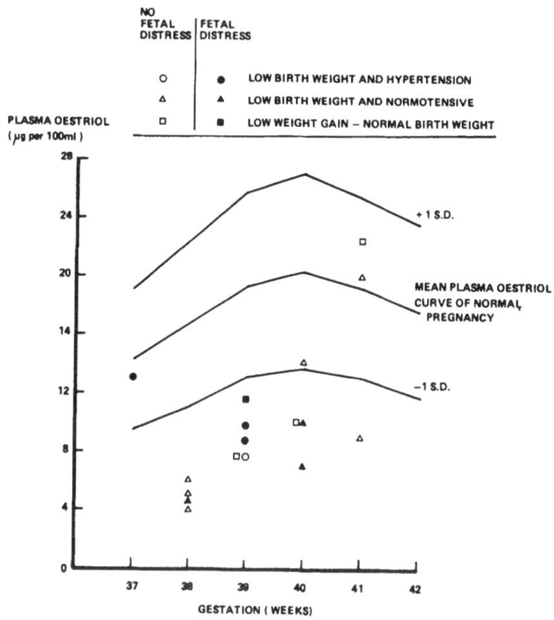

Fig. 8. Plasma oestriol levels correlated with foetal distress, birth weight, blood pressure and maternal weight gain

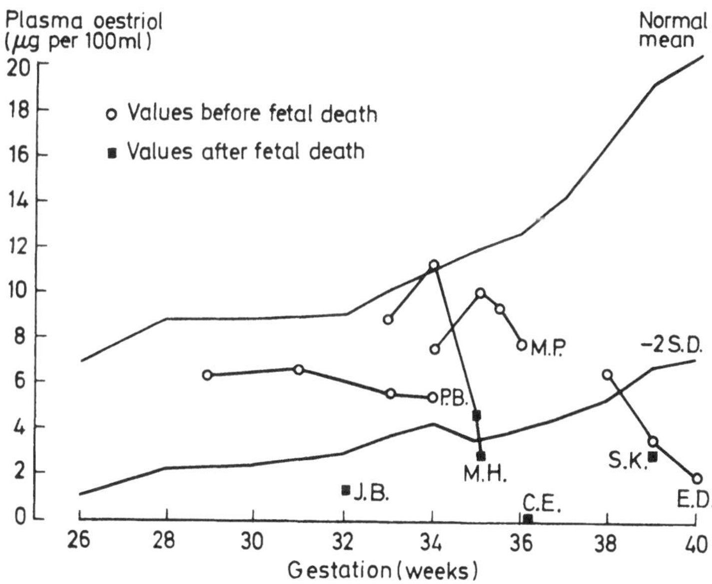

Fig. 9. Plasma oestriol values associated with intra-uterine foetal death

Validity of Cardiotocography in the Control of Feto-Placental Insufficiency. Preliminary Results

G. Agostoni, A. Longatti, A. Parini, F. Scapin, L. De Vito and F. Pianetti

In 12 neonates whose birth-weight was below two standard deviations (Gruenwald values 2), we assessed fetal behaviour during pregnancy by determination of urinary oestriol (by gas chromatography), by hormonal evaluation of vaginal smears and by repeated cardiotocographic tracing analysis (Table 1).

Table 1. Casuistry

Analysis	Cases	Analysis	Mean Number of analysis per case	Mean Number of days between two following analysis
Cardiotocographic tracings	12	138	11.5	2.0
Oestriol	12	79	6.5	3.5
Ormonal evaluation of vaginal smear	12	59	4.9	4.7

Cardiotocographic analysis has been based on a semiquantitative evaluation of the severity of different fetal heart rate patterns 1, 3, 4, 5. (Table 2). The score given to each pattern was multiplied by the frequency of the same pattern found in one tracing (Table 3). We obtained a "total score" which indicates the degree of abnormality of the examined tracing. Finally all recordings have been classified as normal, doubtful or pathological according to the same subjective criterion (Fig. 1).

The oestriol excretion (E_3) has been classified according to the following criteria: normal $E_3 > M-1SD$; doubtful $E_3 > M-2SD$; pathological $E_3 \leq M-2SD$. To ascertain the relationship between the 3 different investigations and fetal behaviour, we studied the correlation between the results of investigations - which have been subdivided into the 3 groups: normal, doubtful and pathological - and the finding, before beginning of the labour, of stained amniotic fluid or fetal death.

Stained amniotic fluid or fetal death is significantly more frequent with foetuses whose tracings are pathological (Fig. 2). Conversely, the persistence of clear amniotic fluid in live foetuses is significantly less frequent when tracings are pathological (Fig. 3). The total scores of the cardiotocographic tracings recorded from "normal" foetuses are distributed in a characteristic way (Fig. 4).

From the analysis of the occurrence of "false-pathological" tests - that is pathological results in normal cases - a good correlation between the 3 different tests is found (Fig. 5).

Table 2. Semiquantitative evaluation of cardiotocographic tracings. Severity score attributed to different fhr patterns

Fhr patterns	evaluation	
Early decelerations Δfhr < 40 bpm	1	
Tipe 1 tracing according to HAMMACHER without contractions	1	
Early decelerations Δfhr ≥ 40 bpm	2	
Tipe 1 tracing according to HAMMACHER with contractions	2	
Variable decelerations Δfhr < 30 bpm	2	
Constant tachycardia or bradycardia	3	
Tipe O tracing according to HAMMACHER without contractions	3	
Variable decelerations Δfhr ≥ 30 bpm	3	
Late decelerations Δfhr < 20 bpm	3	
Tipe O tracing according to HAMMACHER with contractions	4	cumulable
Late decelerations Δfhr ≥ 20 bpm	4	
Late decelerations with tipe O tracing	8	

Also the analysis of the "false-normal" tests correlate well (Fig. 6). It is important to note that the cardiotocographic method gives rise to a lesser number of false-normal results than the other two investigations.

Table 3. Semiquantitative evaluation of cardiotocographic tracings. Total score calculation formula

$$(P_1 \times F_1) + (P_2 \times F_2) + \ldots (P_x \times F_x) = V$$

P = severity score given to the patterns 1, 2, ... x.

F = percental occurence frequency of the patterns 1, 2, ... x in relation to the number of contractions or to the total duration of the tracing

V = total score of the tracing

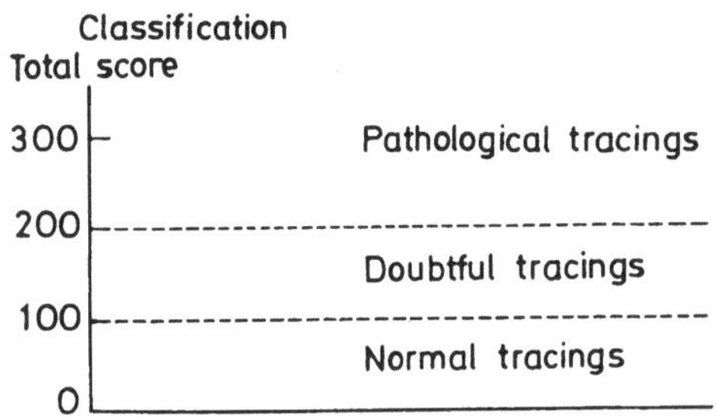

Fig. 1. Classification of tracings. Authors rule

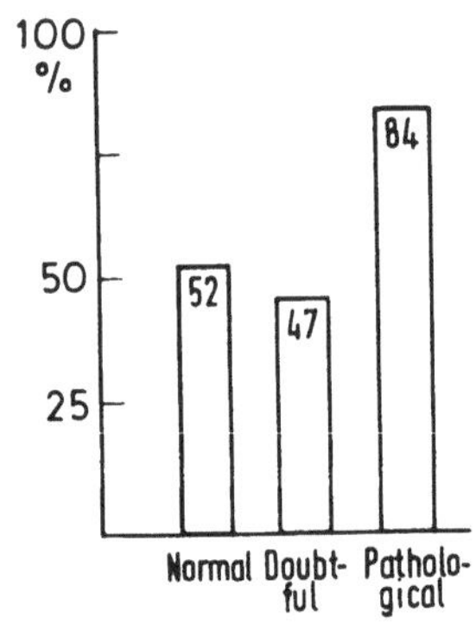

Fig. 2. Percental frequency of stained amniotic fluid or fetal death finding in relation to the 3 groups of cardiotocographic tracings

This analysis supports the value of the cardiotocographic method in the assessment of "risk" foetuses before labour. We present 2 case reports which show the practical value of the method and its advantages over oestriol estimations.

CASE 1 (Fig. 7). Pre-eclamptic state with retarded uterine growth. Measurements were made from the 36th week. Analysis of tracings recorded during the 37th week (Fig. 8) had encouraged us to ignore oestriol fall and we allowed the pregnancy to go on till 39th week. At that stage a Cesarean Section was conducted because of deterioration in the pathological tracings (Fig. 9), although excretion varied little.

CASE 2 (Fig. 10). Pre-eclamptic state with retarded uterine growth and threat of premature delivery. Measurements were made from the 31st week. By the 34th week, although there were no variations in oestriol excretion, pathological tracings (Fig. 11) preceded the finding of stained amniotic fluid, so that inhibition of labour was stopped and delivery induced.

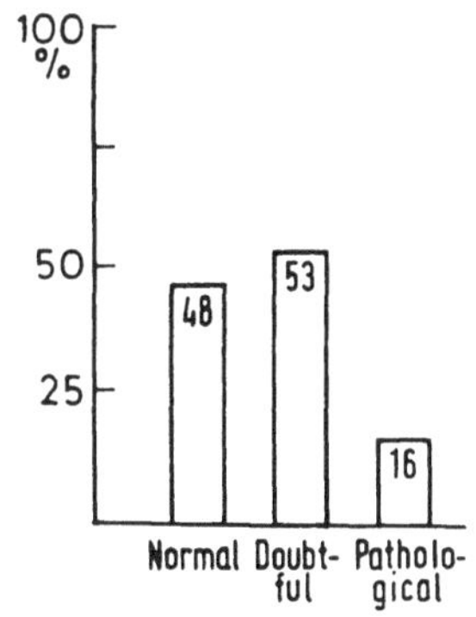

Fig. 3. Percental frequency of persistence of clear amniotic fluid in alive foetuses in relation to the 3 groups of cardiotocographic tracings

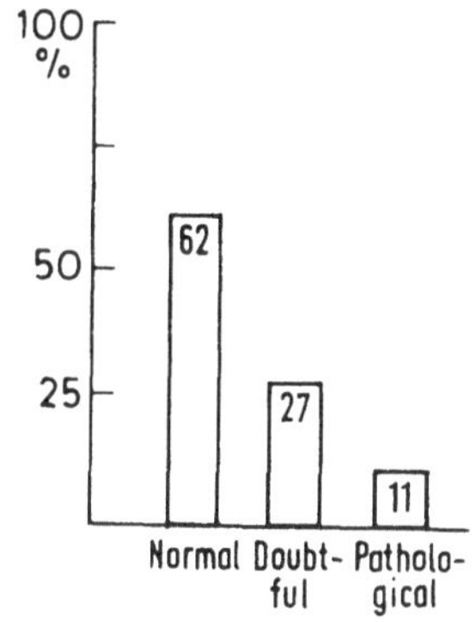

Fig. 4. Percental distribution of "total scores" of all cardiotocographic tracings from "normal" foetuses

To conclude: we suggest that the analysis of the fetal heart rate before labour, in cases of potential fetal distress, is valuable. The limits of the investigation are: 1. uncertain classification of tracings; 2. the consequent subjectivity of the limits between normality and degrees of pathology; 3. the frequency of false-normal results. Regarding the third problem, our experience indicates that more frequent cardiotocographic readings, together with the fetal heart rate and uterine contraction recording for not less than one hour, considerably increase the accuracy of cardiotocography. Variability of results is characteristic of cardiotocography, as it is a technique for giving an immediate assessment of the fetal condition. Therefore each examination should not be considered separately, but in the context of continued supervision. For this reason we judge that the investigation has to be repeated as frequently as the finding abnormalities indicate (Table 4).

With elevated scores (that is more than 400 points) there is no absolute indication for removal of the foetus but for continued intensive observation, similar to the care which is necessary for high risk foetuses during labour.

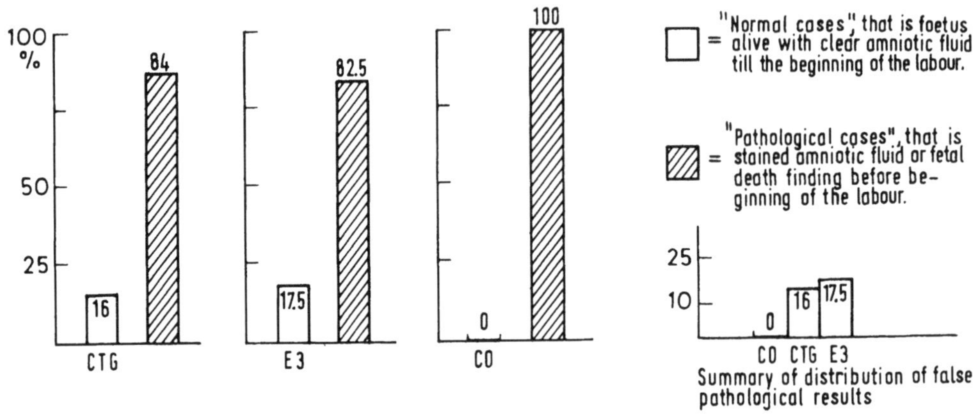

Fig. 5. Percental distribution of pathological tests between "normal" and "pathological" cases

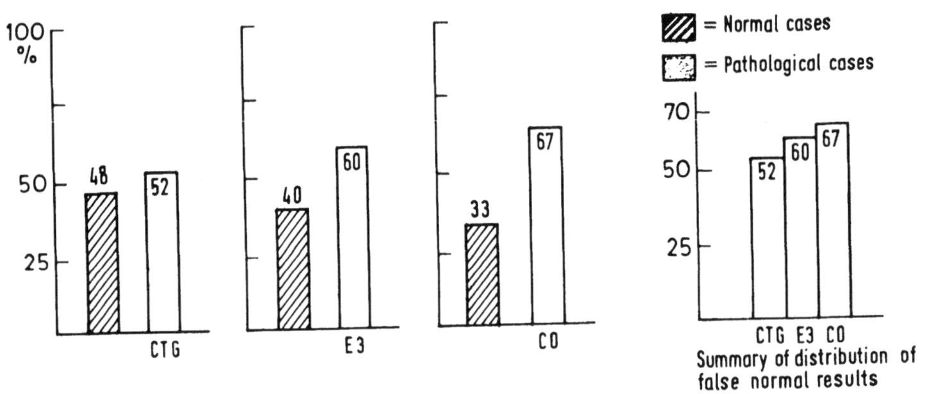

Fig. 6. Percental distribution of normal tests between "normal" and "pathological" cases

Table 4. Practical utilization of fhr recording out of labour

Total score	Classification of tracings	Indication
400	Severe fet. dis.	Continued intensive control
300	Pathological fetal distress	3 Controls per day
200	Alarm	2 Controls per day
100	Doubtful	1 Control per day
0	Normal	1 Control each other day

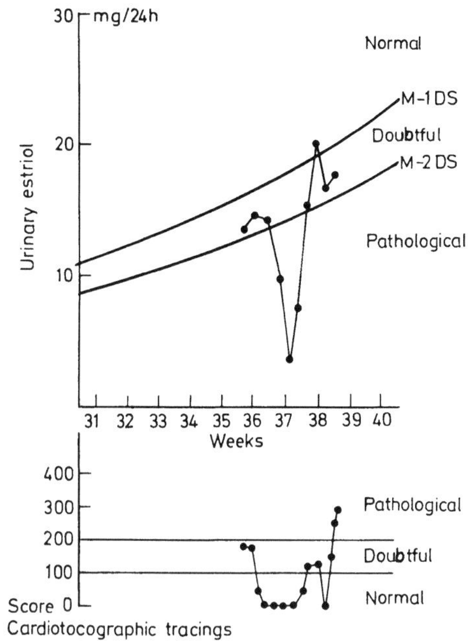

Fig. 7. Case 1. L. W.; age 29; C. C. 8209/71

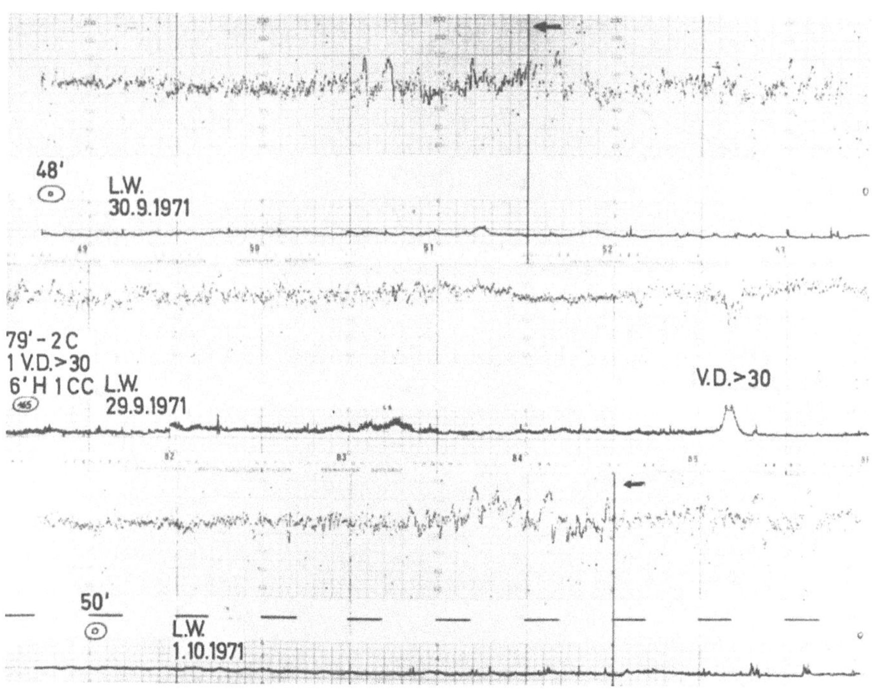

Fig. 8. Case 1. Cardiotocographic tracings of 37th week

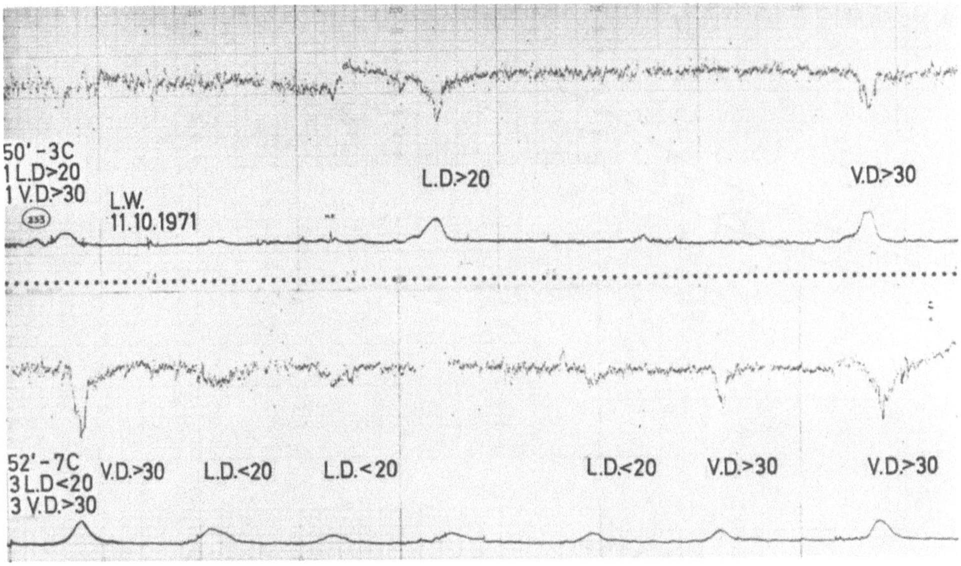

Fig. 9. Case Case 1. Cardiotocographic tracings of 39th week

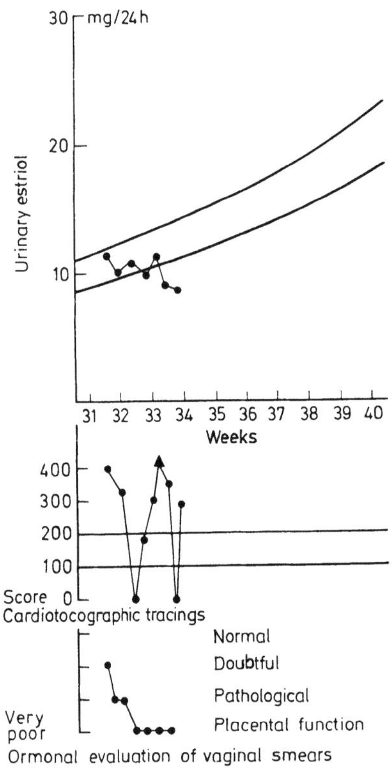

Fig. 10. Case 2

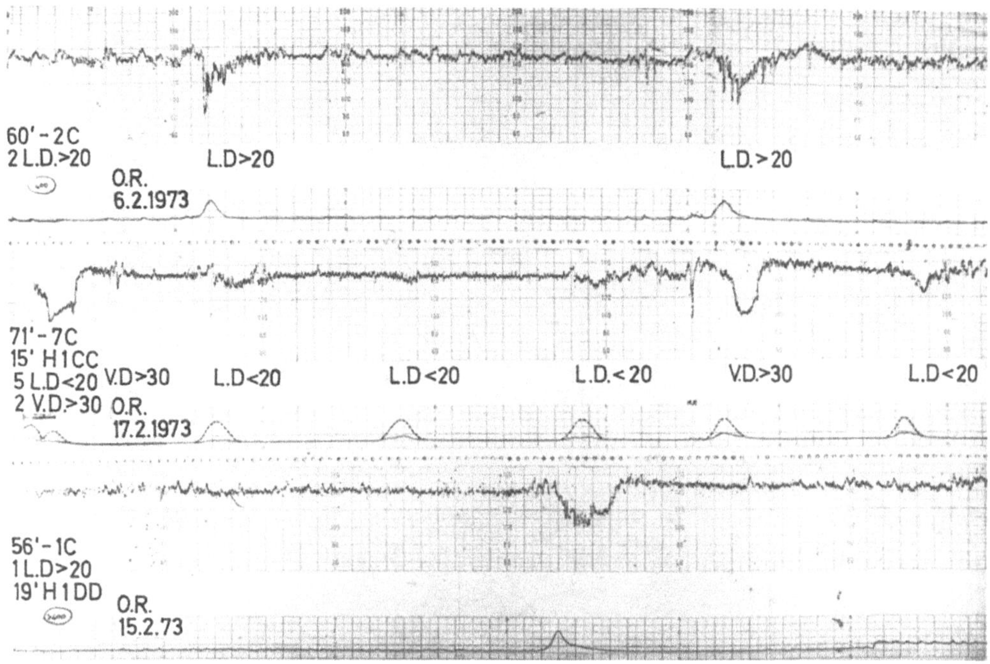

Fig. 11. Case 2. Cardiotocographic tracings of 34th week

The Diagnosis of "Small for Dates" Babies by the Cytological Examination of the Amniotic Fluid

N. S. Athanassiades, A. S. Vrettos, C. Koliopoulos, and P. P. Panayotou

The Diagnosis of "small for dates" babies as compared with those of similar, but appropriate, weight for gestational age, is of great importance because of the different risk and mortality rate between the two groups.

The estimation of fetal maturity by cytological examination of the amniotic fluid was first introduced by ANDERSON and GRIFFITHS (1), BROSENS and GORDON (2), and BROSENS et al. (3). We obtained 112 samples of amniotic fluid from 105 pregnant women at 34 - 40 weeks. The sediment was stained with Nile blue sulphate. If amniotic cells were present this indicated a gestational age of less than 34 weeks and absence of orange staining cells indicated a gestational age of less than 39 weeks (Fig. 1).

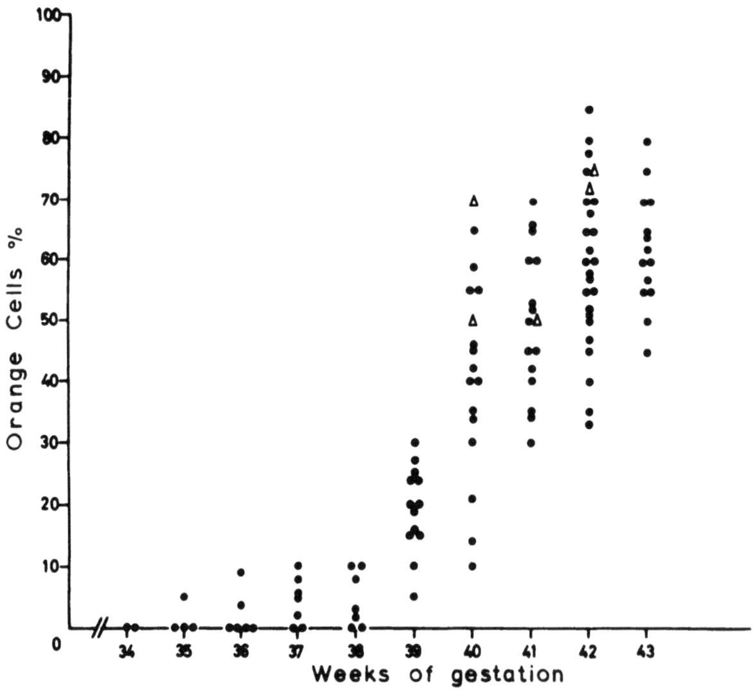

Fig. 1. Orange cell count in relation to weeks of gestation

Orange staining counts of over 20 % suggest a period of gestation over 39 weeks and a count of over 30 % suggest a period of gestation of more than 40 weeks. No correlation was found between orange staining cell percentage and fetal weight (Fig. 2).

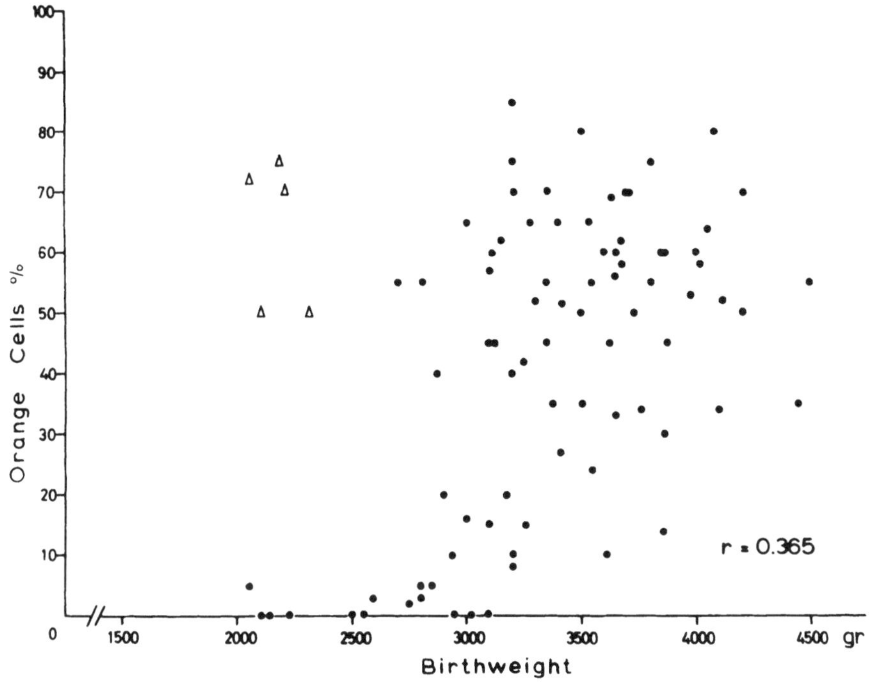

Fig. 2. Orange cell count in relation to birth weight

In a preliminary study we found 5 cases which, calculated from their last menstrual period, were considered full term pregnancies. The cytological examination of the amniotic fluid showed an orange cell count of over 40 % indicating a gestation of more than 40 weeks. At birth the neonates had a weight of less than 2,500 g - i.e. below the tenth percentile of the weight for a gestational age of 40 weeks - and were considered as "small for dates" (4). This observation led us to investigate further the value of cytological examination of amniotic fluid for the diagnosis of retarded intra-uterine growth fetuses.

From the material of our Department we selected 50 cases in labour which, according to their last menstrual period, represented full term pregnancies but by clinical examination had small fetuses. Amniotic fluid was examined cytologically after staining with Nile blue sulphate. Six neonates had a birth weight of less than 2,500 g, the remainder (44) weighing between 2,500 - 2,800 g. All cases had an orange cell count of over 30 % corresponding to full term pregnancies. The 6 cases were considered as "small for dates", because their weight fell below the tenth percentile of the weight for a gestational age of 39 - 40 weeks while showing clinical evidence of 36 - 40 week development.

Figure 3 shows the eleven cases of "small for dates" babies which, although having a weight of less than 2,500 g, had an orange cell count of over 40 %. These findings are in agreement with those of ANDERSON and GRIFFITHS (1) and of SHARP (5).

The results are explained by the fact that the histology of fetal skin is not affected by placental insufficiency. Thus the orange cell count

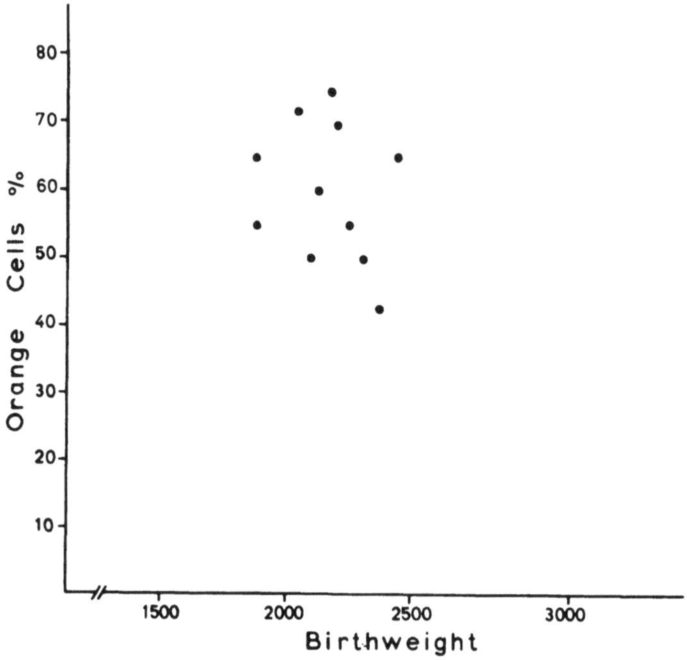

Fig. 3. Orange cell count in relation to birth weight of "small for dates" babies

of the amniotic fluid may have a further application in differentiating the premature fetus from that suspected of being retarded due to placental insufficiency.

References

1. ANDERSON, A. B. M., GRIFFITHS, A. D.: Estimation of duration of gestation by amniotic fluid cytology. J. Obstet. Gynaec. Brit. Cwlth. 75, 300 (1968).
2. BROSENS, I., and GORDON, H. J.: The estimation of maturity by cytological examination of the liquor amnii. J. Obstet. Gynaec. Brit. Cwlth. 73, 85 (1966).
3. BROSENS, I., GORDON, H. J., and BAERT, A.: Prediction of fetal maturity with combined cytological and radiological methods. J. Obstet. Gynaec. Brit. Cwlth. 76, 20 (1969).
4. LUBCHENEO, L. O., HANSMAN, C., DRESSLER, M., and BOYD, E.: Intrauterine growth as estimated from liveborn birth weight data at 24 to 42 weeks of gestation. PEDIATRIOS 32, 793 (1963).
5. SHARP, F.: Estimation of fetal maturity by amniotic fluid extrafoliative cytology. J. Obstet. Gynaec. Brit. Cwlth. 75, 812 (1968).
6. VRETTOS, A. S., KOLIOPOULOS, C., DASCALAKIS, N. et PANAYOTOU, P. P. L'âge de la gestation. Sa détermination par l'examen du liquide amniotic. J. Gyn. Obst. Biol. Repr. 1, 323 (1972).

The Value of the Atropine Test in Therapeutic Orientation during Feto-Placental Insufficiency

G. Brunel and J. L. Vinkler

The treatment of feto-placental insufficiency needs an early aetiological diagnosis and the use of elaborated paraclinic investigations.

Material and Methods

We studied the atropine test in 50 pregnant women during the third term of gestation, using the protocol of IONASCU (4). Correlation were studied with urinary hormonal measurements, cyto-hormonal vaginal smears, biparietal diameter measurements by ultrasonic methods, amniotic fluid study, clinical state of the new-born and systematic examination of the anatomy and pathalogy of the placenta.

Interpretation of the Test

We do not agree with all conclusions of IONASCU (4) and we assumed the following: a normal test implies a latent time less than 15 minutes an increase of F.C.F. of more than 20 per minute, a flattening of oscillations (type 1 or 0). We also define the typical pathological response (absence of fetal response) and the limited response.

Results

The conditions in which we used the nitrogen test are summarized in Table 1.

Table 1

Indications	Number of cases
Overlong pregnancy	21
Small fetus	6
Maternal diabetes	5
Placental endocrine insufficiency	4
Vasculo-renal disease	4
Premature Rupture of Membranes	3
Other indications	7
	total = 50 cases

The results of atropine test are summarized in Table 2.

The fetal response to the atropine test was classified in three ways: normal, pathological and doubtful (the last agrees with intermediate or non typical diagrams).

Table 2. Results of the atropine test in 43 cases

Indications	Result			Total
	Wormal	Pathological	Doubtful	
Overlong pregnancies	10	9	2	21
Small fetus	4	1	1	6
Maternal diabetes	3	2	-	5
Placental endocrine insufficiency	3	-	1	4
Vasculo-renal diseases	1	1	2	4
Premature rupture of membranes	1	1	1	3

Discussion

The value of the atropine test as a standard for therapeutic guidance during feto-placental insufficiency depends on its meaning, its reliability and its harmlessness.

The atropine test is most useful in assaying the respiratory function of the placenta and so allows the detection of anoxia during feto-placental insufficiency. But this test is a poor measure of the endocrine and nutritive functions of the placenta. The test is not entirely reliable. The duration of prediction is not known, but we suggest that 4 days is the maximum because we observed fetal distress 2 days after a doubtful response (a case of false labour) and at 4 days after a normal response (in a case of maternal adreno-cortical insufficiency). When a fully normal response is found, probably there is no fetal anoxia. However, in one case - an elderly primipara with placental insufficiency, meconium staining of the amniotic fluid and a dysmature placenta had a normal atropine response. But when the test is abnormal, fetal distress is almost always present. In one patient we obtained a pathological response but the fetus weighed 3240 g and had a Apgar score of 8 - 10. The mother was a diabetic who went into spontaneous labour at 38 weeks.

We found the best correlations in post-mature infants. When the response is of the doubtful type, reliability is at its worst, because we unexpectedly have had to deliver anoxic neonates and saw dystocia in labour when we had not suspected any abnormalities. We did not treat those patients in whom we had found a doubtful response. Retrospectively we were probably wrong. Atropine was well tolerated by both fetus and mother.

We noted that atropine in high doses exerts an oxytocic-like effect. This is only rarely mentioned by other workers.

Conclusions

The atropine test assesses the respiratory function of the placenta and can warn the obstetrician of fetal anoxia in cases of feto-placental insufficiency. A pathalogical test indicates fetal anoxia and demands active medical or obstetrical treatment.

The doubtful response requires much vigilance and this situation demands a detailed correlative study of the other parameters of feto-placental balance, because we frequently found sub-acute fetal distress in the presence of the doubtful response.

References

1. ORIMAIL, Ph., LUCIANI, M.: Etude du rythme cardiaque foetal pendant grossesse. Epreuve à l'ocytocine et test à l'atropine. Rev. franc. Gynec. 67, 12, 749 - 761 (1972) (bibliographic).
2. HELLMANN, L. M., FILLISTI, L. P.: Analysis of the atropine test for placental transfer in gravidas toxemia and diabetis. Amer. J. Obstet. Gyn. 91, 797 - 808 (1965).
3. HON E. H., BRADFIELD A. M., HESS, O. W.: The electronic evaluation of the fhr . The vagal factor in fetal bradycardia. Am. J. Obst. Gyn. 82, 291 - 300 (1961).
4. IONASCU, D. R.: Dépistage de la souffrance foetale avant le début du travail par une épreuve à l'atropine. Gynec. et Obst. 70, 465 - 475 (1971).
5. JARVINEN, P. A., HIRVONEAU, E.: Value of the intraveneus atropine test as a criterion of placental fondion. J. Obst. Gynec. Brit. Cwth. 71, 740 - 743 (1961).
6. JOHN, A. H.: Placental transfer of atropine and the effect on foetal heart rate. Brit. J. Anaest. 37, 57 - 60 (1965).
7. JUNGE, H. D., LOCH, W.: Die Wirkung von Atropin auf die Herzfrequenz des Feten und des Neugeborenen. Z. Geburtsh. Gynaek. 174, 22 - 25 (1971).
8. OTTENI, J. C., BERTRAND, J. C., FOURNIER, A., PONTONNIER, G.: Médications préanesthétiques. Rapport du XXIIème congrès national d'anesthésie et réanimation. 1972 Librairie ariette.
9. PAINTAR, PH. B., LAURIC, M. D.: Atropine test and postmature pregnancy. Obst. and Gynec. 32, 520 - 524 (1968).
10. RENOU, P., NEWMAN, W., WOOD, C.: Automatic control of foetal heart rate. Am. J. Obst. Gyn. 106, 949 - 958 (1969).
11. RICARDO, L., SCHWAREZ, J. R., NESTOR, L. et al.: Effect of atropine upon uterine contractility induced by artificial cervical dilatation.
12. SANDBERG, F. et al.: The effect of papaverine, atropine, pethidine, relaxin and spasmaverin on the spontaneous motility on different parts of the pregnant and non pregnant uterus. J. Obst. Gyn. Brit. Somm. 68, 1000 - 1007 (1961).
13. SOIVA, K., SALMI, A.: Phenocardiographic studies of the fetal heart rate. Ann. Chir. Gyn. Fem. 48, 5287 - 5298 (1969).

Assessment of the Value of Hormonal Assays and Ultrasonic Measurements in the Management of Placental Insufficiency

R. C. Chef and M. J. Bouche

For the management of fetal high-risk pregnancies, we used different investigational methods (Table 1).

Table 1. Method for the management of fetal high-risk pregnancies

Serial hormonal assays (all the 1 or 2 weeks)	Oestriol Pregnandiol H. C. S. (serum)	(24-hour urine collection)
Dynamic test of placental function (during the 1st and 2nd trimester)	DHEA-S load test	
Serial ultrasonic measurements (all the 1 or 2 weeks)	Biparietal diameter	

In order to assess their value in the management of placental insufficiency (P. I.) and intra-uterine growth retardation (I. U. G. R.), we have reviewed the results of 46 pregnancies divided in 4 groups according to the weight of the neonates on our intra-uterine growth curve and pathological examination of the placentas (Table 2).

Table 2. Material studied. Distribution in 4 groups according to the position of the weight of the neonates on our intra-uterine growth curve and the pathological examination of the placenta.
I. U. G. R. = intra-uterine growth retardation
P. I. = placental insufficiency

	Normal pregnancy	Placental insufficiency without I.U.G.R.	Intra-uterine growth retardation without P. I.	P. I. with I. U. G. R.
Weight of the neonate	Normal	Normal	Below the 10th percentile	Below the 10th percentile
Pathological examination of the placenta	Normal	Pathological	Normal	Pathological
N	29	10	2	5

We have used the following methods:

a) Serial Hormonal Assays

We analysed our results using the method of FRANDSEN et al. (1). The curve is considered normal or pathological according to his profile during the pregnancy (Fig. 1).

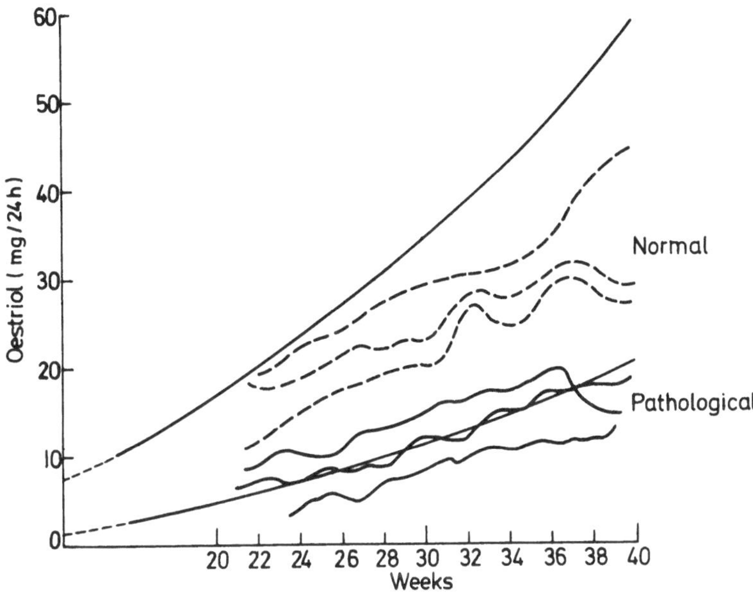

Fig. 1. Serial hormonal assays. Analysis of the results according to FRANDSEN (1)

b) DHEA-S Load Test

We used our method of scoring (2) according to the 24-hour urinary oestriol excretion before the load, the day-to-day variation of the excretion and the DHEA-S conversion rate (Fig. 2).

The score is pathological (danger zone) if it is equal or inferior to 10 during the 2nd trimester or to 15 during the 3rd trimester (Fig.3).

c) Serial Ultrasonic Measurements of the Biparietal Diameter

The curve is abnormal when it falls below the 10th percentile curve of the normal range (Fig. 4).

Score	0	1	2	3	4	5
1	< 1	1-1.9	2-2.9	3-3.9	4-4.9	5-5.9
2	< 0.5	0.5-0.9	1-1.4	1.5-1.9	2-2.4	2.5-2.9

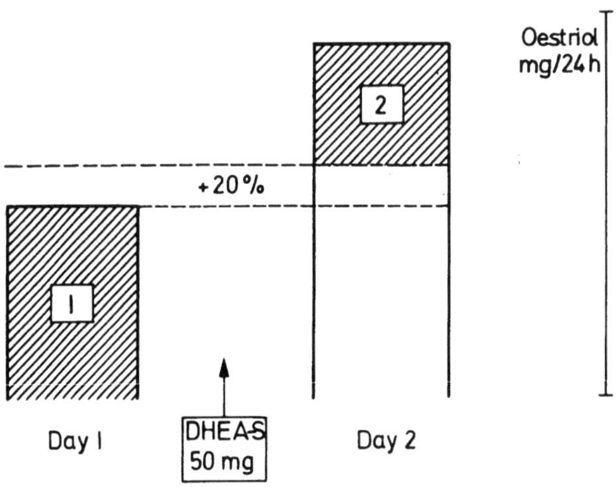

Fig. 2. DHEA-S load test. Analysis of the results according to CHEF (2)

Results (Table 3)

a) Serial Hormonal Assays

1. Oestriol
In the normal pregnancy, the frequency of the normal curve is 93 %. The curve is abnormal in 50 % of the P. I. without I. U. G. R. group, in 100 % of the I. U. G. R. without P. I., and in 80 % of the P. I. with I. U. G. R.

2. Pregnandiol
The results are similar to the first ones except in the I. U. G. R. without P. I. group where the curve is normal.

3. Human Chorionic Somatomammotrophin (H.C.S.)
In the normal pregnancies, an abnormal curve occurs in 17 %. The curve is abnormal in 58 % of the cases of P. I. without I. U. G. R. and in all cases of P. I. with I. U. G. R. In the I. U. G. R. without P. I. group, the curve was always normal.

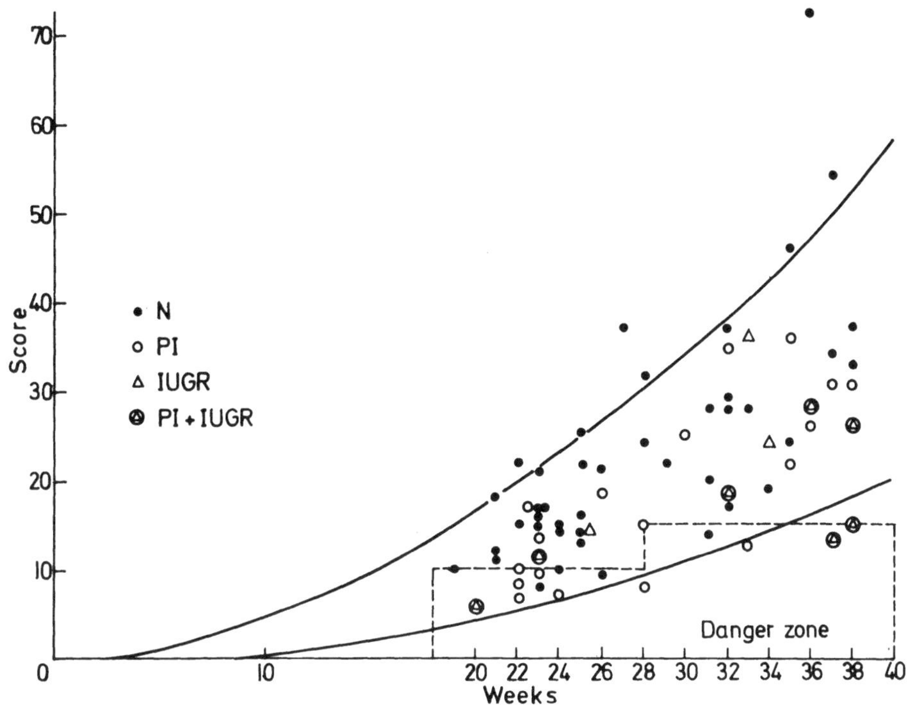

Fig. 3. DHEA-S load test. Results in the 4 groups

b) DHEA-S Load Test

This test is normal in 87 % of the normal pregnancies and in all cases of I. U. G. R. without P. I. It is abnormal in 45 % of the cases of P. I. without I. U. G. R. and in 43 % of the cases of P. I. with I. U. G. R.

c) Serial Ultrasonic Measurements of the Biparietal Diameter

The curve is normal in the normal pregnancy and the P. I. without I. U. G. R. The abnormal curve is found in 50 % of the I. U. G. R. without P. I. group and in 40 % of the I. U. G. R. with P. I. group.

Conclusions

The predictive valve of the serial hormonal assays is very high if the placental function is quite normal (normal pregnancy, I.U.G.R. without P. I.) or very abnormal (P. I. with I. U. G. R.); when this function is moderately reduced (P. I. without I. U. G. R.), the variability diminishes the value of the investigation.

The DHEA S load test does not seem very useful in the diagnosis of the P. I. In the P. I. without I. U. G. R. group the variability is the same (45 %) as in those of the serial hormonal assays (45 to 58 %) and in the P. I. with I. U. G. R. group it is less reliable (43 % and 80 to 100 %).

Table 3. Frequency of the normal (▭) and pathological (▨) results in the 4 groups.
I. U. G. R. = intra-uterine growth retardation
P. I. = placental insufficiency

	Oestriol		Pregnandiol		H. C. S.		DHEA - S		Biparietal diameter	
	normal	pathological	normal	pathological	normal	pathological	normal	pathological	normal	pathological
Normal pregnancy (n = 29)	93	7	96	4	83	17	87	13	100	
Placental insufficiency (without I.U.G.R) (n = 10)	50	50	60	40	42	58	55	45	100	
I. U. G. R. (without P. I.) (n = 2)		100	100		100		100		50	50
P. I. with I. U. G. R. (n = 5)	20	80	20	80		100	57	43	60	40

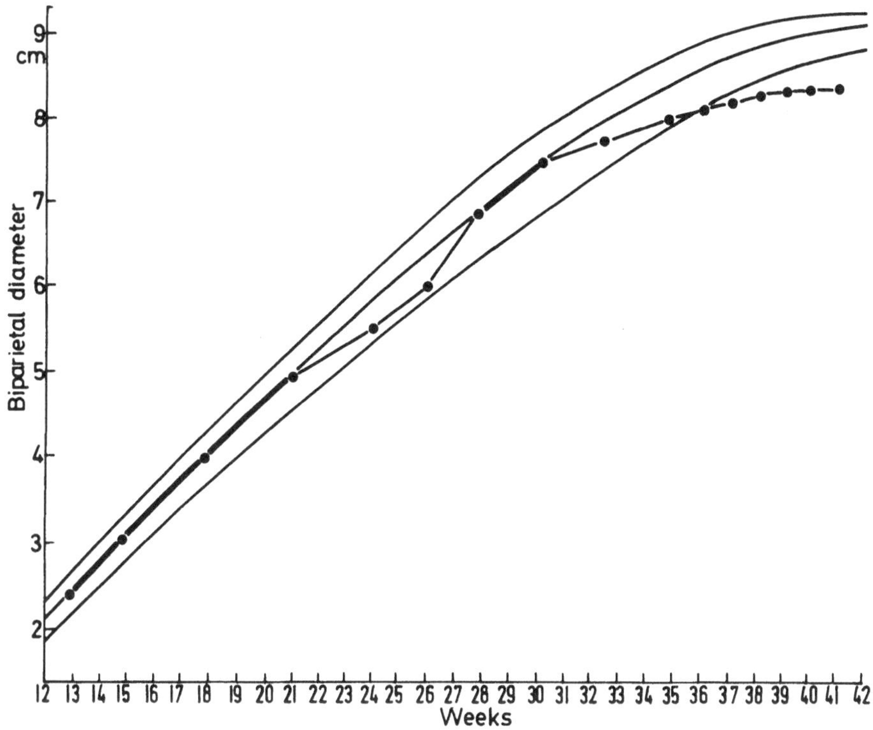

Fig. 4. Ultrasonic measurements of the biparietal diameter. Normal zone and example of pathological curve I. U. G. R. = from a case of intra-uterine growth retardation

The serial ultrasonic measurements of the biparietal diameter allows repetitive assessment of brain growth. The curve is normal when this growth is normal (normal pregnancy and P. I. without I. U. G. R.). In the I. U. G. R. group the normal growth of the biparietal diameter allows one to verify that normal growth is taking place. When the curve is normal, the prognosis of subsequent cerebral function is good, if the curve is abnormal, the prognosis is poor.

References

1. FRANDSEN, V., JORGENSEN, P. I., SVENSTRUP, B.: The adventures of one thousand and one obstetrical patients assessed by oestriol excretion. Annals of clinical research 2, 354 - 364 (1970).
2. CHEF, R., LAMBOTTE, P.: Valeur pronostique du test de surcharge au DHEA-S pratiqué avant la 25e semaine de la gestation. International symposium "Treatment of dangerous conditions in the fetus" - 12 et 13 mai 1972.

Human Placental Lactogen as an Index of Placental Function: Plasma Measurements in Normal and Pathological Pregnancies

G. Culucci, G. C. Englaro, G. C. Tosolini, F. Di Chiara, E. Desole, and L. Franzolini

The object of this work is to confirm the importance of measuring the serum concentration of human placental lactogen (HPL) as a clinical index of placental function.

Material and Methods

470 serum samples were collected from 129 pregnant women to measure HPL. We used the double antibody assay method followed by centrifugation of the precipitate. The results are expressed as µg /ml and were corrected to the Scalvo standard. The kits used were manufactured by Sorin.

Results

With serial determinations of 56 normal pregnancies we plotted a curve which shows a constant rise from the 7th week of gestation to the 37th, and a moderate fall until delivery. The HPL concentrations in abnormal pregnancies were compared with our normal range (Fig. 1).

We measured HPL in 30 threatened abortions: the cases in which abortion was averted show increasing HPL values while those cases ending in spontaneous abortion showed low levels or levels which decrease rapidly. This confirms the prognostic value of HPL in threatened abortion (Fig. 2).

We measured the HPL concentration in four cases of placental insufficiency with intra-uterine fetal death (Table 1). HPL values were below the confidence limits, before fetal death. In 2 cases, HPL values increased after fetal death. In 1 case, HPL was measured about 3 weeks after fetal death and was still present in the serum. We suggest that HPL measurements provide a good parameter of placental function, but are unreliable in abortion. More statistics are necessary to confirm our figures.

In three cases of hyperemesis the HPL levels were normal. In 20 cases of hepatic dysfunction during the third trimester, HPL values fell within the lower limits of the normal range. The 6 most serious cases were below it (Fig. 3).

We were only able to examine four cases of pre-eclamptic toxaemia. In all cases HPL levels were low. In 9 cases of feto-maternal isoimmunization (7 anti-Rh and 2 anti-A) HPL values were variable, without a clear and constant correlation with haemolytic disease of the newborn (Fig. 4). Plasma levels of HPL were measured in 5 cases of prolonged pregnancy (Table 2). In cases (1, 2, 3) with low values of HPL, the fetuses were dystrophic and the placenta under weight. In cases 4 and 5 where HPL values were within normal limits, normal weight fetuses were born and the placenta was normal in weight. HPL concentration may be shown to be of value in prolonged, but otherwise normal, pregnancies to differentiate them from those pregnancies with an ageing placenta.

Table 1. Five intra-uterine fetal death due to primitive placental insufficiency

	Intra-uterine fetal death	Neonatal weight	Placental weight	Serum HPL	Serum Progesterone	Urinary estrogens	Histologic finding
1	during labor 38 weeks	1300 g 38 weeks	300 g numerous infarcts	37 weeks 3.21 µg/ml 38 weeks 2.60 µg/ml 38 weeks 2.55 µg/ml	75.0 ng/ml	12.0 mg/24 h	sclerohyalinosis hypotrophy of the villi
2	30 weeks	950 g macerated 33 weeks	150 g	29 weeks 1.70 µg/ml 30 weeks 1.68 µg/ml 32 weeks 2.60 µg/ml	75.0 ng/ml 82.5 ng/ml 50.0 ng/ml	11.2 mg/24 h 4.8 mg/24 h	fibrinoide necrosis hypotrophy of the villi
3	27 weeks	550 g macerated 31 weeks	230 g	30 weeks 3.28 µg/ml 31 weeks 1.93 µg/ml			fibrinoide necrosis hypotrophy of the villi
4	31 weeks	450 g macerated 32 weeks	200 g partial detachment and numerous infarcts	27 weeks 0.88 µg/ml 29 weeks 1.03 µg/ml 30 weeks 1.25 µg/ml 31 weeks 1.38 µg/ml 32 weeks 1.36 µg/ml 32 weeks 2.00 µg/ml	22.0 ng/ml 28.0 ng/ml 46.0 ng/ml 32.0 ng/ml 36.0 ng/ml	 6.2 mg/24 h 2.4 mg/24 h 3.0 mg/24 h	fibrinoide necrosis hypotrophy of the villi
5	33 weeks	260 g macerated 34 weeks	160 g	32 weeks 2.65 µg/ml 33 weeks 2.70 µg/ml 34 weeks 3.20 µg/ml	75.0 ng/ml 84.0 ng/ml	2.8/24 h	fibrinoide necrosis hypotrophy of the villi

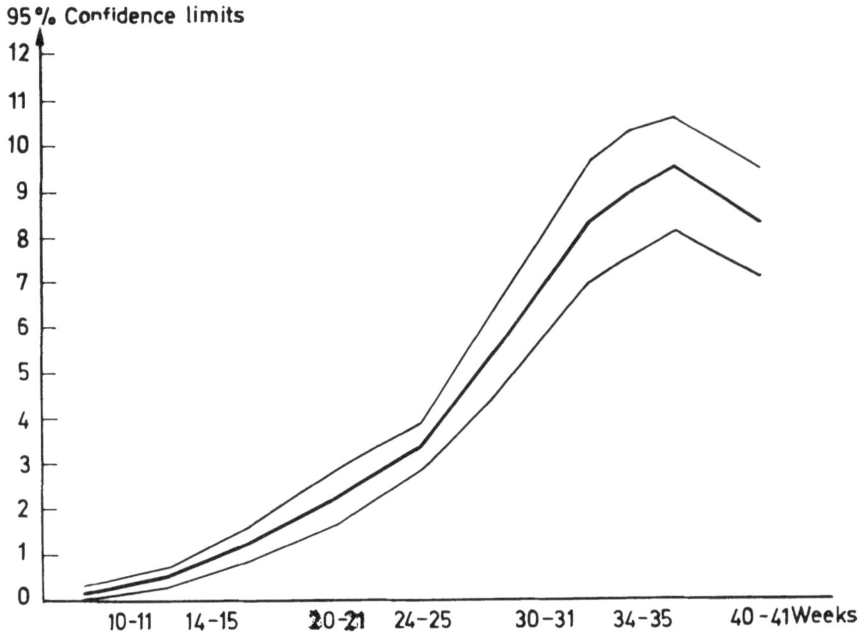

Fig. 1. Plasma levels of HPL 95 % confidence limits

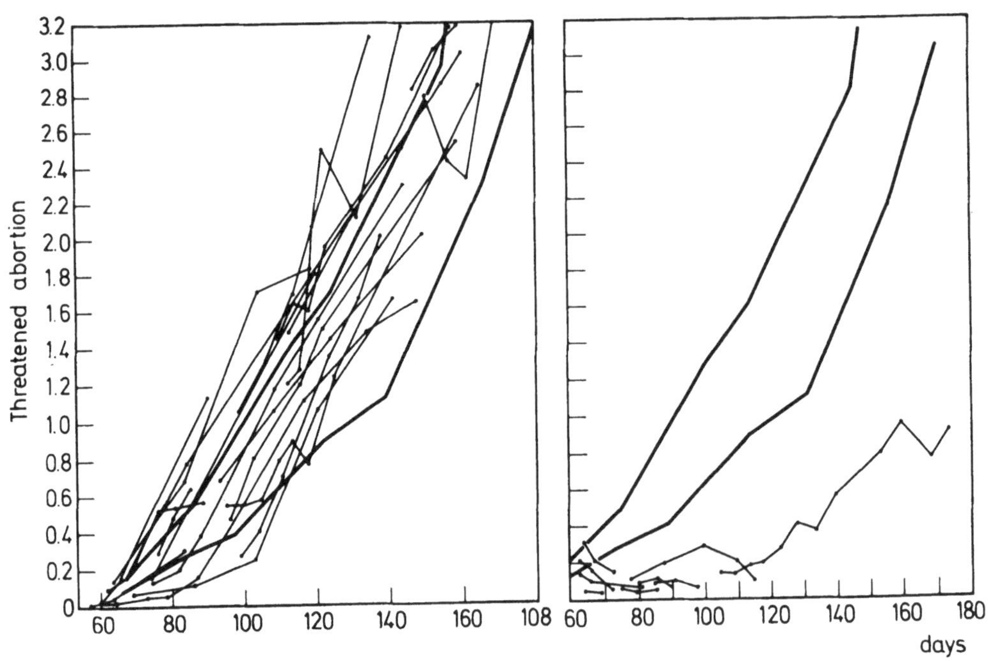

Fig. 2. HPL plasma levels in cases of threatened abortion, resolved favourably (left side) and ending in spontaneous abortion (right side)

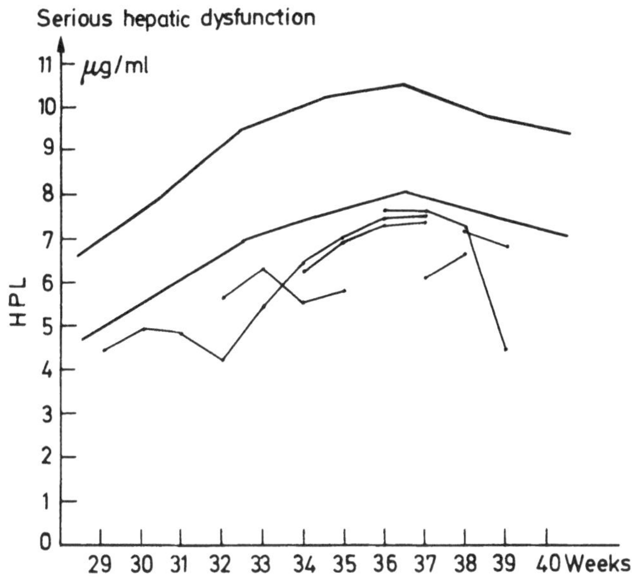

Fig. 3. Plasma levels of HPL in 6 cases of serious hepatic dysfunction

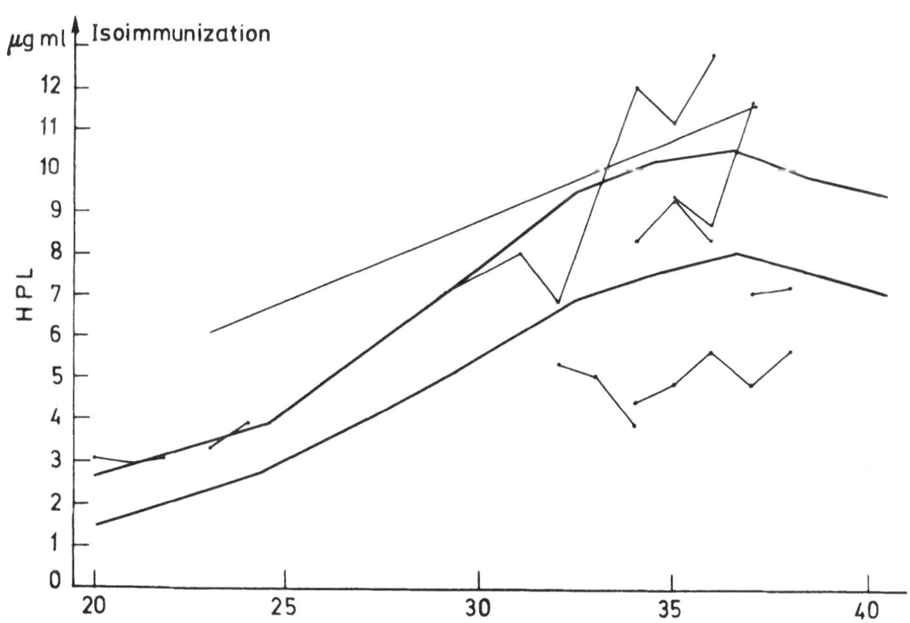

Fig. 4. Plasma levels of HPL in 9 cases of feto-maternal isoimmunization

Table 2. Plasma levels of HPL in prolonged pregnancy

Week		weight of fetus	weight of placenta	HPL (Ng/ml)
1	42	2650 g	310 g	6.15 µg/ml
2	42	2750 g	300 g	4.40 µg/ml
3	42	3000 g	380 g	3.40 µg/ml
4	42	4200 g	600 g	10.50 µg/ml
5	42	3850 g	560 g	9.50 µg/ml

References

AUBERT, M. L., NERI, P., GENAZZANI, A. R., COCOLA, F., FELBERT, J. P.: Methodological aspects of the radioimmunassay of human chorionic somatomammotropin (HOS or HPL) Ann. Sclavo 12/5 - 6, 689 (1970).

COHEN, M., DOMONT, M. BERTRAND, J.: Les grossesses a risque êlevê. Valeur pronostique et limites au dosages plasmatiques de la somatomammotrophine chorioque humaine (MCS). J. Gyn. Obst. Biol. Repr. I, 697 - 713 (1972).

COCOLA, P., GENAZZANI, A. R., NERI, P.: A critical evaluation of the double antibody radioimmunoassay of HCS for use in clinical practice. Folia Allergologica 18.6, 518 - 531 (1971).

GENAZZANI, A. R., COCOLA, F.: Il dosaggio radioimmunologico della somatomammotropina corionica umana (HCS) in gravidanze fisiologiche e patologiche. Atti Congr. su metodi radioimmunologici in endocrinologia. Milano 18 - 19 maggio, pagg. 193 - 215 (1971).

GENAZZANI, A. R., COCOLA, F., CASOLI, M., MELLO, G., NERI, P., FIORETTI, P.: L'importance des traux de HCS comme index de fonctionalité placentaire. Ann. Sclavo 12/5 - 6, 714 - 724 (1970).

GENAZZANI, A. R., COCOLA, F., NERI, P., FIORETTI, P.: Human chorionic comatomammotropin (HCS) plasma levels in normal and pathological pregnancies and their correlation with the placental function. Acta Endocrinolo. suppl. 167, vol. 71 (1972).

FIORETTI, P., GENAZZANI, A. R., COCOLA, F., SCARSELLI, G., MELLO, G.: Correlazione tra trofismo fetale alla nascitae concentrazione plasmatica materna di somatomammotropina corionica (HCS). Min. Gin. 24/12, 609 (1972).

NIVEN, P. A. R.: I livelli del lattogeno placentare come guida alla prognosi della minaccia d'aborto. Bryt. Med. J. (1972)

SPELLICY, W. N., CARLSON, K. L., BIRK, S. A.: Dynamics of HPL. Am. J. Obst. Gyn. 96/8, 1164 (1966).

SPELLICY, W. N., TEOH, E. S., BUNI, W. C., BIRK, S. A., MC. CREARY, S. A.: Valve of HPL in managing high-risk pregnancies. Am. J. Obst. Gyn. 109/4 588 (1971).

NIVEN, P. A. R., LANDON, J., CHARD, T.: Placental lactogen levels as a guide to autcome of threatened abortion. Brit. Med. J. 3, 799 - 801 (1972).

EMERSON, K. Jr., SELENKOW, H. A., SAXENA, B. N.: Serum placental lactogen (HPL) levels as an index of placental function. The New England J. Med., 281/5, 225 (1969).

SAXENA, B. N., REFETOFF, S., EMERSON, K., SELENKOW, H. A.: A rapid radioimmunoassay for human placental lactogen. Applicationto normal and pathologic pregnancies. Am. J. Obst. Gyn. 101/7, 874 - 885 (1968).

SPONA, J., JIANISCH, H.: Diagnosi dell'insufficienza placentare mediante analisi radioimmunologiche della HCG e dell'HPL del siero Wiener Klin. WSchi 84, 385 (1972).

Human Choriogonadotropin, Choriosomatomammotrophin and Fetal Nutrition

P. G. Crosignani

Normal fetal nutrition is largely dependent on normal placental development and on normal placental function. Fetal malnutrition is most frequently caused by deterioration in placental perfusion or by reduction in the exchange area. It has been shown that there is a relationship between normal choriogonadotropin (HCG) and choriosomatomammotrophin (HCS) production, and integrity of placental function. In the intact placenta, HCG secretion appears proportional to the number of cytotrophoblastic cells (1), while serum HCS shows a definite relationship with placental weight (2). These observations suggest a possible association between circulating HCG and HCS and fetal nutrition.

Abortion

About 70 % of pregnancies with threatened abortion have little alteration in the placental function, and the embryo keeps on feeding and growing. If bleeding occurs, both birth-weight and placental weight are decreased (3) and about one third of the cases will abort at this stage. In the first circumstance, the values of radioimmunoassayable HCG and HCS are normal; in the second, the normal or already low levels of the two hormones fall rapidly (4).

Post-term Pregnancy

There is no change in HCG concentration between the 41st and the 42nd weeks, but significantly lower HCS concentrations in the latter pregnancy age-group have been found (6.13 $\pm$ SD 0.34 and 4.70 $\pm$ SD 0.26 μg/ml). The reduction in placental activity in prolonged pregnancy is known often to produce poor conditions for fetal nutrition; the parallel lowering of HCS concentration seems similarly related to worsening of placental function, while that of HCG does not.

Diabetes

Patients treated with elevated amounts of insulin showed normal levels of HCG and normal or low HCS concentrations. Abnormally high levels of HCG have been found in cases of gestational diabetes and in severe diabetic patients with poor metabolic control. In the latter subjects, pathologically elevated HCS levels have been observed.

The well controlled diabetic mothers all had normal weight babies, but it seems notable that, dividing these women in two groups, on the basis of their HCS levels, there is a significant difference of the fetal weight at delivery.

The high HCG concentration supports the idea that the excess of chorionic gonadotropin is associated with a failure of villous maturation

	Range HCS	Low HCS
Cases	9	5
Birth weight		
- mean	3536 g	2976 g
- range	3250 - 3900 g	2700 - 3430 g
Mann-Whitney "U" tests: $p < 0.01$		

(1). Maternal serum HCS concentration probably parallels syncytotrophoblastic mass, and it is known that the number of cells in the placenta of untreated diabetics is greater than in the normal ones, while normal or even low placental mass or activity is related to the insulin available rather than to the severity of the diabetic state (6).

Toxaemia

In 43 toxaemic patients we observed abnormally elevated levels of HCG in 21 subjects and low HCS values in 16. In the "high HCG group" 7 intra-uterine fetal deaths occurred and 7 still-births were observed in "low HCS group". In 12 cases the two abnormalities were associated and the still-birth rate was 50 %. HCG elevation probably measures the reactive hyperplasia of cytotrophoblastic cells to hypoxia (5).

The reason why serum HCS levels appear to correlate well with fetal well-being is still unknown.

References

1. FOX, H., in: CROSIGNANI, P. G., PARDI, G., editors: Fetal Evaluation during pregnancy and labour, p. 33. New York and London; Academic Press (1971).
2. SAXENA, B. N., EMERSON, K., SELENKOW: New Engl. J. Med. 281,225 (1969).
3. PECKHAM, C. H.: Obstet. Gynec. 39, 48 (1972).
4. CROSIGNANI, P. G. NENCIONI, T.: Excerpta Med. Congr. Series 244, 239 (1971).
5. FOX, H.: Amer. J. Obstet. Gynec. 107, 1058 (1970).
6. POWELL, E. D. V., CAULFIELD, J. B., FIELD, R. A.: Diabetes 16, 227 (1967).

The Clinical Value of the Placenta Lactogen in the Monitoring of Feto-Placental Disfunction

F. W. Dittmar, P. Tykal, and W. Schmidt

The experiences from the last time show an increasing value of human placenta lactogen (HPL) in the monitoring of risk-pregnancies. In the University Woman Hospital and School of Midwife of Kiel since many years beside traditional monitoring methods (like Estriol, pregnandiol, chorion gonadotrophin determination), estimation of human-placenta-lactogen in serum is performed.

Radioimmunoassay technique with double antibody system (Sorin) was used for HPL determination. Precipitated HPL was separated with centrifugation. Up to now were 520 determination of HPL in 80 patients performed; in order to accuracy threefold determination were performed. The hormon determinations were mostly regularly performed from 6th months of pregnancy and they were compared with a group of normal pregnancies.

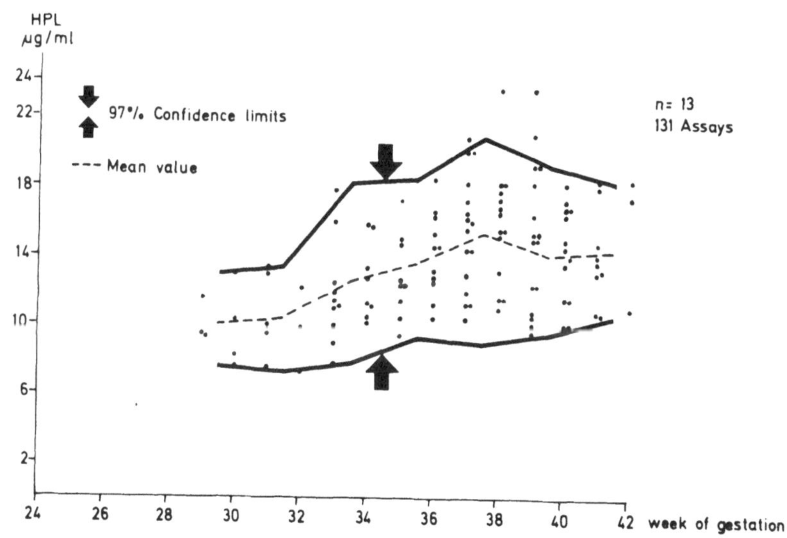

Fig. 1. Normal pregnancy

Fig. 1 shows the confidence limit of the normal HPL levels in serum. The maximum of HPL production rate appears according our studies in the 37th week of pregnancy; and than the fall is connected, t. m. concentration decreasing till 40 weeks of pregnancy is reached. The group of risk pregnancies were divided as follows: EPH-Syndrom, diabetes mellitus, Rh-incompatibility, adipositas per magna, stage after abortus habitualis, gemini, jeopardy of intra-uterine fetal death and placenta insufficiency.

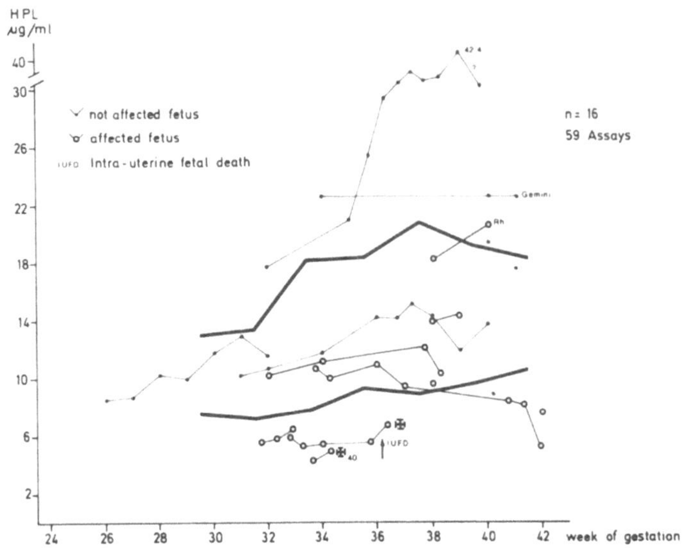

Fig. 2. EPH-Syndrom

Fig. 2 demonstrates the serum HPL concentration in EPH-gestosis. Significant is here a low HPL concentration in serum. In these pregnancies were neonates under the delivery in more danger. The lowest HPL concentration were in pregnancies with retardation of fetal weight (Dystrophy) or pregnancies in which intra-uterine fetal death occured. Higher levels were found in gemini or Rh-incompatibility complicated with gestosis.

Fig. 3 shows the HPL concentration in pregnancies with Rh-incompatibility. This value are in the lower part of the normal range. They tend to decreasing of concentration. The neonates marked with circle received blood-exchange post partum.

The monitoring of diabetic pregnancies (Fig. 4) with HPL determination in serum seems us to be less reliable. This value are almost in normal range. In cases with sharp fall of HPL value or long time constant low HPL value was prompt preterminal ending of pregnancy necessary or the intra-uterine fetal death occurred. The HPL concentrations was low in cases with retardation of fetal growth, in contrary high in pregnancies with big-babies.

Summarized, we can comment:

1. Regulary determination of HPL concentration in serum for monitoring of risk-pregnancies can be recommended.
2. This method seems to be reliable for monitoring of EPH-gestosis, if these is regulary end continuously performed.
3. In cases of intra-uterine, fetal retardation (chronical, nutritiv placenta insufficiency), were the HPL value extreme low and this monitoring method seems to be especially reliable.
4. High levels were suspected for gemini or severe cases of erythroblastosis or for diabetes mellitus.

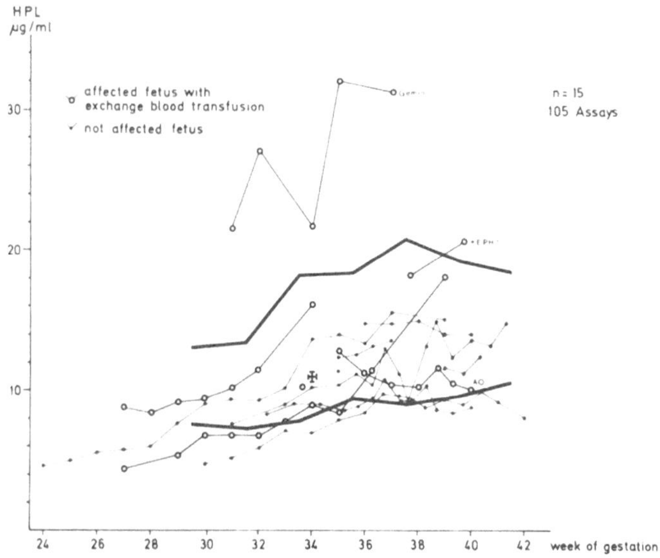

Fig. 3. Rhesus incompatibility

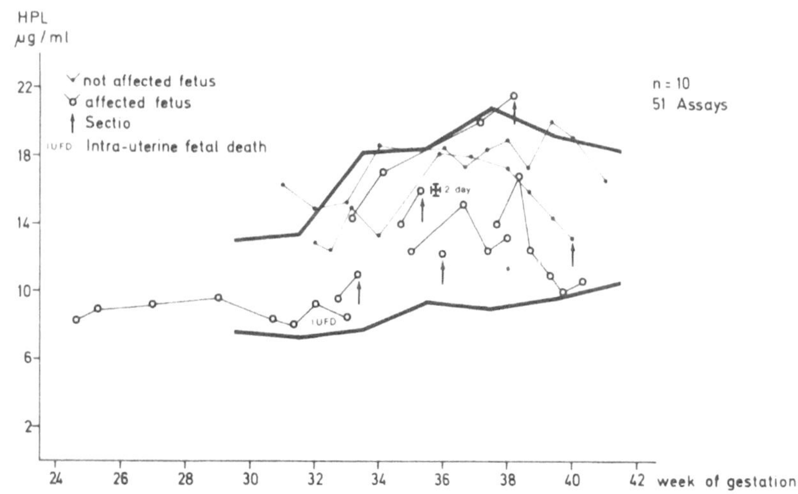

Fig. 4. Diabetic pregnancy

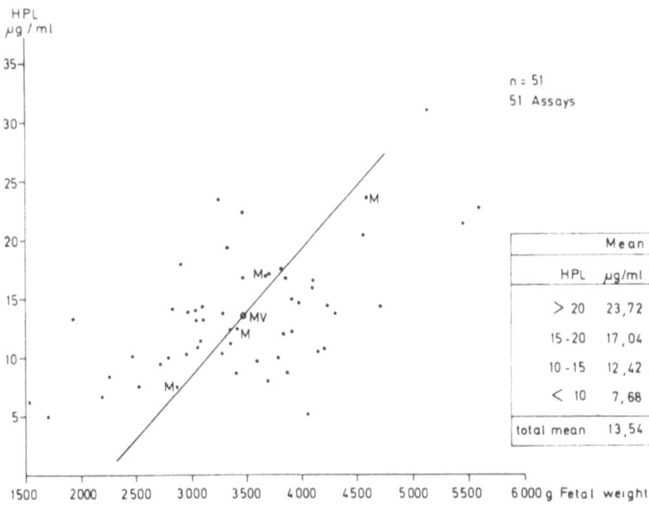

Mean value			
HPL	µg/ml	Fetal weight	n
> 20	23,72	4572 g	6
15-20	17,04	3686	9
10-15	12,42	3386	25
< 10	7,68	2868	11
total mean	13,54	3466	51

Fig. 5. Fetal weight and serum HPL levels in the last 5 days before delivery

Amniotic Fluid Analysis in Placental Insufficiency

A. Dražančić, Jasna Ivić, and I. Kuvačić

The measurement of orange polygonal cells (BROSENS and GORDON 1966) and of creatinine (PITKIN and ZWIREK 1967) in the amniotic fluid, have proved to be useful in predicting fetal maturity. There are few reports concerning amniotic fluid glucose concentration; value of 20 to 30 mg/100 ml have been reported as normal. SCHREINER (1963) observed the decrease of amniotic fluid glucose concentration from 48.1 (± 23.6) mg/100 ml between the tenth to sixteenth weeks to 22.2 (± 23.2) mg/100 ml in the last weeks of pregnancy. The same author found a significant decrease to 12.1 (± 9.4) mg/100 ml in toxaemia.

The aim of our investigations was to establish in placental insufficiency and especially in those cases with intra-uterine growth retardation (together with a group of diabetic pregnancies) whether both the number of orange polygonal cells and creatinine concentration were abnormal. We also measured amniotic fluid glucose concentration.

Materials and Methods

The orange cells were determined in 354 specimens from 242 normal pregnancies (the control group), in 41 specimens from 32 pregnancies with intra-uterine growth retardation (infants born less that the 10th percentile for gestational age) and in 31 specimens from 14 diabetic pregnancies. The cells were counted in fresh specimens stained by the Nile-blue sulphate and by the PAPANICOLAOU methods.

Creatinine was measured, by the GORDON method, in 432 specimens from 294 normal pregnancies, in 44 specimens from 37 pregnancies with intra-uterine growth retardation and in 31 specimens from 14 diabetic pregnancies.

Glucose was estimated, by the glucose-oxidase method, in 177 specimens from 148 normal pregnancies, in 32 specimens from 28 pregnancies with intra-uterine growth retardation and in 40 specimens from 10 diabetic pregnancies.

Included in the control group were normal pregnancies with social or psychiatric indications for termination, pregnancies without any sign of pathology and also pregnancies with Rh-immunisation but with normal glucose tolerance.

Results

Table 1 shows the mean values and 2 standard deviations of the orange cells in the three groups of pregnancies. In Fig. 1, the mean values are plotted against gestational age. From the table and figure a progressive increase in the number of orange cells in all three groups, from 33rd to 42nd week, can be seen. No significant difference between the three groups in separate two-weeks intervals was established.

Table 1. Orange polygonal cells (mean values ± 2 standard deviations) in separate two week groups in the control group, placental insufficiency with intra-uterine growth retardation of the fetus and in diabetic pregnancies. The number of estimations are bracketed

	Weeks of pregnancy				
	33 - 34	35 - 36	37 - 38	39 - 40	41 - 42
Control group	1.66±1.23 (16)	8.44±10.12 (31)	26.20±25.30 (98)	50.25±26.70 (136)	63.19±24.60 (73)
Intra-uterine growth retardation	4.57±6.75 (7)	4.0 ± 5.55 (6)	21.56±28.20 (9)	39.21±25.24 (14)	59.60±31.80 (5)
Diabetes mellitus	0.57±0.53 (7)	5.71± 8.20 (14)	28.00±26.71 (10)	-	-

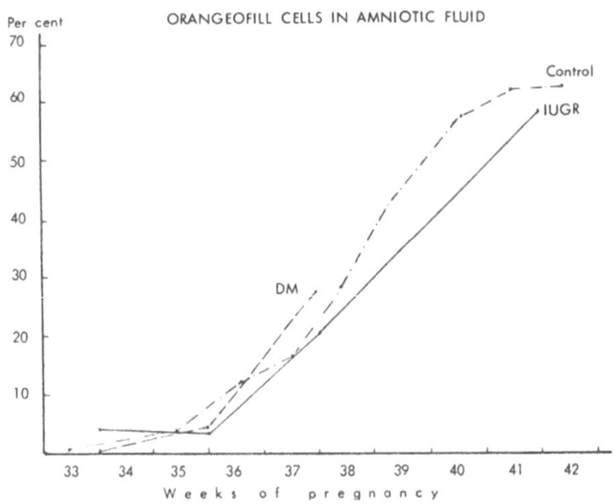

Fig. 1. Mean values of orange polygonal cells in the amniotic fluid. Abscisse: weeks of pregnancy, ordinate: polygonal cells per cent. Control - normal pregnancies, I. U. G. R. - pregnancies with intra-uterine growth retardation of the foetus, DM - diabetic pregnancies

In Table 2, the mean values and 2 standard deviations of the amniotic fluid creatinine concentrations are presented. The progressive increase in the control group and in diabetic pregnancies is evident. In the group with intra-uterine growth retardation, high values, over 2 mg/ 100 ml, in the 33 - 34 and 35 - 36 week period were found. In Fig. 2, the progressive linear rise of creatinine concentration in the control group and in diabetic pregnancies is shown, whereas a U-shape curve in pregnancies with intra-uterine growth retardation was found.

Table 3 shows the mean values and 2 standard deviations of the glucose concentrations in the amniotic fluid of the control group.

There is a progressive decrease in the mean value from 65.25 (±12.1) in the 8 - 12 week period to 21.65 (± 4.56) in the 21 - 24 week period. The mean glucose concentration remains fairly constant to the end of

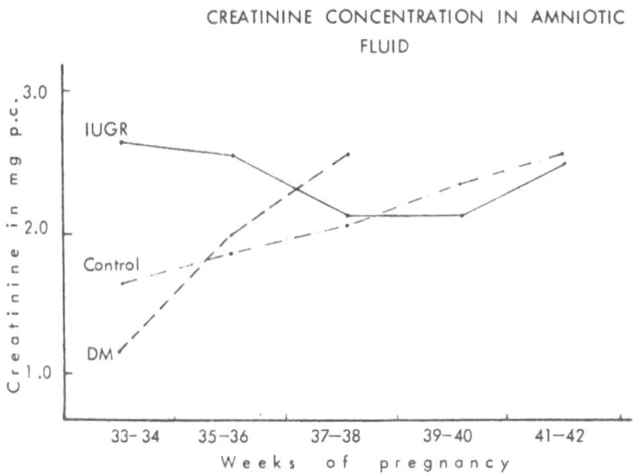

Fig. 2. Mean values of creatinine concentration in the amniotic fluid. Abscisse: weeks of pregnancy, ordinate: creatinine in mg/100 ml. Control - normal pregnancies, I. U. G. R. - pregnancies with intra-uterine growth retardation of the foetus, DM - diabetic pregnancies

Table 2. Creatinine concentration in mg/100 ml (mean values ± 2 standard deviations) in two week groups in the control group of normal pregnancies, placental insufficiency with intra-uterine growth retardation of the fetus and in diabetic pregnancies. $^{+}t = 3.10$, $p < 0.01$. $^{++}t = 2.25$, $p < 0.05$. The number of estimations are bracketed.

	Weeks of pregnancy				
	33 - 34	35 - 36	37 - 38	39 - 40	41 - 42
Control group	1.58±0.62 (32)$^{+}$	1.83±0.69 (52)$^{++}$	2.04±0.67 (130)	2.32±0.80 (155)	2.55±0.97 (73)
Intra-uterine growth retardation	2.55±1.04 (6)$^{+}$	2.45±1.09 (9)$^{++}$	2.09±0.67 (10)	2.09±0.96 (14)	2.69±1.64 (5)
Diabetic pregnancy	1.1 ±0.28 (7)	1.93±0.60 (15)	2.45±0.48 (9)	-	-

Table 3. Glucose concentrations in mg/100 ml (mean values ± 2 standard errors) in the amniotic fluid of normal pregnancies. The number of estimations are bracketed.

Weeks of pregnancy							
Z 12	13 - 16	17 - 20	21 - 24	25 - 28	29	30	31
65.25_12.10	47.20_14.34	28.01_4.41	21.65_4.56	23.58_9.43	-	23.50	24.60
(8)	(4)	(27)	(14)	(6)	(0)	(2)	(1)

Weeks of pregnancy							
Z 32	33	34	35	36	37	38
26.03	16.01_8.67	20.20	16.32_12.45	17.35_15.82	15.96_8.85	13.28_4.37
(3)	(7)	(2)	(6)	(4)	(7)	(27)

Table 3. (continued)

Weeks of pregnancy				
Z 39	40	41	42	
5.22±3.14 (21)	4.87±2.67 (22)	1.67±1.99 (9)	0 (7)	

the 36th week. An abrupt fall occurs at the 39th week and by the 42nd week glucose is absent from the amniotic fluid.

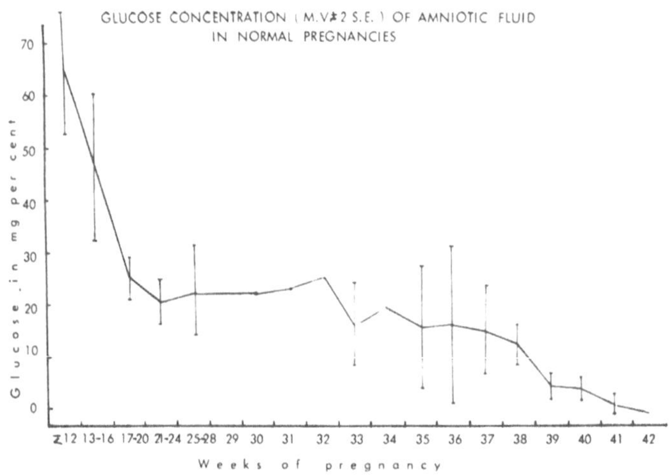

Fig. 3. Mean values and 2 standard errors of glucose concentration in amniotic fluid in normal pregnancies. Abscisse: weeks of pregnancy, ordinate: glucose in mg/100 ml

In Table 4 the mean values and 2 standard deviations in the control group together with the cases with intra-uterine growth retardation and the diabetic cases are presented.

There are statistically significant differences between the mean values in the control group compared with the group with intra-uterine growth retardation up to the period of 39 - 40 weeks, and between the control group and the diabetic group. In Fig. 4, the mean values are plotted against the weeks of pregnancy.

Fig. 5 shows incidence of amniotic fluid specimens with negative glucose in two-week periods, in the control, the placental insufficiency and the pre-eclampsia groups. From the diagram it can be seen that an absence of amniotic fluid glucose in the control group does not occur befor the 37 - 38th weeks, but in the group with placental insufficiency it may be absent by the 33rd or 34th week. In the group with placental insufficiency the percentage is high by 33 - 34 weeks and persists to the end of the pregnancy. In normal pregnancies the incidence only becomes high after the 40th week.

Table 4. Glucose concentration in mg/100 ml (mean values ±2 standard deviations) in two weeks groups in the control group of normal pregnancies, placental insufficiency with intra-uterine growth retardation of the fetus and in diabetic pregnancies.
$^{+}t = 3.61$, $p < 0.01$. $^{++}t = 1.48$, $p > 0.05$

	Weeks of pregnancy				
	33 - 34	35 - 36	37 - 38	39 - 40	41 - 42
Control group	16.94±10.71 (9)	16.89±11.90 (10)	13.72±10.30 (34)+	5.04±6.53 (43)++	0.99±1.37 (16)
Intra-uterine growth retardation	0 (3)	7.13± 9.47 (4)	1.22± 2.48 (9)+	2.29±3.99 (14)++	0 (2)
Diabetic pregnancy	46.44±14.02 (9)	44.89±28.37 (14)	21.49±18.17 (17)	-	-

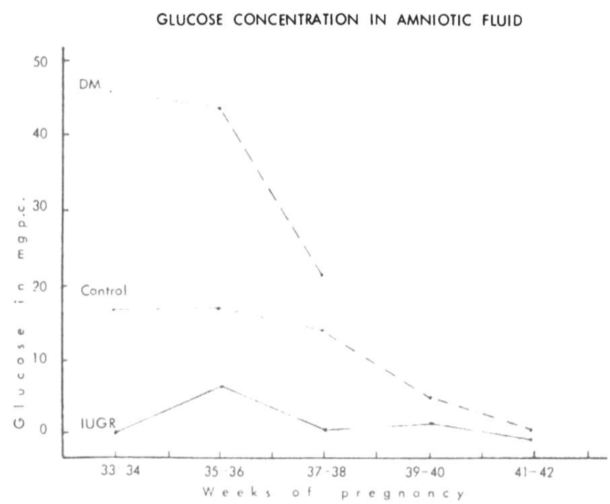

Fig. 4. Mean values of glucose concentration in amniotic fluid. Abscisse: weeks of pregnancy, ordinate: glucose in mg/100 ml. Control - normal pregnancies, IUGR - pregnancies with intra-uterine growth retardation of the foetus, DM - diabetic pregnancies

Discussion

The progressive increase in the orange cell count in the amniotic fluid in pregnancies with intra-uterine growth retardation (the values of which correspond to the control group of the same gestational age, in spite of the small-for-dates infants), agrees with known somatic and neurological maturity (MINKOWSKI) of the small-for-dates infants.

The significantly higher concentration of the amniotic fluid creatinine in the 33 - 34 and the 35 - 36 week periods, in the cases with intra-uterine growth retardation, is presumably the result of exaggerated fetal catabolism. In the cases with pronounced intra-uterine growth retardation, the neonates were under the 5th percentile for gestational age.

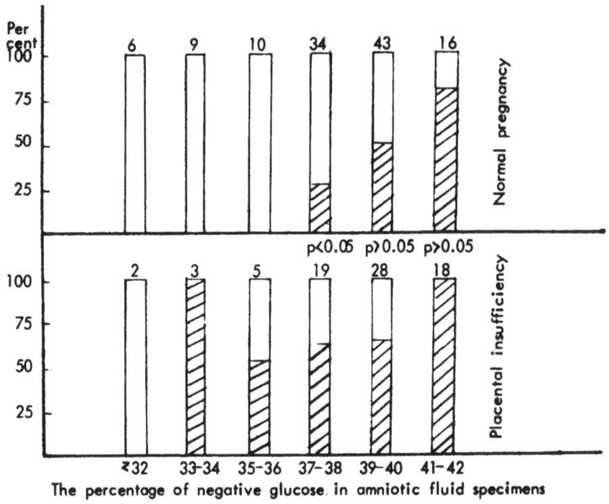

Fig. 5. Amniotic fluid glucose concentration in two-weeks periods of pregnancies. On the top of each column the number of estimations. Shaded fields: the percentage of "absent" findings. Top of the figure: control group of normal pregnancies. Bottom of the figure: pregnancies with placental insufficiency (pre-eclampsia and cases with intra-uterine growth retardation of the foetus)

The decreased amniotic fluid glucose concentration in the pregnancies with intra-uterine growth retardation (and not infrequently the absence of the glucose in the amniotic fluid), is of special interest. Experimental placental insufficiency often leads to fetal hypoglycaemia and depletion of fetal hepatic glycogen stores (OH et al.). This work parallels the clinical observations, in patients with placental insufficiency, of neonatal hypoglycaemia (CORNBLATH et al., NELIGAN et al., BROWN and WALLIS) and the diminished glycogen stores demonstrated in stillborn children (SCOTT).

The estimation of fetal blood glucose concentration could be of prognostic value, but unfortunately is not measurable during pregnancy. The amniotic fluid glucose concentration is the reflection of the glucose gradient: mother → fetus → amniotic fluid, and therefore seems to represent the fetal blood glucose concentration and glycogen stores.

From the practical point of view, a reduction of absence of glucose in the amniotic fluid in patients carrying a small fetus could substantiate the diagnosis of intra-uterine growth retardation. In the cases of pregnancies near term or post-term, absent amniotic fluid glucose could be an additional sign of danger to the fetus, as is suggested by low oestriol values, meconium-stained liquor or fetal heart-rate deceleration measured by cardiotocography. When amniotic fluid glucose is correlated with pH values of the neonates (Table 5), those neonates with absent amniotic glucose have a lower pH than those with an amniotic glucose of more than 10 mg/100 ml. This helps to substantiate the prognostic value of amniotic fluid glucose estimations. The significant decrease of the pH value from the first stage of labour to the time of delivery, in the cases with absent amniotic fluid glucose, and persistence of the normal pH value between the first stage to the time of delivery in the cases with normal amniotic fluid glucose, add weight to the prognostic value.

Table 5. Fetal and neonatal pH values (M. V. ±2 SD) in cases with absent and normal amniotic fluid glucose. The number of estimations are bracketed. $^{+}t = 4.69$, $p < 0.01$. $^{++}t = 0.74$, $p > 0.05$

		Fetus Cervix 23 cm	Neonates
Amniotic Fluid Glucose	Absent	$7.33 \pm 0.68^{+}$ (26)	$7.20 \pm 0.11^{+}$ (21)
			$p < 0.02$
	> 10 mg	$7.35 \pm 0.06^{++}$ (4)	$7.32 \pm 0.08^{++}$ (8)

Summary and Conclusion

In pregnancies with chronic placental insufficiency with intra-uterine growth retardation of the foetus, the diabetic pregnancies and the control group of normal pregnancies, there was no difference in the orange polygonal cell count in the amniotic fluid.

An abnormally high amniotic fluid creatinine concentration in the pregnancies with intra-uterine growth retardation occurs by the 33rd week, possibly due to exaggerated fetal catabolism.

The amniotic fluid glucose concentration decreased gradually from 65 (±12) mg/100 ml at 8 - 12 weeks, to 21 (± 4.5) mg/100 ml by 21 - 24 weeks, persisted unaltered to the 36th week, and then abruptly falls to zero by 42 weeks. In diabetic pregnancies the values are elevated. In pregnancies with chronic placental insufficiency we have found lowered concentrations and not infrequently absence of glucose in the amniotic fluid. The reduced or absent glucose is a measure of fetal intra-uterine growth retardation and may suggest neonatal hypoglycaemia.

References

1. BROSENS, I., GORDON, H.: J. Obst. Gynaec. Brit. Cmwlth., 73, 88 (1966).
2. BROWN, R. J. K., WALLIS, P. G.: Lancet, 1963, I 1278.
3. CORNBLATH, M., ODELL, G. B. LEVIN, E. Y.: J. Pediat., 55, 545 (1959).
4. MINKOWSKY, A.: Proc. 2nd Europ. Cong. Perinatal Medicine, London 1970, S. Karger, 203 - 209.
5. NELIGAN, G. A., ROBSON, E., WATSON, J.: LANCET, 1963, I 1282.
6. OH, W., D' AMOUIO, M. D., YAO, L. L., HOHENAUER, L.: Am. J. Obstet. Gynec., 108, 415 (1970).
7. PITKIN, R. M., ZWIREK, S. A.: Am. J. Obstet. Gynec., 98, 304 (1967).
8. SCHREINER, W. E., GRUBER, A.: Zbl. Gynäk., 85, 304 (1963).
9. SCOTT, J. M.: Arch. Dis. Childhood, 40, 317 (1965).

Thermostable Alkaline Phosphatases in Feto-Placental Insufficiency

J. Gombert, J. R. Giraud, X. Bareau, and D. Reiss

Thermostable alkaline phosphatases, produced by the placenta and probably taking part in phosphate ion transfer, are held to be an index of placental function.

1500 measurements have been made; 636 of which were made during normal pregnancies.

The 636 measurements made during normal pregnancies are presented in Fig. 1.

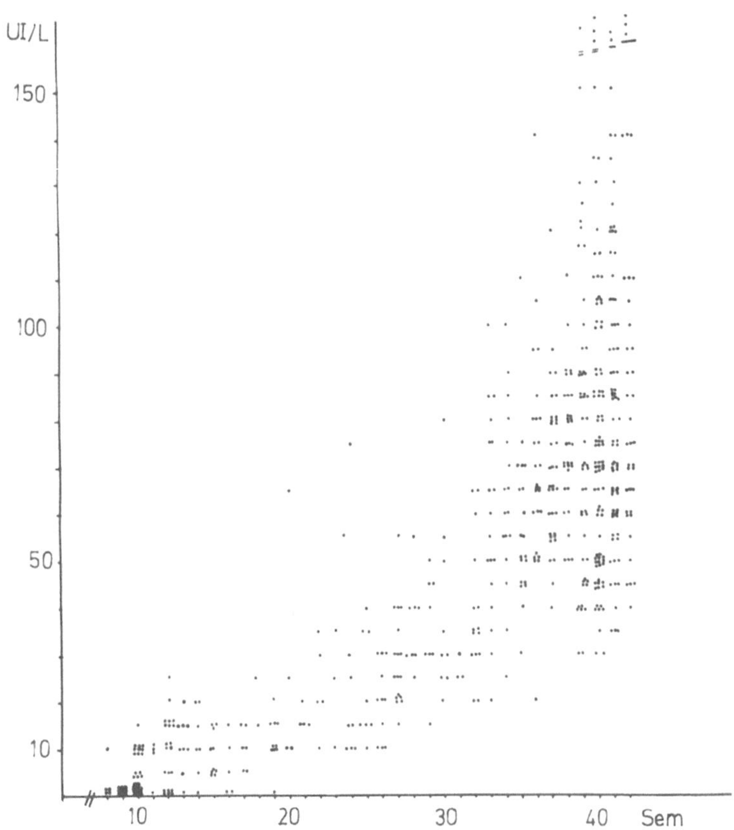

Fig. 1

We were thus able to establish a range of normal values between the 5th and 95th percentiles (Fig. 2).

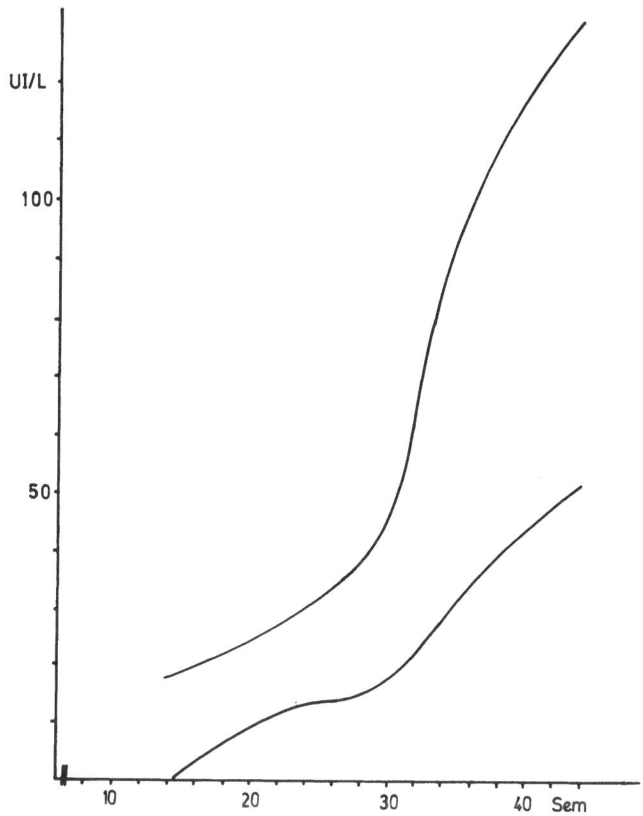

Fig. 2

The course of pathological pregnancies was followed by referring this graph. We have found that multiple measurements are of more value than a single measurement.

In the following examples, we have represented:
in a dotted line the moderate cases;
in solid lines the severe cases, usually ending with Caesarian section;
in an open circle the living new-borns;
in a black circle the still-borns.

These pregnancies were supervised with the usual clinical and biological methods. Thermostable alkaline phosphatase assays were rarely taken into account for therapeutic reasons, and when so, only as a minor contribution.

Pregnancies with Diabetes Mellitus

In the two still-born cases, values are low. In the case where a very important break in the curve occurs, the decision to interrupt the pregnancy was made on evidence of a previous still-born infant, a fall of urinary oestriol values and, also, the change in phosphatases' levels.

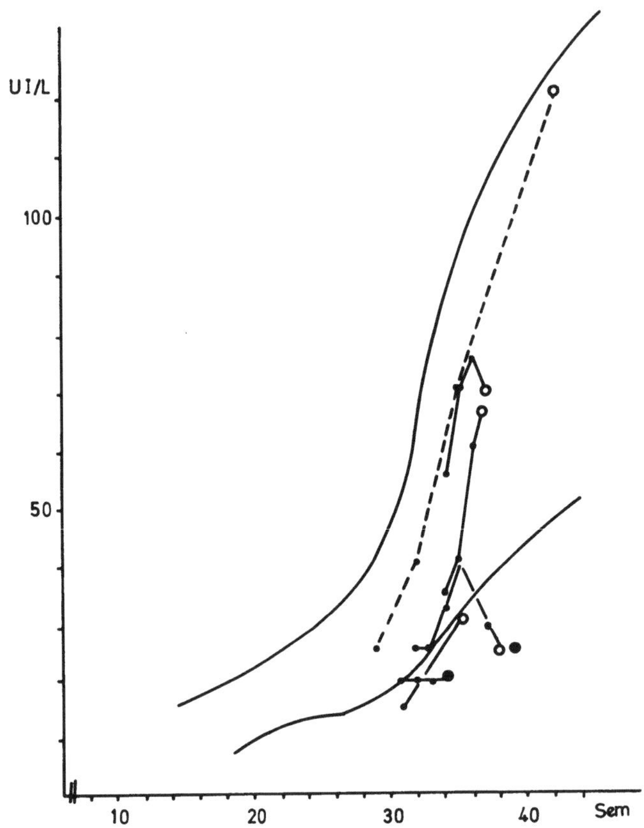

Fig. 3

Pregnancies with Pre-eclampsia

In two out of the three pregnancies with still-born infants, the values were low.

We have followed the course of 4 very severe cases by repeated assays.

In the first case, there was a full-term spontaneous labour. The low but slowly increasing levels showed a placental insufficiency, but the gradual increase was reassuring.

In the second case, there was a premature spontaneous labour; the break in the curve suggested a placental insufficiency, also supported by oestriol levels.

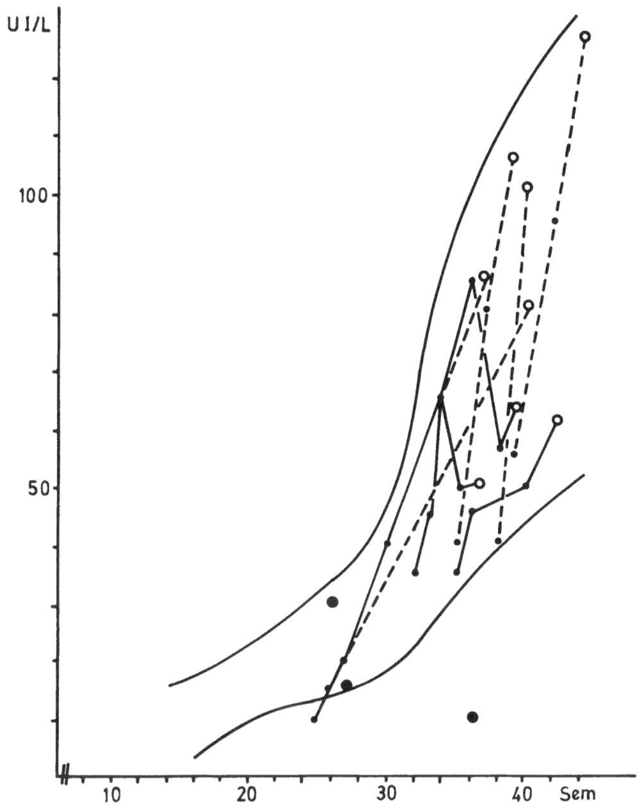

Fig. 4

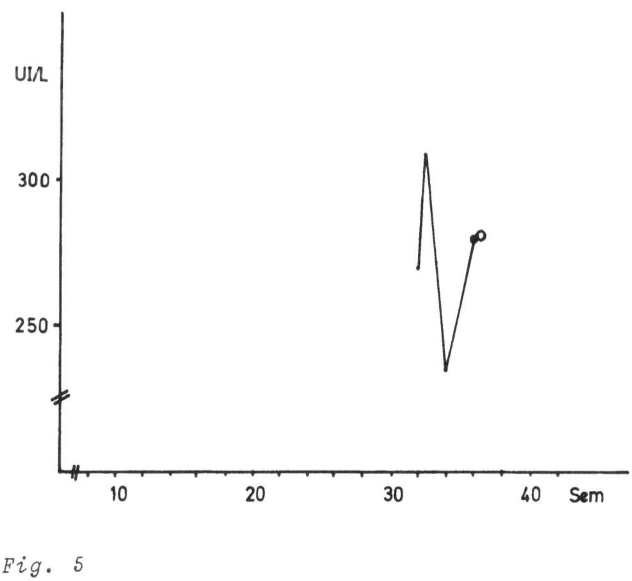

Fig. 5

In the third case, a Caesarian section was performed because of the agreement between the clinical features, the oestriol values and the break of phosphatase curve.

The fourth patient had eclampsia at 32 weeks, controlled by medical treatment and followed by spontaneous labour at 35 weeks. The phosphatases' curve was serrated, but never entirely broken. In this case, the great increase in values is perhaps related to the severity of hypertension, as reported by some authors (Fig. 5).

Conclusions

We have shown that thermostable alkaline phosphatases are an index of placental function.

Their concentration can be a useful test for abnormal pregnancies, especially in diabetes mellitus and pre-eclampsia. The failure of value to rise and, particularly, the break in the curve, must lead one to suspect feto-placental dysfunction.

The Insulin Tolerance Test (I.T.T.) as a Basis for the Therapy of Placental Insufficiency

S. Friedman and J. A. Goldman

The pseudo-diabetogenic properties of H. P. L., and the role it plays in the metabolic process which aims to meet the fetal requirements of carbohydrates, have been well-documented.

In "placental insufficiency" a decrease occurs in the secretion of H. P. L. and insulinase by the placenta, while at the same time the secretion of insulin by the pancreas remains more or less at the same level. This should bring about a decrease in glucose tolerance and increased sensitivity to insulin, so that there is less glucose available for the fetus.

On the basis of this concept, for the past few years our treatment of "idiopathic" placental insufficiency has been that of daily intravenous infusions of hypertonic glucose. An improvement in fetal growth has been noted in several cases.

A difficulty encountered in the application of this therapy has been the lack of a reliable method for the evaluation of the severity of placental dysfunction and of the results of treatment as expressed in the parameters of metabolism, placental function and fetal prognosis.

It was the object of our study to test the validity of the above theory by determining whether or not there is indeed a decrease in insulin tolerance in cases of placental insufficiency. Furthermore, we wished to establish whether the I. T. T. performed in pregnancy can serve as a reliable test of placental function, and whether it is of value in monitoring fetal growth and well-being, as well as in indicating the results of our treatment with glucose infusions.

Insulin tolerance was determined in three groups of women:
a) 20 women in the 3rd trimester of normal pregnancy admitted to the department because of false labour pains, premature rupture of membranes, etc.
b) 20 women in the 3rd trimester of pregnancy with a diagnosis of placental insufficiency.
c) The women in group b, a year or two following delivery.

After the withdrawal of a blood sample for the determination of fasting blood glucose, insulin was injected intravenously. Additional blood samples were then taken every 10 - 15 minutes for a period of two hours following the injection.

In the patients with placental insufficiency (group b), treatment was started with infusions of 1000 ml of hypertonic glucose. In b group the insulin tolerance test was repeated after two to three weeks of treatment. The results of this study clearly showed that there is a decrease in insulin tolerance, and in the fasting blood levels in cases of placental insufficiency as compared to the results obtained in normal pregnancy.

There is a correlation between the changes in the I. T. T. and improvement or further deterioration in the fetal growth retardation. By studying the I. T. T. curve and comparing it to the mean curve of normal pregnancy, it is possible to estimate the state of placental dysfunction and to monitor the results of any particular treatment.

Radioimmunologic Determination of Plasma Estriol in Pregnancy with a Specific Antiserum to Estriol

H. J. Künzig and W. Geiger

By immunising rabbits with a mixture of an estriol -C 2- and estriol -C 4- albumin conjugate (1) we could obtain an antibody to estriol, which showed no crossreaction with various steroids and phenolic derivates (Fig. 1).

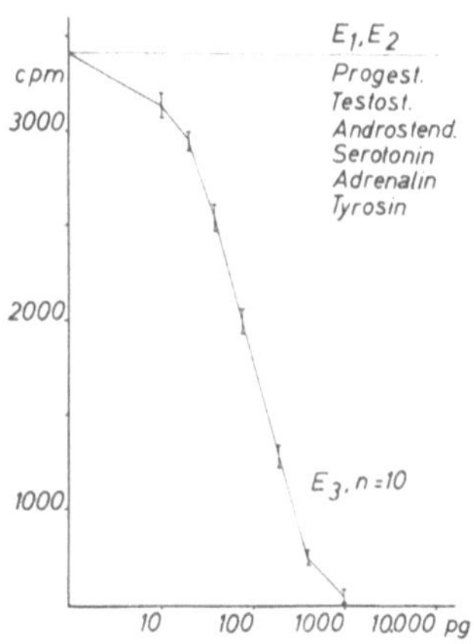

Fig. 1. Cross-reaction of various steroids and phenolic derivates with estriol-antibody

This antibody could be used in a radioimmunoassay for plasma estriol with no preceeding chromatographic separation steps necessary.

0.1 ml plasma were extracted once with ether and evaporated to dryness. After dissolving the extract with ethanol an aliquot was transferred to disposable glass tubes for the radioimmunoassay (Table 1). By shortening the time of incubation to 75 min., no detectable increase of binding could be observed after this time, numerous plasma samples can be assayed in one day.

The estriol content of each sample was determined from a standardcurve, which was linear between 20 and 500 pg. (Fig. 1). The precision, assessed by serial determinations, was between 5 and 10 %, the mean recovery of radioactive hormone 99 ± 8.1 %.

The measurement of plasma estriol has a big advantage over urinary determinations. Besides saving of time an error in urine collection can be eliminated, which may lead to misjudgement of a high risk prenancy (Fig. 2). Plasma from unselected patients showed an increase of unconjugated estriol, which amounts to apr. 10 % of plasma estriol, from 2.9 ng/ml around the 20th week to 16.6 ng/ml at term. The absolute values vary widely from (Fig. 3) patient to patient.

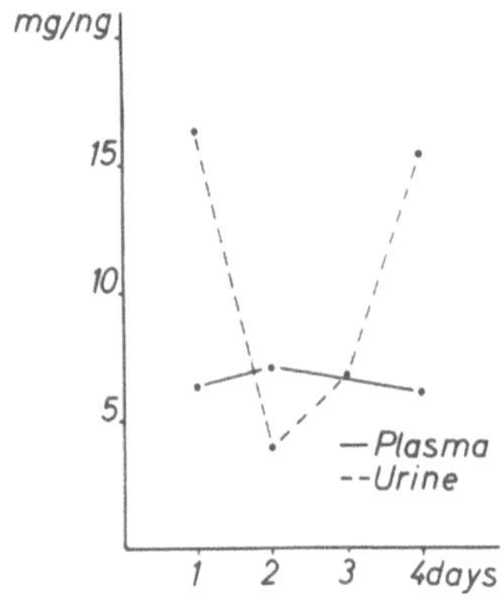

Fig. 2. Plasma- and urinary estriol in case of a sampling error of 24 h urine

Table 1. Flow diagram of method

Method
0.1 ml PLASMA
↓
ETHER EXTRACTION
1 x 10 ml
↓
DRIED ETHER EXTRACT
+
1 ml ETHANOL
↓
R I A
0.1 ml DRIED ETHANOL + 0.1 ml PBS, PH 7.0
0.2 ml GAMMA-GLOBULIN
0.1 ml ESTRIOL ANTISERUM
0.1 ml ^{3}H - ESTRIOL (1.8 x 10^{-9} mol)
↓
INCUBATED
45 min. ROOM T $\underline{\overset{o}{\rightarrow}}$ 30 min. 4° C, or 8 - 16 h, 4° C
+
0.5 ml DEXTRAN - COATED CHARCOAL
10 min. 4° C
↓
CENTRIFUGATION
10 min. 4° C
↓
0.75 ml INCUBATION MEDIA
+
14 ml COUNTING SOL.
COUNTED FOR ^{3}H - COUNTS

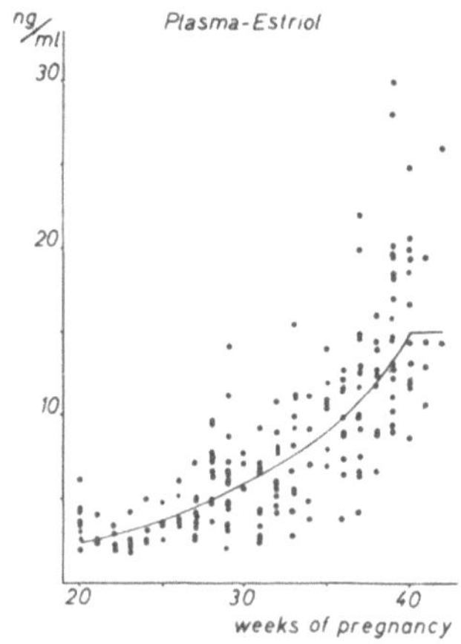

Fig. 3. Plasma estriol levels in normal pregnancy. The calculated average values are indicated by the solid line

There is a marked rise of plasma estriol in the last trimenon of pregnancy, as it has been shown already for urinary estrogens.

The results of serial determinations in eight normal patients at varying stages of gestation show diurnal variations, with no persistent pattern (Fig. 4).

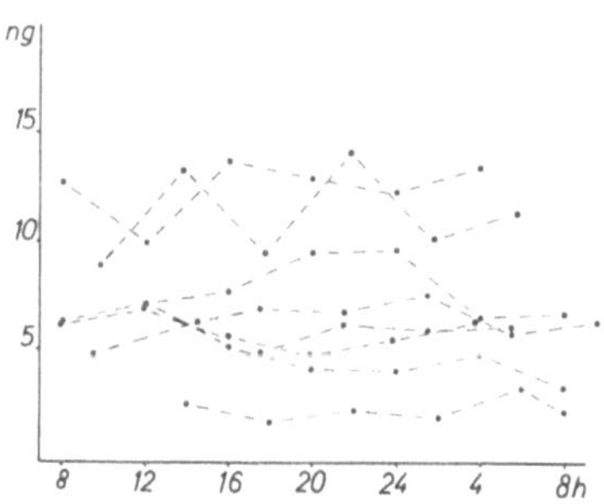

Fig. 4. Diurnal variation of plasma estriol in 8 different patients

A mean coefficient of variation of 18.4 % was obtained, the maximum being 27.3 %. Subnormal values of plasma estriol were found in patients with placental insufficiency; serial assays showed either no increase or even a decline of the plasma levels (Fig. 5).

The low values in plasma and urine correlated significantly, $p < 0.05$ (Fig. 6).

Fetal growth retardation could be demonstrated with ultrasound in a forty-one year old para 5 in the 32th week of gestation. The urinary estriol level rose from 5.7 mg/24 h at this time to a maximum of 13.8 mg/24 h at term. After a decline to 11.1 mg estriol /24 h and the

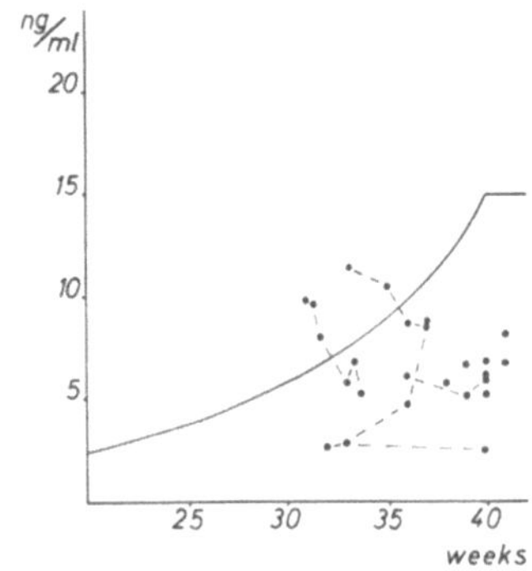

Fig. 5. Plasma estriol in placental insufficiency

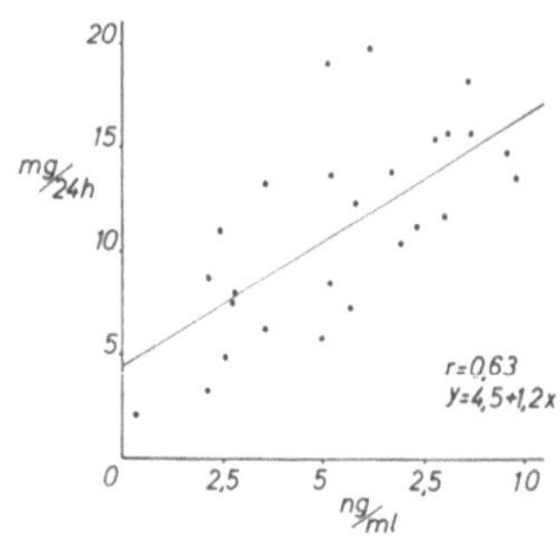

Fig. 6. Relationship between estriol concentration in plasma and urine in placental insufficiency

detection of discoloured amniotic fluid, labour was immediately induced. A 2790 g "small for date baby" was delivered. The plasma estriol curve was virtually flat throughout the course of the study, the values being 2.6 ng/ml in the 32th week of gestation and 2.4 ng/ml shortly before delivery (Fig. 7).

Two patients with severe pre-eclampsia, leeding to intra-uterine death in the 30th week of pregnancy, showed an early decline of the plasma estriol values. In another case of suspected fetal death no measurable estriol values could be obtained (Fig. 8).

The limited number of the cases studied so far don't allow definite conclusions; nevertheless this radioimmunoassay system is a very practible tool for the control of the abnormal pregnancy, since only 0.1 ml plasma is needed and the estriol level can be determined in a very short time. Serial determinations of plasma estriol increase the liability of this method as an index of fetal well being, just as urinary estriol assays do. Moreover plasma determinations allow controls within shorter time intervals then possible with urinary estrogen determination including sampling of a 24 h specimen.

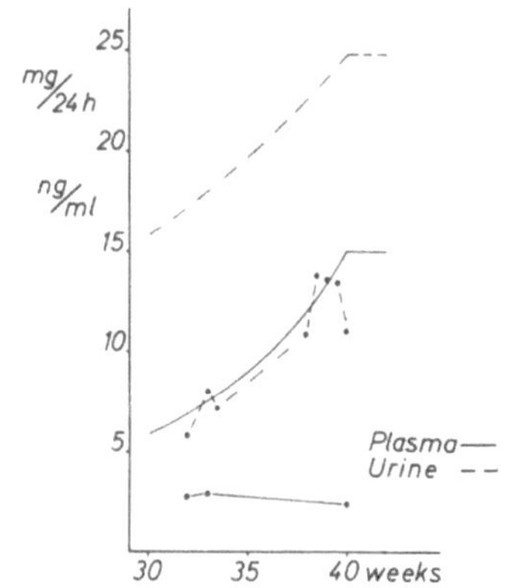

Fig. 7. Serial determination of plasma and urinary estriol in a case of placental insufficiency

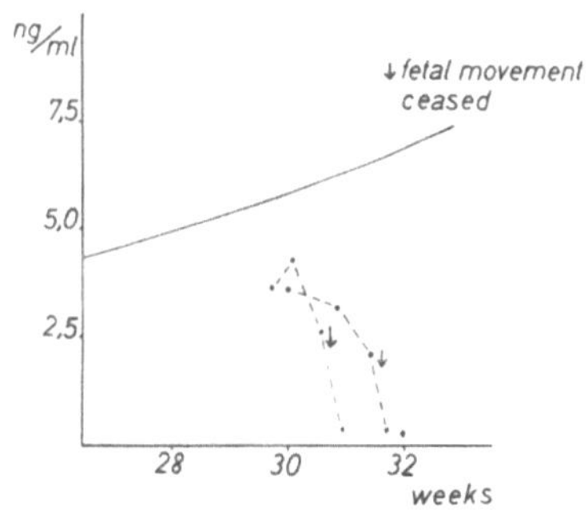

Fig. 8. Plasmaestriol in fetal death

The antigen was kindly supplied by Prof. P. W. JUNGBLUT (Max-Planck-Institut für Zellbiologie, Wilhelmshaven)

1. JUNGBLUT, P. W.: Symp. der Deutschen Ges. f. Endokrin. Berlin Heidelberg: Springer 1970.

Some Parameters of Feto-Placental Insufficiency

F. Santi, G. M. Lamedica, G. Rossi, M. Scafidi, and E. Porro

Oestriol determination in urine has been shown to be a reliable method for monitoring feto-placental function. Other laboratory tests seem to correlate well with the perinatal clinical condition of the fetus.

(HPL) Human placental lactogen and heat-stable alkaline phosphatase (HSAP) are claimed to have a particular relevance regarding placental function, as both of them are synthesized in the placenta.

In order to verify the clinical usefulness of these biochemical tests, we have studied one hundred pregnant women, seventy-one of whom were normal, twenty-one pre-diabetic, and eight with Rh-immunization. We have performed about six hundred determinations of oestrogens and about one hundred of both HPL and HSAP. Oestrogen values (Fig. 1, 2, 3) are given as mg/g of urinary creatinine. This method was chosen in order to minimise the errors inherent in urine collection.

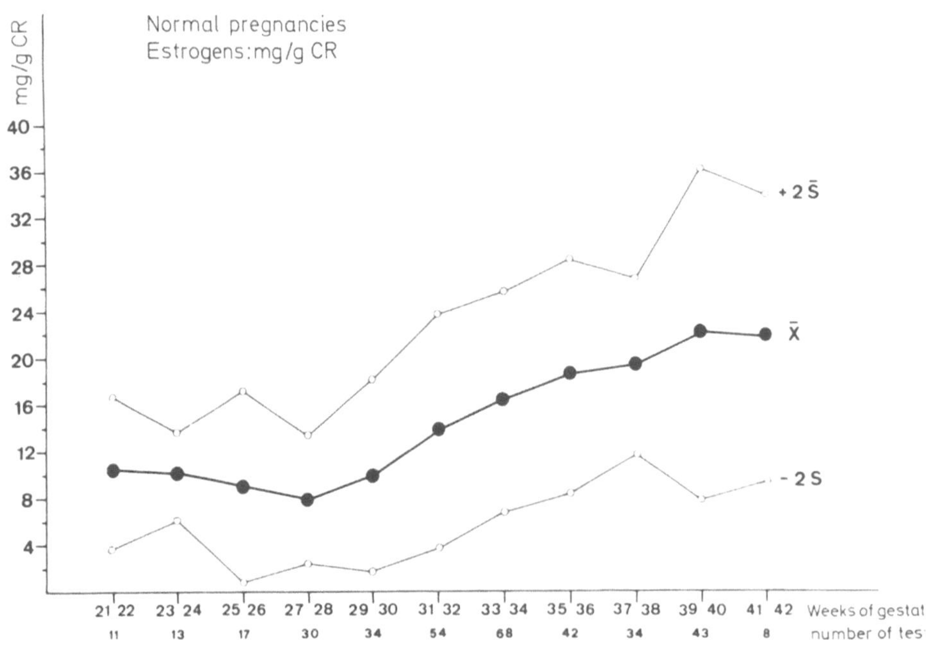

Fig. 1

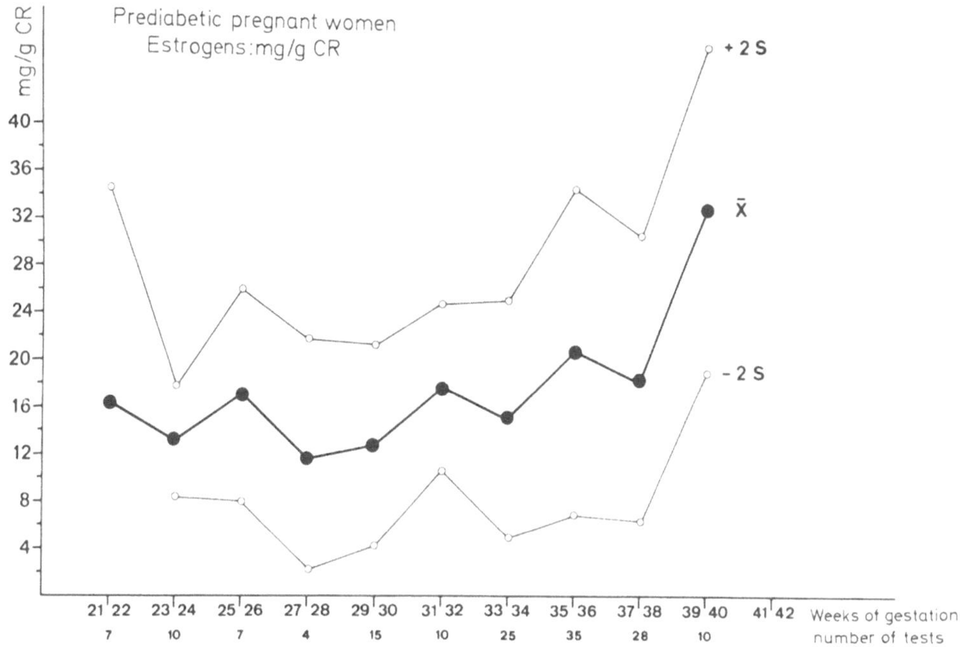
Prediabetic pregnant women
Estrogens:mg/g CR
mg/g CR
+2 S
X̄
-2 S
Weeks of gestation
number of tests

Fig. 2

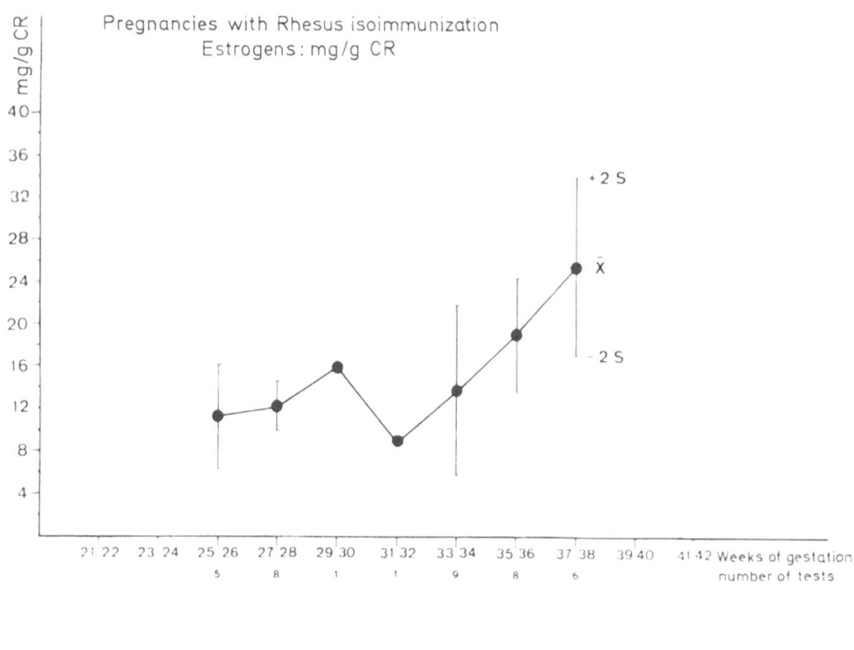
Pregnancies with Rhesus isoimmunization
Estrogens: mg/g CR
mg/g CR
+2 S
X̄
-2 S
Weeks of gestation
number of tests

Fig. 3

The results of HPL and HSAP measurements are shown in Fig. 4 - 7. The cases of Rh-immunization studied are too few for any statistical analysis. With reference to the pre-diabetic subjects, the variance analysis demonstrated a significant ($P < 0.01$) difference between these subjects and the normal ones up to 28th week of pregnancy, as well as an insignificant ($P > 0.05$) one after that time.

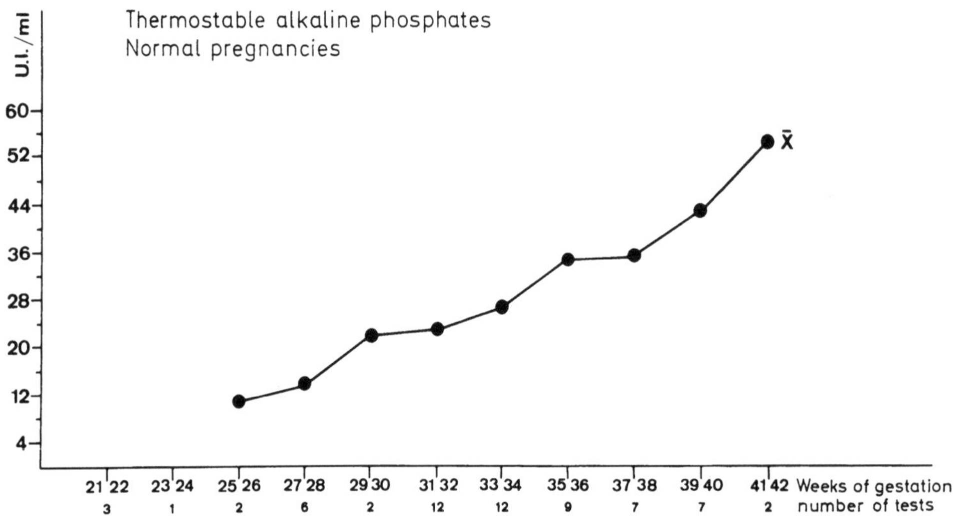

Fig. 4

All three parameters studied have had a discriminant ability but chiefly, HPL. Further data are needed to confirm these observations.

In our clinic we saw a case in which the tests were very useful both clinically and therapeutically. The patient (Fig. 8), a diabetic and asthmatic had three abortions at the 32nd week. Oestrogen concentrations decreased at the 29th week and fell below the lower limit of normal (-2 s) at the thirty-first week. Both HPL and HSAP were also sub-normal. On the basis of these results, suggesting a severe placental insufficiency, and having considered the case history, as well as having found a normal L/S ratio, a Caesarean section was performed.

A pregnant patient (Fig. 9) suffered from a periodic icterus of unknown origin. Her former pregnancy resulted in neonatal death. A familiy history revealed several inter-uterine or neonatal deaths in relatives. In this case our measurements were always in the normal range, and they allowed us to delay the delivery until the 35th week.

In conclusion, our data supports the clinical usefulness of oestrogen excretion, HPL and HSAP determination, preferably performed at the same time.

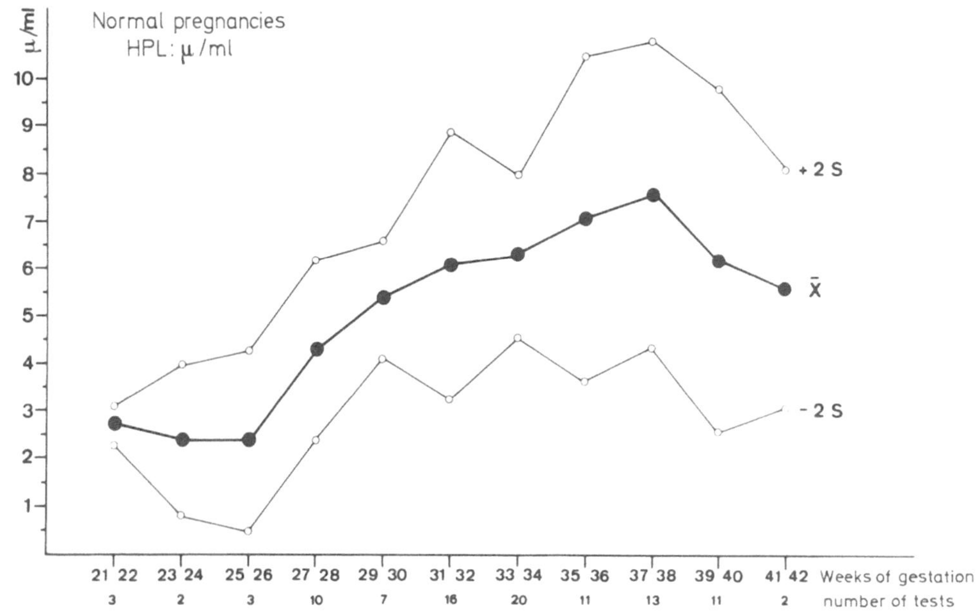
Normal pregnancies
HPL: μ/ml
μ/ml
10
9
8
7
6
5
4
3
2
1
+2 S
x̄
-2 S
21 22
23 24
25 26
27 28
29 30
31 32
33 34
35 36
37 38
39 40
41 42
Weeks of gestation
3
2
3
10
7
16
20
11
13
11
2
number of tests

Fig. 5

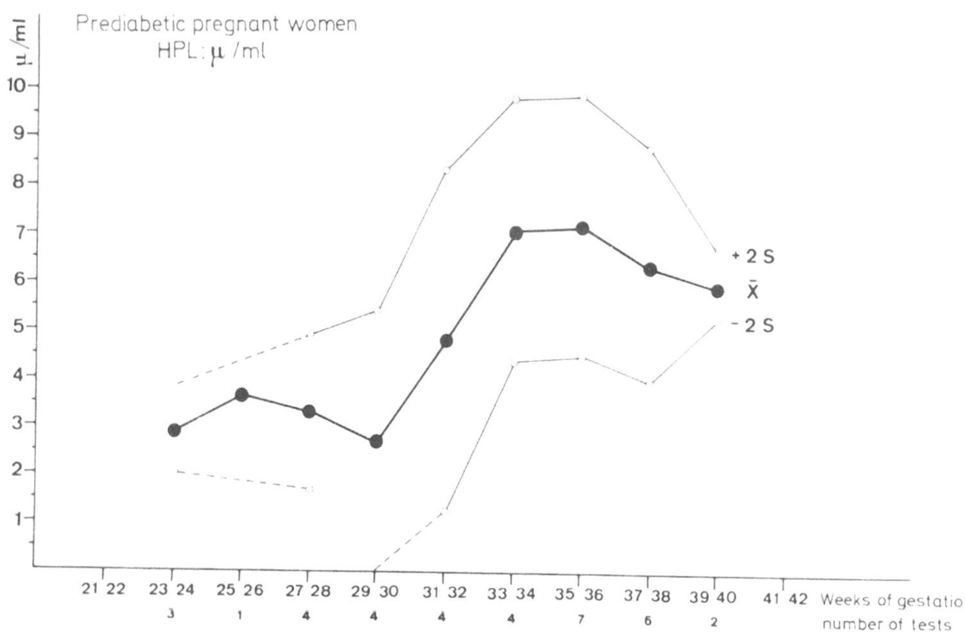
Prediabetic pregnant women
HPL: μ/ml
μ/ml
10
9
8
7
6
5
4
3
2
1
+2 S
x̄
-2 S
21 22
23 24
25 26
27 28
29 30
31 32
33 34
35 36
37 38
39 40
41 42
Weeks of gestation
3
1
4
4
4
4
7
6
2
number of tests

Fig. 6

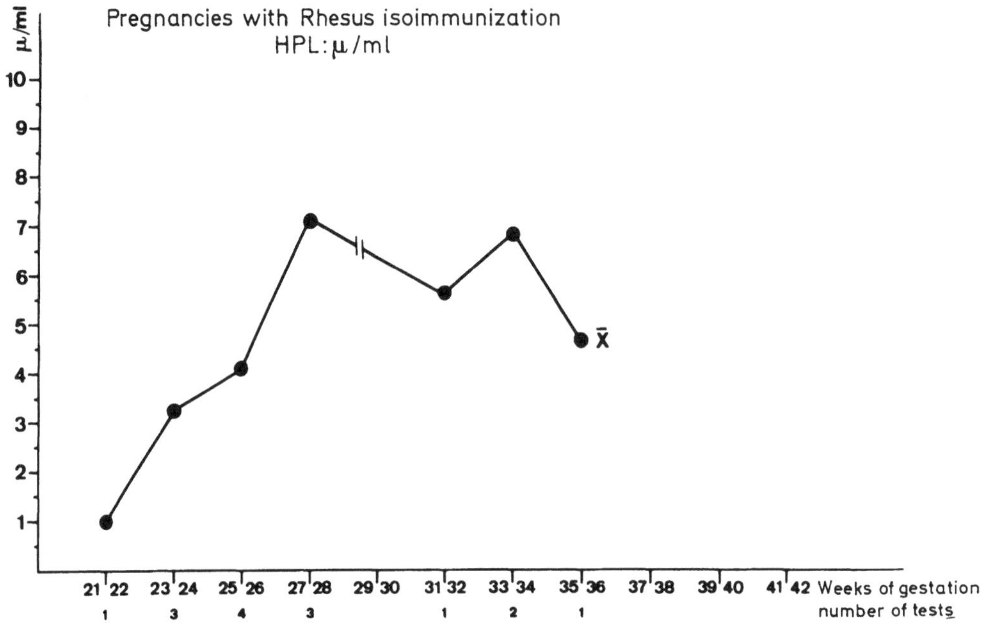
Pregnancies with Rhesus isoimmunization
HPL: μ/ml
μ/ml
10
9
8
7
6
5
4
3
2
1
x̄
21 22
23 24
25 26
27 28
29 30
31 32
33 34
35 36
37 38
39 40
41 42
Weeks of gestation
1
3
4
3
1
2
1
number of tests

Fig. 7

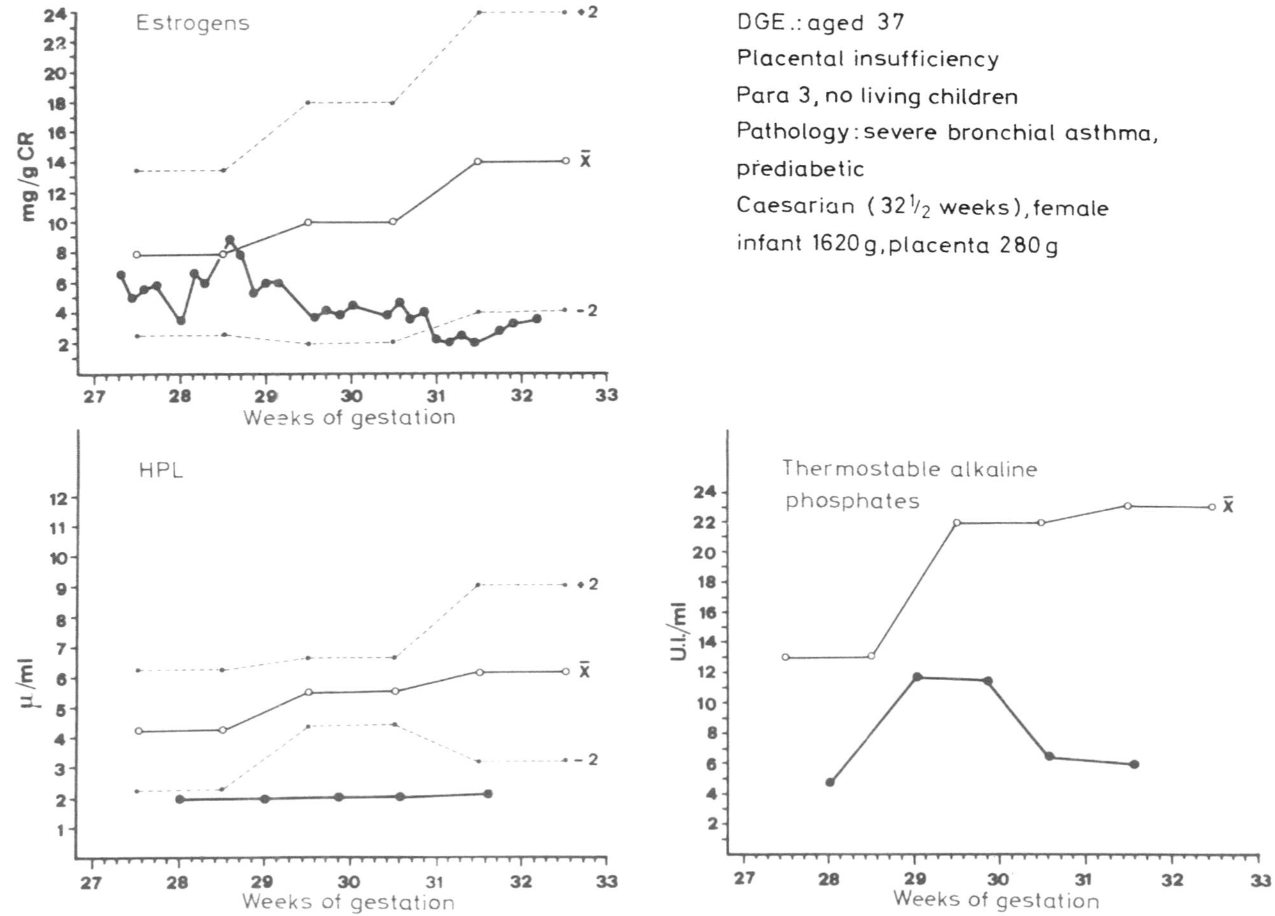
Estrogens
mg/g CR
24
22
20
18
16
14
12
10
8
6
4
2
+2
x̄
-2
27
28
29
30
31
32
33
Weeks of gestation
DGE.: aged 37
Placental insufficiency
Para 3, no living children
Pathology: severe bronchial asthma,
prediabetic
Caesarian (32 1/2 weeks), female
infant 1620 g, placenta 280 g
HPL
μ/ml
12
11
10
9
8
7
6
5
4
3
2
1
+2
x̄
-2
27
28
29
30
31
32
33
Weeks of gestation
Thermostable alkaline
phosphates
U.I./ml
24
22
20
18
16
14
12
10
8
6
4
2
x̄
27
28
29
30
31
32
33
Weeks of gestation

Fig. 8

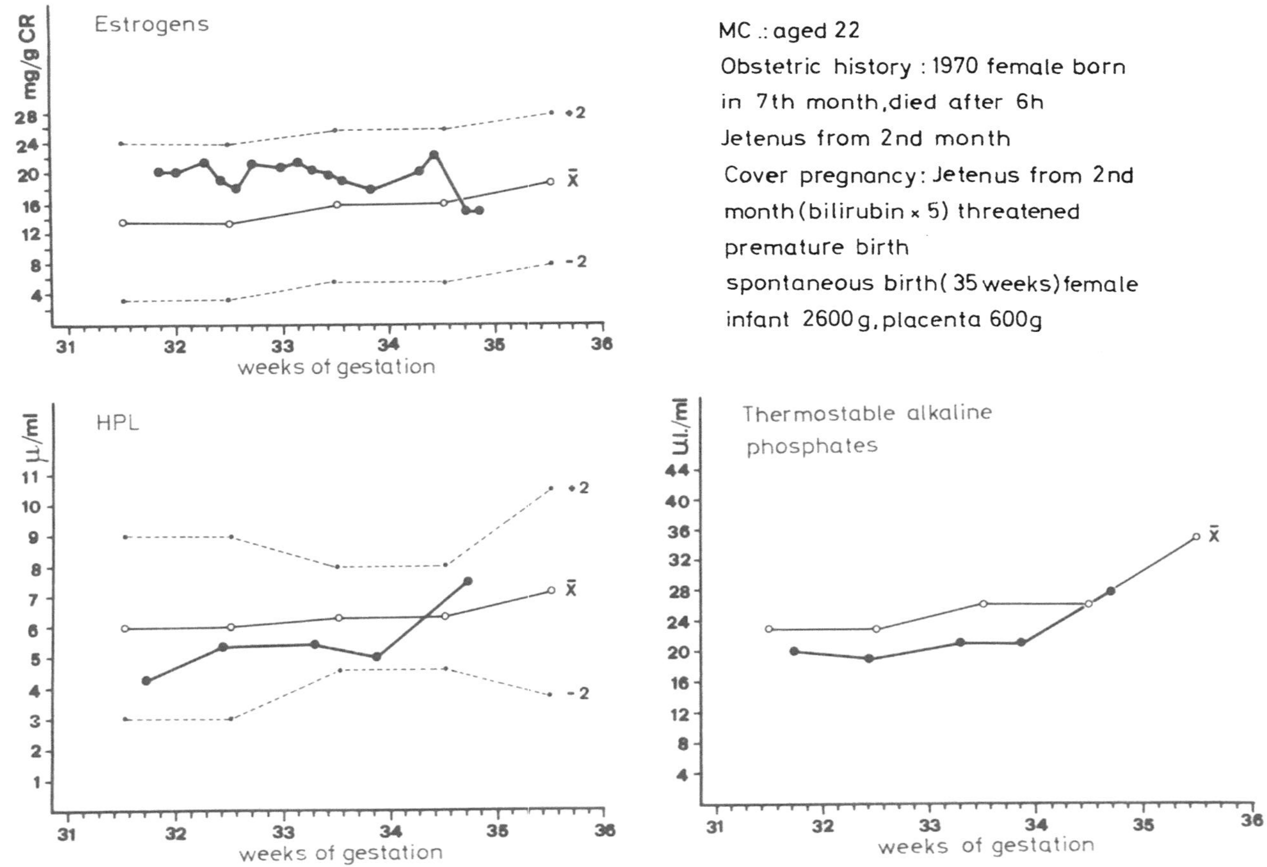
Estrogens
mg/g CR
28
24
20
16
12
8
4
+2
x̄
-2
31
32
33
34
35
36
weeks of gestation
MC .: aged 22
Obstetric history : 1970 female born
in 7th month, died after 6h
Jetenus from 2nd month
Cover pregnancy: Jetenus from 2nd
month (bilirubin × 5) threatened
premature birth
spontaneous birth (35 weeks) female
infant 2600 g, placenta 600g
HPL
μ/ml
11
10
9
8
7
6
5
4
3
2
1
+2
x̄
-2
31
32
33
34
35
36
weeks of gestation
Thermostable alkaline
phosphates
U.I./ml
44
40
36
32
28
24
20
16
12
8
4
x̄
31
32
33
34
35
36
weeks of gestation

Fig. 9

Urinary Estriol as a Therapeutic Guide of Feto-Placental Failure in the Vasculo-Renal Hypertensive Syndrome of Pregnancy

A. P. Mirescu

100 pregnant women with the vasculo-renal hypertensive syndrome (VRHS), 60 % of whom it existed in before pregnancy, have been investigated in the Obstetric Institute "Filantropia" of Bucarest. Another 100 normal women after the 24th week of gestation were also examined as controls.

For the purpose of the study, the following parameters were considered: the cytology of the vaginal smear, the urinary levels of estriol and pregnandiol (according to the method of BROWN) and their connection with the growth degree of the newborn.

It has been observed that the estriol urinary levels present gradually steeper curves, in accordance with the gestational age in the normal subjects, while in pregnant women with VRHS the excretion curves appear flattened.

The results are summarized in the following table:

	Controls		V. R. H. S.	
Parameters considered	Range	Mean value	Range	Mean value
Total estrogens	10.2 - 28	18.8	16 - 27.6.0	20.2
Estriol	9.0 - 21.6	16.0	16.6 - 20.3	18.3
Pregnandiol	18.6 - 31.2	27.8	24.8 - 36.0	31.0
17-KS	4.6 - 11.1	9.7	8.1 - 19.6	12.5

In comparison with the estriol urinary levels, the vaginal cytology shows a significant elevation of the KI index, inversely related to the decreasing values of the urinary estriol.

30 % hypotrophy fetuses, according to the LUBCENKOE GRUENWALDI tables based on weight standards, have been observed in the patients with VRHS, while the levels of urinary estriol appeared directly related with the hypertension severity and the importance of the vasculo-renal syndrome.

Since multiple estrogen determinations revealed a sharp decrease of their urinary excretion, we decided accordingly the lines of our therapeutic behaviour: in 2 cases with medical induction and 6 cases with Caesarian section we managed to rescue 8 hypotrophyc newborns. The placental examination showed in these cases white infarctions, hyalinization and fibrinoid depositions. Postnatal growth appeared to be normal. In two cases the data on urinary estriol were not available in due time, so it was impossible to arrange a timely operation and the fetuses died *in utero.* The values of the estriol excretion were anyway very low.

Diagnosis of Fetal Maturity by Biochemical and Cytological Studies

F. Santi, G. M. Lamedica, E. Cevasco, L. Ambrosini, and E. Porro

The evaluation of fetal maturity is usually necessary when abnormal conditions, such as placental insufficiency, gestosis and isoimmunisation necessitate the introduction of premature labour. The same evaluation is also useful in elective cesarean sections.

Various determinations in amniotic fluid are claimed to have a reliable relationship with the pathological state of the fetus. Among these, uric acid, creatinine, lecytine/sphingolyeline ratio (L/S ratio) and cytological examinations are considered to be the most useful.

We have collected this data to verify usefulness and to find optimal combinations, if any.

82 samples of amniotic fluid were examined. They were withdrawn by 68 amniocenteses from 39 women suffering from any of the disturbances reported in Table 1. The remaining samples were obtained at amniorexis.

Table 1. Cases subjected to amniocentesis

	Patients
Diabetes	9
Rh-Isoimmunisation	10
Men. of premature delivery	8
Polyhydramnios	2
Placental insufficiency	3
Elective cesarean section	3
Jaundice in pregnancy	1
Pretermissed labour	1
Suspicion of malformation	2
	39

In order to minimize the risk, amniocentesis was performed after labour was interrupted by administering orciprenaline or isoxuprine. In our hands, amniocentesis never induced labour nor caused neonatal death. Fetal death only occurred in two cases judged too risky for amniocentesis. These mothers delivered at 35.2 weeks (2.400 g) and at 31 weeks (1.500 g). These observations suggest a larger use of amniocentesis in risk pregnancy.

Table 2. Cases, frequency and gestation weeks in which the amniocentesis was performed

		Weeks of gestation				
	No.	20	20 - 27	28 - 34	35 - 36	36
Isoimmunisation	39	1	11	13	8	6
Maturity	27			4	7	16
Prenatal diagnosis of malformation	2			1		1
	68	1	11	18	15	23

The cytology of amniotic fluid was evaluated in 24 samples from 18 women. Our results, although obtained from a limited number of samples, confirm previous reports on dye uptake and morphology of amniotic cells while pregnancy is progressing.

The values of L/S ratio, uric acid and creatinine are expressed in Tables 3, 4 and 5. Tables 6, 7 and 8 show the figures obtained in three patients who were subjected to repeated amniocentesis because of immunisation.

Table 3. L/S ratio found in all subjects studied

Weeks of gestation													
19	20	21	22	23	24	25	26	27	28	29	30	31	32
0.5	0.5		0.45	1		1	1.24	1	0.85	1.77		2.15	1
				1.47		1	0.8	1.1	1.8	0.43		1.28	1.94
				1								2.5	2.3
													3
													0.5

Weeks of gestation								
33	34	35	36	37	38	39	40	41
1.68	1	2	2.5	1.27	2.7	2.51	3.5	2.7
1.78	3	2.45	1.91	3	3.5	2.05		6.7
3	2.70	2.23	2.28	2.70	4	3.5		2.56
2.65	3	2.05	2.05	3	3.5	4.88		2.40
3.05	3.3	3.1	4.2	3.3	1.75			2.05
	3	2.86		3	1.85			3.70
	3.05	1.32		3.05	5.45			
		2.5			1.51			
					3.5			
					2.67			
					3.5			
					2.32			

Table 4. Creatinine in amniotic Fluid (mg %) found in all subjects studied

Weeks of gestation												
18	19	20	21	22	23	24	25	26	27	28	29	30
	0.49	1.01		0.58	0.97	0.86	0.94	0.35	1.06	1.4	1.4	1.41
	0.65				0.97		0.73	1.07	0.82	1.4		
					0.78							

Weeks of gestation										
31	32	33	34	35	36	37	38	39	40	41
1.42	1.86	1.85	2.30	2.30	2.45	3.00	3.75	3.75	3.08	1.48
0.89	0.78	2.00	1.90	2.15	2.35	1.78	2.45	3.6		3.60
1.18	1.88	1.94	1.38	2.25	2.60	2.25	3.60	3.78		3.05
		1.63	2.35	2.35		2.37	2.35	2.05		1.65
		1.28	2.60	0.86		3.20	1.50			2.70
		2.15		1.08		2.75	3.55			3.03
				1.80			3.87			
							2.78			
							3.91			
							2.65			
							3.15			
							4.80			

Table 5. Uric acid in amniotic Fluid (mgr %) found in all subjects studied

Weeks of gestation											
19	20	21	22	23	24	25	26	27	28	29	30
5.3	4.4		6.45	6.15	6.65	8.9	4.73	7.75	6.00	9.65	5.30
5.45				5		4.95	6.25	5.7	5.18	6.20	
				2.45					6.55		
				6.75							

Weeks of gestation										
31	32	33	34	35	36	37	38	39	40	41
11.30	6.15	10.70	2.62	13.50	6.80	13.50	10.50	12.30	5.70	19.00
7.60	7.80	10.80	9.20	9.60	10.60	9.20	10.80	12.00		15.00
6.60	6.85	5.60	5.80	10.00	10.70	7.60	9.80	8.80		6.80
7.80		7.05	10.00	6.55		8.80	10.50	6.50		12.20
		7.50	7.80	8.80		14.50	7.15			
		5.00	5.10	6.10		9.20	10.90			
				6.15			14.00			
							10.10			
							13.00			
							9.00			
							14.20			

Table 6. Uric acid, creatinine and L/S Ratio determined in a case (B.O.) which, although Rh-immunised by previous pregnancies, was clinically normal and delivered a normal Rh-negative fetus.

Weeks	Uric Acid mg %	Creatinine mg %	L/S ratio
25	8.90	0.94	1.00
27	7.75	1.05	1.00
29	9.65	1.40	1.77
31	11.30	1.42	2.15
33	10.70	1.85	1.68
35	13.50	2.30	2.00
37	13.50	3.00	1.27
39	12.00	3.75	2.05

Table 7. Uric acid, creatinine and L/S ratio values found in a Rh-immunised woman (B. A. M.)

Weeks	Uric Acid mg %	Creatinine mg %	L/S ratio
32	6.15	1.86	1.10
34	2.62	2.30	1.00
36	6.80	2.45	2.50
37	9.20	1.78	3.00
39	8.80	3.60	3.50

Table 8. Uric acid, creatinine and L/S ratio values found in a Rh-immunised woman (C. A. M.)

Weeks	Uric Acid mg %	Creatinine mg %	L/S ratio
32	10.80	2.00	1.78
34	9.20	1.90	3.00
35	9.60	2.15	2.50
36	10.60	2.35	2.10

Previously we had never practised amniocentesis but now we are convinced of its diagnostic value.

None of our subjects delivered a fetus who developed the respiratory distress syndrome and showed a L/S ratio lower than 1.9. Uric acid and creatinine showed increasing concentrations although in a less constant way than L/S ratio. They seem to be useful as a subsidiary measurement.

Radioimmunological Determination of Human Placental Lactogen (HPL), Cystynyloaminopeptidase (CAP) and Daily Excretion of Urinary Oestriol in the Diagnosis of Chronic Placental Insufficiency

A. Cekański and P. Skalba

The data from literature on the subject and our experiments confirm the usefulness of the determination of human placental lactogen (HPL) and cystynylaminopeptidase (CAP) in the diagnosis of placental insufficieny.

These methods, though they seem to be inferior to the determination of the excretion of urinary oestriol, which measures the efficiency of the feto-placental unit, allow one to recognise early chronic placental insufficiency.

Material and Methods

26 pregnant women with suspected chronic placental insufficiency have been examined in the last weeks of pregnancy. Among these cases there were 12 with EPH-gestosis, 4 with chronic pyelonephritis, 8 with pathologically prolonged pregnancy and 2 with hypoplacentosis.

HPL was determined in plasma by means of radioimmunoassay applying the technique of double antibodies, CAP was determined by means of the enzymatic method with l-cysteinodi-beta naphtylamid as a substrate.

In all patients the daily urinary oestriol excretion has been estimated by means of the BROWN-ITTRICH method. Oestriol and CAP have been remeasured several times at three or four-day intervals. Radioimmunoassay determination of HPL was carried out on CAE-CEN-SORIN kits.

Results and Comment

The mean value of HPL determined by radioimmuno assay in the plasma of healthy pregnant women in the last weeks of normal pregnancy was 11.000 ng/ml, the standard deviation S = 2000.

In the group of previously diagnosed placental insufficiency, the mean value was RI - HPL = 6000 ng/ml, the standard deviation S = 1200.

The mean level of CAP in healthy pregnant women is 5.45 IU with standard deviation S = 1.2. In the group of placental insufficiency it was 3.1 IU with a standard deviation of 0.7. A low level of CAP, with a tendency towards even lower values with each subsequent examination together with delayed labour, always carried a bad prognosis.

In these cases the decreased excretion of oestriol lower than 10 mg/24 hours was observed and required the termination of pregnancy. This occurred in 26 % of our patients. With the remaining number of pregnant women the level of oestriol in the daily collection of urine averaged 16.4 mg/24 h (S = 2.5) with daily oscillation never exceeding 20 %.

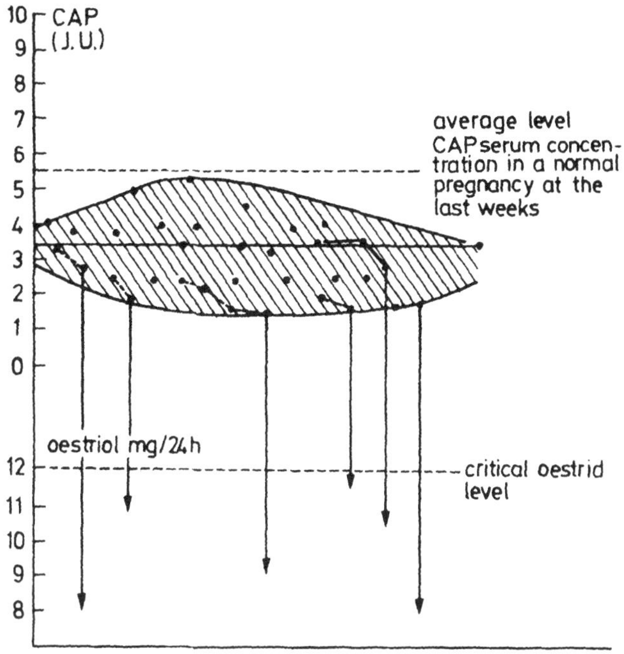

Fig. 1

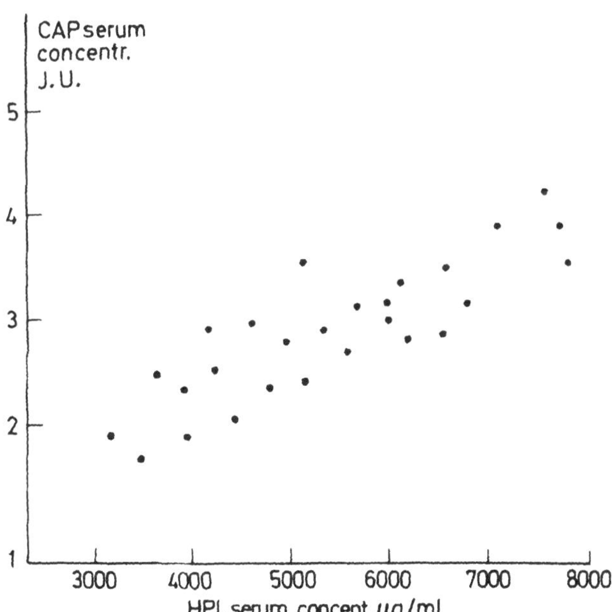

Fig. 2. Scattered diagram of HPL and CAP correlation

The correlation between the levels of HPL-CAP was also estimated. The coefficient of correlation was 0.62 which proves the existence of such correlation.

Table 1

	Number of cases	X H P L - ng/ml	X C A P - J U	Oestriol mg/24 h
Healthy pregnant women	35	11.000 S = 2.000	5.45 S = 1.2	12 - 24
Pregnant women with chronic placental insufficiency	26	6.000 S = 1.200	3.1 S = 0.7	< 10/26 %/ 16.4 S = 2.5

To summarise, the determinations of both HPL and CAP is an important factor in the evaluation of the placental activity. These two determinations, together with the determining of daily oestriol, seem to be sufficient for the diagnosis of chronic placental insufficiency.

Oestriol as Guide in the Treatment of Feto-Placental Insufficiency: Possibilities and Limits

P. Spanio, G. P. Mandruzzato, M. C. Sabbati, F. Nisi, M. Macchia, and C. Persello

Among the numerous biological parameters which are considered useful to assay the function of the feto-placental unit, the assay of urinary oestriol is widely accepted.

The reasons leading to the choice of this particular procedure are the low cost and the precision and speed of administration. In addition, the medical literature on this subject is very large and the excretion of oestriol has been studied in almost all possible obstetrical situations.

However, by limiting our interest to the conditions of feto-placental insufficiency which, if chronic, implies a considerable retardation in growth, it is obviously important, from both diagnostic and therapeutic aspects, to establish whether there is a significant correlation between the value of oestriol and the weight of the foetus and placenta.

Opinions on this issue are far from being in agreement. Besides those authors who have found a correlation between fetal weight and the daily excretion of oestriol, there are others who deny or question this relationship. We report the results obtained from an analysis of 214 cases.

Materials and Methods

214 specimens of urine were assayed.

The oestriol was measured according to BROWN and COYLE (1963) in 24-hour urine samples obtained within 4 days of delivery of a live foetus.

Cases of multiple pregnancies, of stillbirths, of pathological pregnancies (toxaemia, diabetics etc.) were excluded.

The analysis was carried out at the University of Trieste's Calculus Centre using a computer 600200CDC. The correlation coefficient between the following data was looked for: weight of newborn baby - oestriol, Log. weight - oestriol, Log. oestriol - Log. weight.

From the 214 pregnancies, 109 males and 105 females were obtained. The data when correlated produced a correlation coefficient close to 0.45 (Table 1).

An interpolation of the observed data was also attempted by using a polynomial instead of a straight line regression, but this produced an even greater scattering of values. We also sub-divided our cases according to gestational age and in so doing obtained a better correlation coefficient for the 39th week, $R = 0.65$, whereas for the weeks 40, 41 and 42 the correlation coefficient was remarkably lower. (Table 2).

Table 1

Weight/E	Correlation	0.45570	
Log. weight/E		0.43911	
Log. E/weight		0.46477	All cases N = 214
Log. E/ log. weight		0.46160	
Weight/E		0.45317	
Log. weight/E		0.44290	Males N = 109
Log. E/weight		0.47213	
Log. E/ log. weight		0.47013	
Weight/E		0.45254	
Log. weight/E		0.42813	Females N = 105
Log. E/ weight		0.45763	
Log. E/ log. weight		0.44804	

Table 2

39th week	weight - E	0.65368	N = 21
40th week	weight - E	0.33150	N = 55
41st week	weight - E	0.45182	N = 52
42nd week	weight - E	0.34130	N = 40

Discussion and Results

The correlation coefficients obtained can be considered statistically significant (higher than 0.254 for samples of 100 and more) but do not allow a sufficiently precise approximation of the weight to be predicted.

An exception is the correlation coefficient of the 39th week which is considerably higher. The results for the weeks beyond the 39th are particularly unsatisfactory and this can be quite easily interpreted. The oestriol excretion only approximately predicts the fetal or newborn weight. It is possible that an improvement in correlation may be obtained by considering the average of 2 or more samples over a 24-hour period in order that the large variability (up to 28 %) in oestriol excretion can be eliminated.

However, in the context of chronic feto-placental insufficiency, and the consequent retarded fetal growth, oestriol has a rather valid significance. The problem is to establish the degree of accuracy of prediction given by the investigation.

Finally, what should be profitable is to determine whether the foetus departs considerably from the medium weight, and in particular, whether there also exists figures near -2 SD of the weight of the pregnancy age.

The method permits a good approximation, especially if the correlation coefficients are calculated for every week of pregnancy, as well as the relative regression line on which the prediction computation can be based.

Conclusion

On the basis of this first investigation which we intend to expand, and in agreement with other writers, we conclude that:

1. There is only slight correlation between the 24-hour oestriol excretion and the weight of the foetus and placenta.
2. This correlation does not increase when logs. instead of numbers are used.
3. The correlation appears to increase significantly when considering the regression lines / pregnancy week before the 40th.
4. Even though oestriol excretion does not supply precise data for the prediction of weight, it is of help in the diagnosis and treatment of retarded growth, particularly when very low values are found.

References

1. BJÖRO, K.: Acta Endocrinologica Suppl. 161 (1972).
2. BOMPIANI, A., DELL ' ACQUA, S., MANCUSO, S., MENINI, E.: Atti Soc. it. ost. Ginec. Vol LIV 219 Milano (1970).
3. BREBOROWICZ, H., KRZYWINSKA, F., PISARSKI, T.: Am. J. Obst. Gynec. 91, 1107 (1965).
4. COYLE, M., BROWN, J.: J. Obst. Gynaec. Brit. Cwlth. 70, 225 (1963).
5. KLOPPER, A., BILLEWICZ, W.: J. Obst. Gynaec. Brit. Cwlth. 70, 1024 (1963).

The Comparative Studies about the Estriol and HPL Production Rate in the Risk-Pregnancies

P. Tykal, F. W. Dittmar, and L. Schapher

In order to recognize the pathophysiology of pregnancy concentration of serum HPL and Estriol production rate in 24 h urin were compared.

Radioimmunoassay technique with double antibody system for HPL determination and method of BROWN for Estriol determination were used in this study.

This comparative studies were performed in 80 risk-pregnancies. They were compared with the equal group of normal pregnancies. The following risk-pregnancies were studied: EPH-syndrom, Diabetes mellitus, Rh-incompatibility, Adipositas per magna, Abortus habitualis, retardation of intra-uterine fetal growth (Placenta insufficiency) and Gemini.

Estriol and HPL determination were regularly and continuously performed from the 28 week of pregnancy.

First slide shows the HPL concentration in serum and Estriol excretion in 24 h urin in EPH-Gestosis. Both, hormon HPL and Estriol are in the lower part of the normal range. Severe cases of Gestosis are associated with decreasing and fail to define.

In cases of Rh-incompatibility is the fall of Estriol excretion indicator for fetal distress in utero. The HPL levels are mostly in the lower part of the normal range. They show no decreasing. In the severe cases with affected foetus they tend to increase sharply.

The next slide compares determination of both hormons in diabetic pregnancies. The fall of Estriol excretion indicates to preterminal ending of pregnancy. In contrary HPL concentration seems to be less reliable. HPL is in spite of already occuring fetal distress in utero in the upper part of the normal range and it shows no decreasing of serum concentration.

Interesting seems us to be correlation of HPL and Estriol with placental weight. Small placental weight is associated with the low hormon levels. As well as were found low hormon concentrations in multiple infarction of placenta. In case of retardation of fetal weight in utero were extrem low concentration of HPL.

There was no correlation in the monitoring of pregnancy with amnioscopy and hormon levels, t. m. the presense of meconium in the amniotic fluid was not always identical with the lower concentration of HPL or Estriol.

Summary: Both monitoring methods give satisfactory results, they complete one another.

Estriol seems to be reliable for monitoring of pregnancies complicated with Gestosis, Rh-incompatibility and diabetes mellitus.

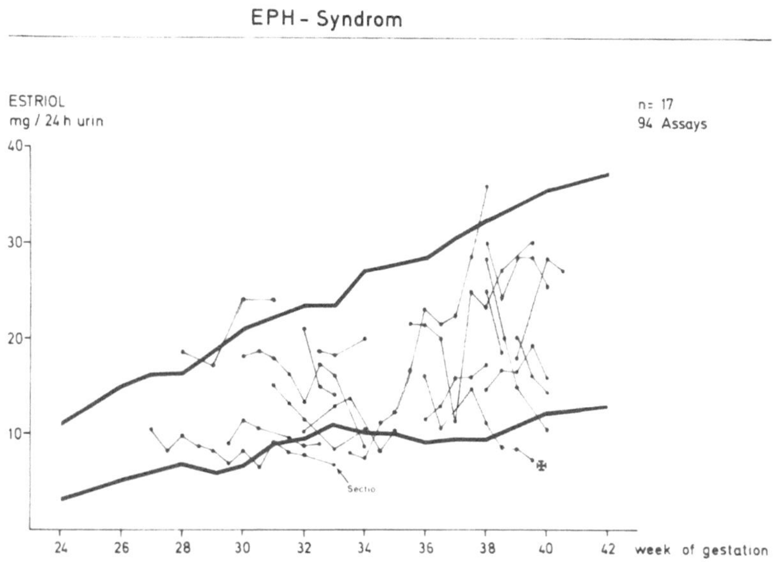
EPH - Syndrom
ESTRIOL
mg / 24 h urin
n= 17
94 Assays
40
30
20
10
Sectio
24
26
28
30
32
34
36
38
40
42
week of gestation

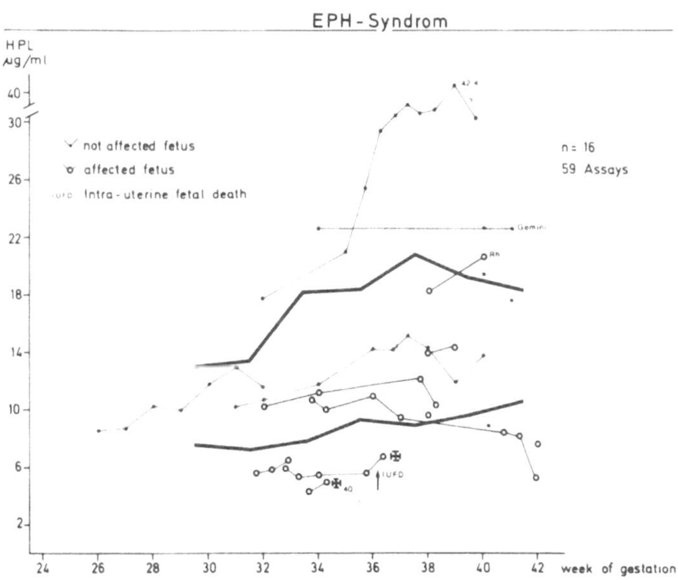
EPH - Syndrom
HPL
µg/ml
40
30
26
22
18
14
10
6
2
not affected fetus
affected fetus
Intra - uterine fetal death
n= 16
59 Assays
Gemini
Rh
IUFD
40
24
26
28
30
32
34
36
38
40
42
week of gestation

Fig. 1

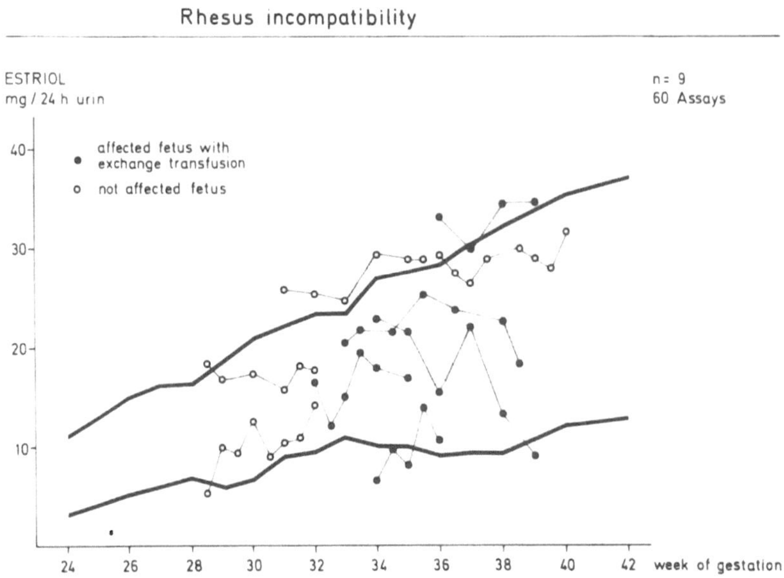
Rhesus incompatibility
ESTRIOL
mg / 24 h urin
n = 9
60 Assays
affected fetus with exchange transfusion
not affected fetus
40
30
20
10
24
26
28
30
32
34
36
38
40
42
week of gestation

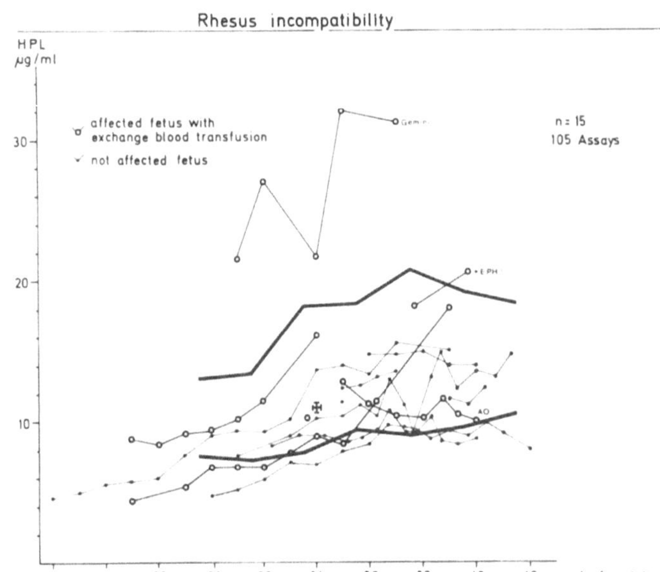
Rhesus incompatibility
HPL
µg/ml
affected fetus with exchange blood transfusion
not affected fetus
n = 15
105 Assays
30
20
10
24
26
28
30
32
34
36
38
40
42
week of gestation

Fig. 2

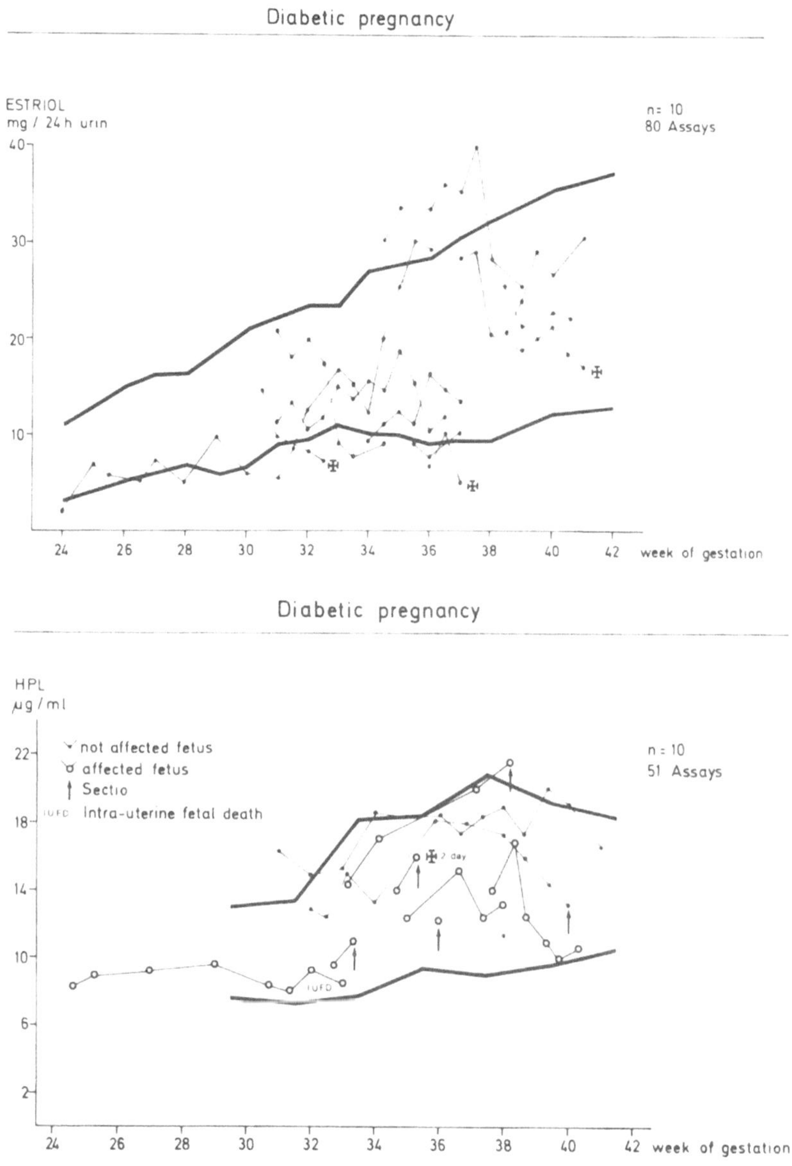
Diabetic pregnancy
ESTRIOL
mg / 24 h urin
n: 10
80 Assays
40
30
20
10
24
26
28
30
32
34
36
38
40
42
week of gestation
Diabetic pregnancy
HPL
µg / ml
not affected fetus
affected fetus
Sectio
IUFD Intra-uterine fetal death
n : 10
51 Assays
22
18
14
10
6
2
IUFD
24
26
28
30
32
34
36
38
40
42
week of gestation

Fig. 3

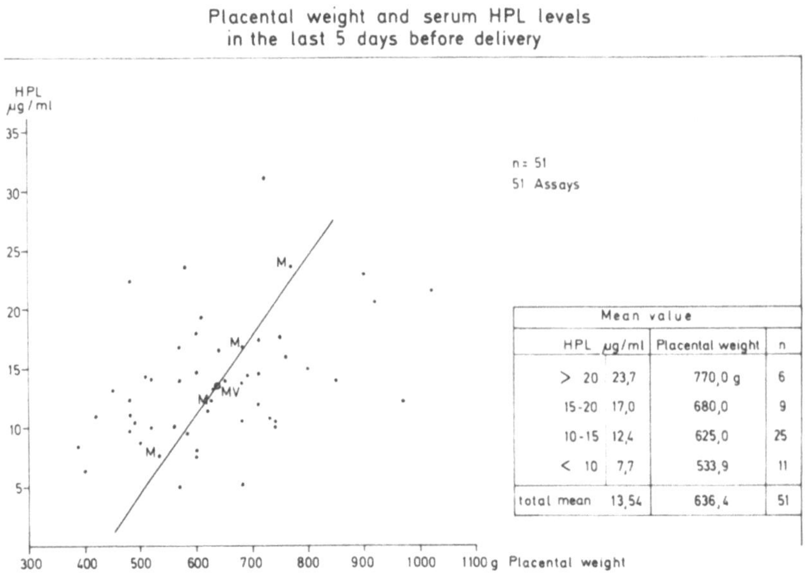

Mean value			
HPL µg/ml		Placental weight	n
> 20	23,7	770,0 g	6
15-20	17,0	680,0	9
10-15	12,4	625,0	25
< 10	7,7	533,9	11
total mean	13,54	636,4	51

Fig. 4

The HPL concentration was especially reliable in the monitoring of retardation of foetal weight in utero p. e. due to severe EPH Gestosis.

In case of jeopardy of intra-uterine fetal death the HPL fall occurs first and later follows decreasing of Estriol excretion.

The Pathology of Feto-Placental Insufficiency in Hypertensive Pregnancy

W. B. Robertson, I. A. Brosens, and H. G. Dixon

Introduction

In seeking a rational approach to the pathology, and hence the treatment, of dysmaturity attributable to placental insufficiency, it may be a good idea to reflect carefully upon the pathology of one cause of placental insufficiency where there is now a better understanding of the morphological lesions associated with placental disease and consequent fetal dysmaturity. The term placental insufficiency is perhaps an unfortunate one as, to many, it implies intrinsic disease of the placenta itself whereas in a large proportion of cases of "small-for-dates" babies the ultimate cause will probably be found to be due to defective interaction between fetal and maternal tissues in the uterus. In hypertensive disease of pregnancy it is now generally agreed that the critical defect is to be found on the maternal side of the placenta, with due allowance being made for the undetermined part played by fetal tissues in the aetiology of pre-eclampsia. This being so it is obvious that we must look for lesions in the maternal blood vessels supplying the placenta that can be related to lesions in the placenta to explain the undernutrition of the fetus and its frequent hypoxia. In the same way we concentrate our attention on the coronary arteries to explain the myocardial lesions of ischaemic heart disease.

Regrettably, despite the detailed work done by many people (HAMILTON and BOYD, 1960; HARRIS and RAMSEY, 1966; BROSENS and DIXON, 1966; BOYD and HAMILTON, 1967; BROSENS, ROBERTSON and DIXON, 1967; GRUENWALD, 1972) in recent years, few reproductive biologists, obstetricians and pathologists have more than a rudimentary knowledge of the anatomy of the maternal vascular supply to the human placenta and little knowledge of the fascinating way that trophoblast establishes haemochorial placentation by its action on the maternal vessels.

Utero-placental Arteries in Normal Pregnancy

If we are to understand something of the pathology of the maternal spiral arteries we must have, first of all, a very clear picture of the normal appearances of these vessels during pregnancy, and it must be emphasized that normal in this context is not the normal that a vascular pathologist uses as his point of reference.

In the non-pregnant uterus of the young woman the spiral arteries are the terminal branches of the uterine radial arteries, their origin lying just proximal to the myometrial-endometrial junction; as their name indicates they are tortuous, an essential anatomic feature to ensure adaptability during the menstrual cycle and pregnancy. They are muscular arteries, 200 to 300 microns in diameter, with a thin endothelialised intima, prominent musculo-elastic media and connective tissue adventitia (Fig. 1). This is the picture of normality that the pathologist has in mind when he is assessing arterial lesions anywhere in the body.

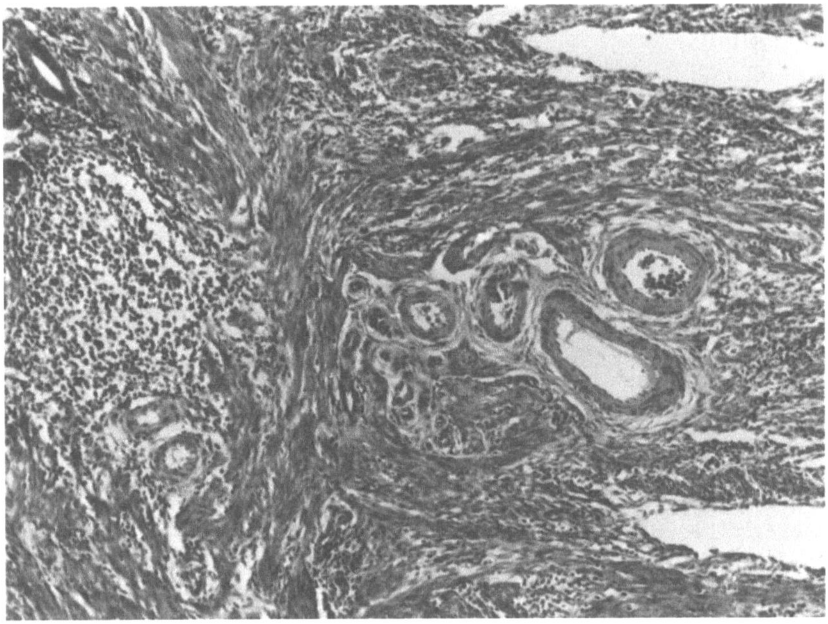

Fig. 1. Normal spiral artery in the non-pregnant uterus at its entry from the myometrium (right) to the endometrium (left). X 125

In stark contrast the normal spiral artery in the placental bed during pregnancy presents a very different picture (Fig. 2). The word normal has to be emphasized, for, as will presently become apparent, without vessels like these to supply the placenta, and hence the fetus, the pregnancy would probably be abnormal. If allowance is made for the artifactual collapse, the consequence of biopsy and processing procedures, it will be appreciated that the lumen is considerably larger than that of spiral arteries in the non-pregnant uterus. Arteries of this dimension must be elaborated if the blood supply is to be increased from the few millilitres per minute for the endometrium in the non-pregnant uterus to the calculated half-a-litre per minute required for the fetus and placenta in the third trimester of pregnancy. The distensibility of the artery has been achieved by partial destruction of the musculo-elastic media, in much the same way that aneurysms are formed, and its replacement by fibrinoid material and connective tissue. This alteration of the morphology and function of the spiral arteries in the placental bed we have called "physiological changes" (BROSENS, ROBERTSON and DIXON, 1967) on the reasonable grounds that they are an essential feature of normal pregnancy. It follows that the physiological changes in the spiral arteries must become the baseline for studying pathology in these same vessels, the true utero-placental arteries, during pregnancy.

To understand how the physiological changes are brought about we must go back to early pregnancy. After implantation the cytotrophoblast shell rapidly proliferates in and through the decidualized endometrium. Maternal capillaries and venules are invaded and later the decidual terminations of the spiral arteries in what is to be the placental bed (Fig. 3). The trophoblast at this early stage of placentation appears

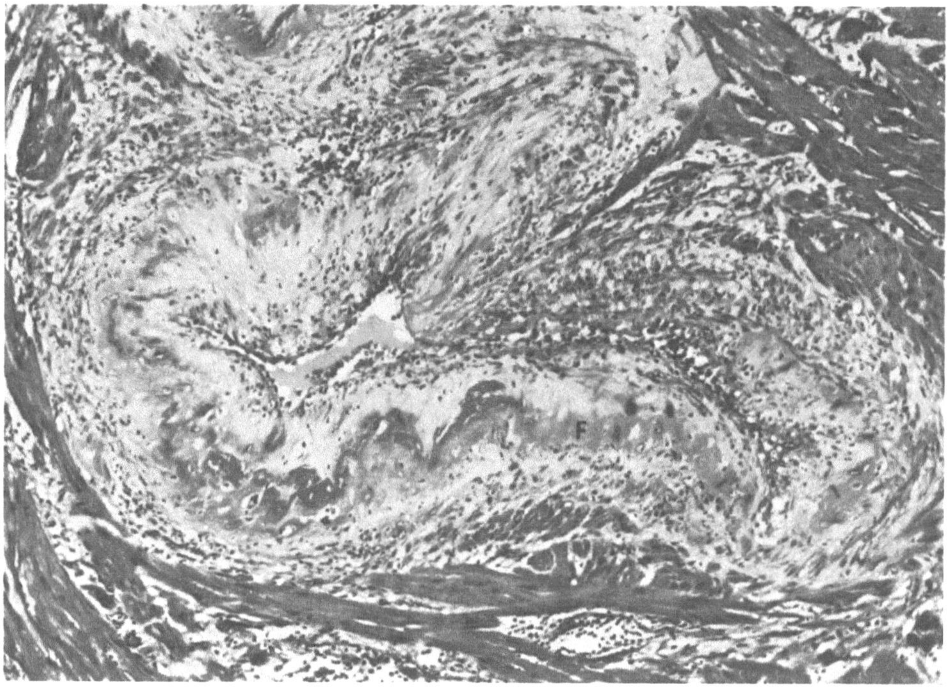

Fig. 2. Placental bed biopsy at 36 weeks gestation: fully developed physiological changes in the myometrial segment of a spiral artery. Artifactual collapse of artery but note convoluted fibrinoid layer (F) containing a few degenerate trophoblasts and mild round cell infiltrate around the artery. X 125

to replace the endothelium and it also infiltrates the musculo-elastic media. This latter feature is associated with the deposition of fibrinoid material in the vessel wall, there being an inverse relation of the amount of fibrinoid to musculo-elastic tissue. The proliferating trophoblast has now breached the main arteries and veins to establish a direct blood supply to, and drainage from, the developing placenta.

As placentation progresses trophoblast extends through the basal decidua and by the twelfth week is well established in the inner third of the myometrium. The spiral arteries are also colonized by the infiltrating trophoblast (Fig. 4) and the trophoblastic action on the walls of these arteries continues quite deeply into the myometrium (Fig. 5); by the twenty-eighth week of gestation it may even have reached the terminations of the radial arteries. Fig. 2 shows the fully-developed physiological changes that can be seen in spiral arteries in a biopsy of the placental bed in the last weeks of normal pregnancy. The final result is the conversion of the spiral arteries of the placental bed to a series, somewhere in the region of 100 to 150 in all, of distended, tortuous and funnel-shaped vessels opening into the intervillous space (Fig. 6). As might be expected the spiral arteries near the centre of the placenta show the most extensive changes while those near the periphery show the least and, of course, the spiral arteries outside the placental bed terminate in the decidua parietalis and show no evidence

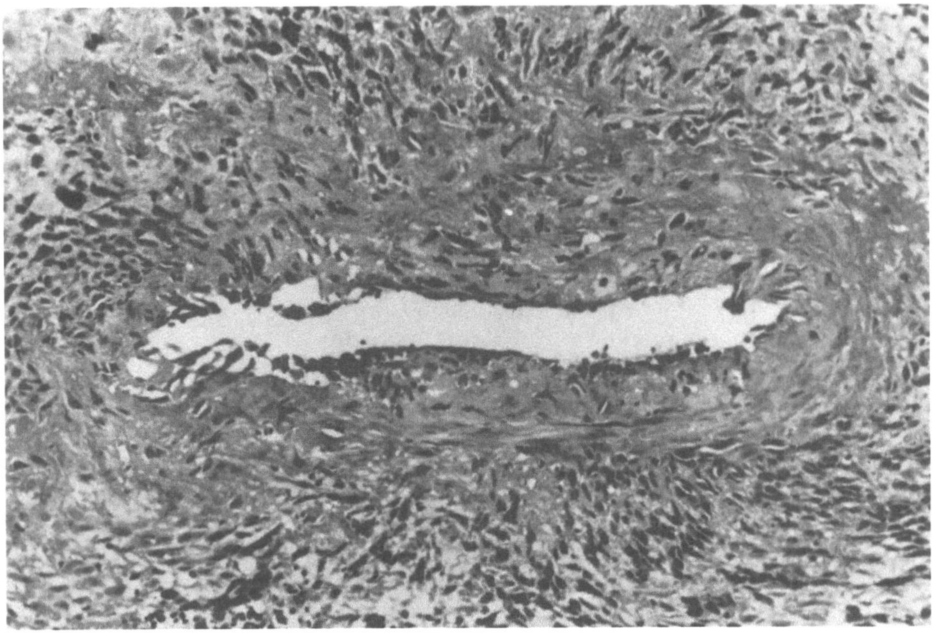

Fig. 3. Post-abortion curettage: decidual spiral artery infiltrated by mononuclear cytotrophoblast. Trophoblast appears to replace the endothelium and there is deposition of fibrinoid material in and around the artery wall. X 160

of physiological changes since there is no trophoblast infiltration. Another class of artery seen in the placental bed are small branches, about 100 microns or less in diameter, of the radials or spirals which are called basal arteries; they do not communicate with the intervillous space but supply only myometrium, terminate in the decidua basalis and hence do not undergo physiological changes.

It has been established (MOLL and KÜNZEL, 1972) that, in animal haemochorial placentation, there is a marked drop in peripheral vascular resistance in the placental bed whereas in ephithelio-chorial placentation the normal peripheral resistance is maintained. In human pregnancy there is almost certainly a reduction of peripheral resistance in the placental bed as a result of the physiological changes in the spiral arteries. Peripheral vascular resistance in arteries is determined by vasomotor influences acting on the muscular or musculo-elastic tissue in the vessel wall. The loss of much of this responsive tissue in arteries which have undergone physiological changes must lead to a loss of resistance, distension of the vessel walls and hence greater conductance, in other words increased blood flow, in the intervillous space.

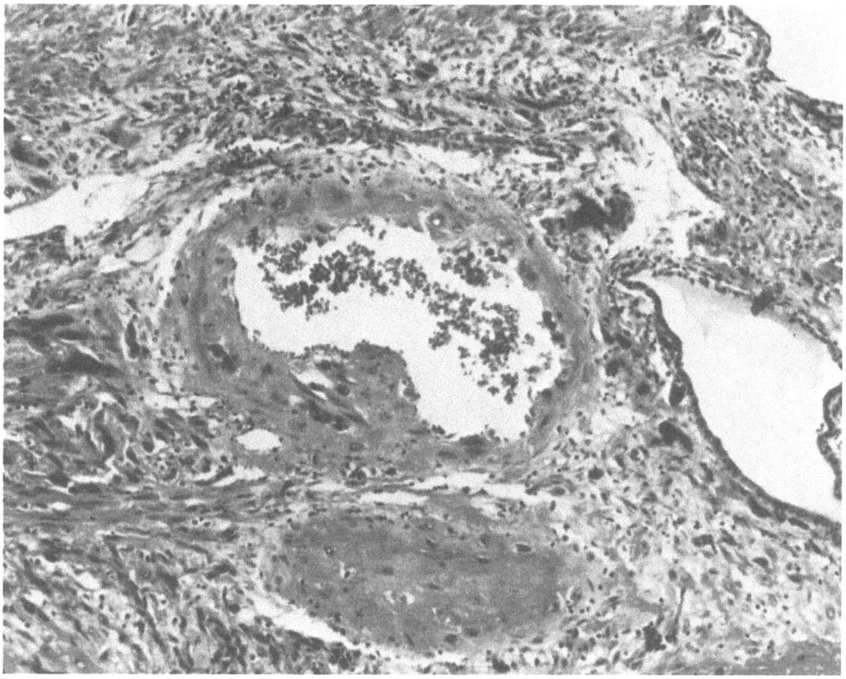

Fig. 4. Hysterectomy specimen at 12 weeks gestation: spiral artery at deciduo-myometrial junction with cytotrophoblast and fibrinoid deposition in the artery wall. Endometrial gland (right) and syncytial giant cells around the artery. X 125

Vascular Lesions in Hypertensive Pregnancy

In systemic hypertension there is known to be increased peripheral resistance in arteries throughout the body but the mechanism producing this increased resistance is unknown. There is evidence from clinical studies (BROWNE and VEALL, 1953; DIXON, BROWNE and DAVEY, 1963) that the uterus shares this defect in hypertensive pregnancy.

In essential hypertension changes ultimately develop in the arterial system. Apart from the increased incidence of atherosclerosis in large arteries (ROBERTSON and STRONG, 1968) there are the classical lesions of hyaline change and arteriosclerosis in small arteries, usually best seen in the kidney. In pregnant women with essential hypertension one would not, perhaps, expect to see similar lesions in the arteries of the placental bed. The hypertension is usually mild or moderate in degree and of relatively short duration as the women are young. It is therefore surprising to find that lesions do occur in the spiral arteries of the placental bed in association with essential hypertension and they may be quite severe. Although hyalinisation of small arteries is rare, hyperplastic arteriosclerosis of the myometrial segments of the spiral arteries is a frequent finding, the degree depending on the

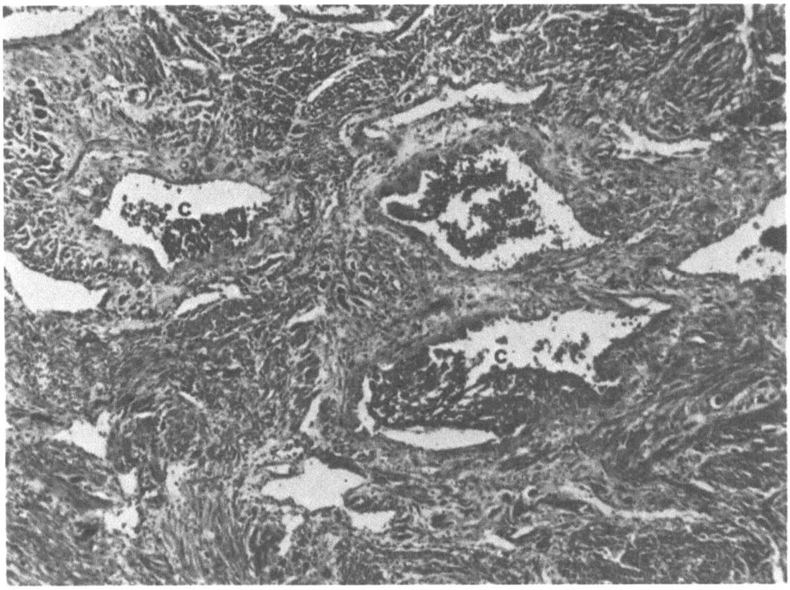

Fig. 5. Hysterectomy specimen at 16 weeks gestation: cytotrophoblast (C) in the lumens and walls of spiral vessels in the myometrium with development of the vascular physiological changes. X 60

severity of the hypertension. The lesions illustrated in Fig. 7 were found in the placental bed of a parous woman of 35 who was known to have had a moderate degree of essential hypertension, with blood pressure readings in the region of 180/110 mm Hg., for about three years prior to the pregnancy from which the biopsy came. The myometrial spiral arteries show marked medial and intimal hyperplasia with luminal stenosis and it is scarcely surprising that, with the onset of pre-eclampsia, caesarean section had to be performed because of hypoxia in a small infant.

When systemic hypertension is of the accelerated or malignant form a different lesion is seen in small arteries, again usually seen best in the kidney. It is a fibrinoid arterio- or arteriolonecrosis and, while it may be the direct result of rapid changes in haemodynamics, there are probably other factors involved in its pathogenesis. In many respects, though by no means in all, pre-eclampsia can be regarded as the analogue of malignant hypertension in pregnancy, and, in fact, we do find an analogous lesion in the intra-uterine arteries of women with pre-eclampsia (Fig. 8). In its fully developed form there is acute fibrinoid necrosis of the vessel wall, infiltration of the damaged wall by lipophages and a mononuclear cellular infiltrate in and around the affected artery. This lesion was first described by HERTIG (1945) and was fully investigated by ZEEK and ASSALI (1950) who gave it the name "acute atherosis" because of its lipid component, by which name it is

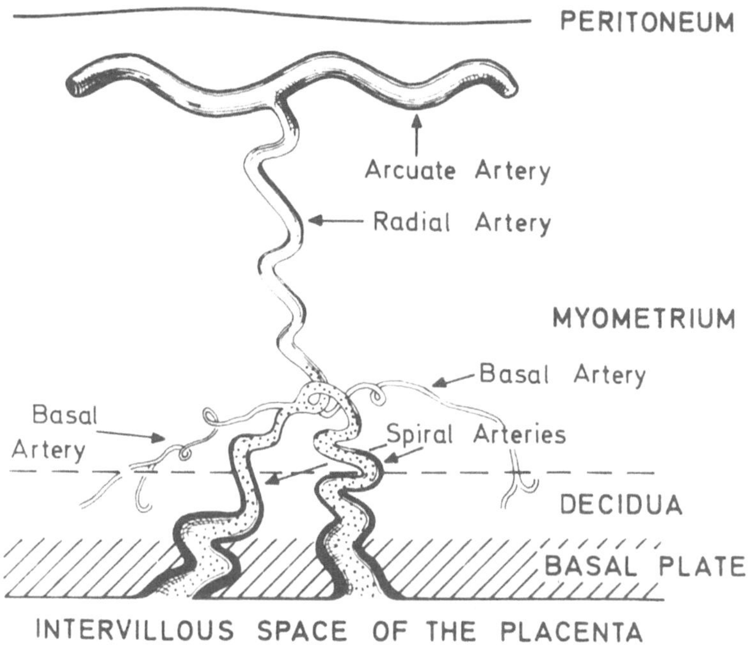

Fig. 6. Diagram illustrating the established blood supply to the mature placenta

now generally known. These lesions are seen most clearly in the arteries of the decidua parietalis adjacent to the placental bed as there are no physiological changes in these small vessels to confuse the picture.

Acute atherosis is also found in the spiral arteries of the placental bed, particularly at the myometrial-decidual junction (Fig. 9), but here the fibrinoid necrosis tends to be less pronounced and the foam cells with fibroblastic proliferation more prominent. The arteriopathy may extend into the decidual segments of the utero-placental arteries but the antecedent physiological changes, having already converted these segments into what are virtually fibrinoid tubes, tend to dominate the picture. When typical atherosis is seen in the decidua basalis it is much more likely to be seen in the small terminations of the basal arteries.

When pre-eclampsia complicates essential hypertension, as would be anticipated, we find a mixture of hyperplastic arteriosclerosis, reflecting the pre-existant hypertension, and acute atherosis associated with the pre-eclampsia (Fig. 10). In the example of atherosis illustrated, which is from the same biopsy as Fig. 7, there is almost total destruction of a myometrial segment of the spiral artery with near occlusion of the lumen. With this spectrum of disease in the spiral arteries one must expect more frequent development of occlusive thrombosis (Fig. 11) with infarction of the decidua and the area of the fetal pla-

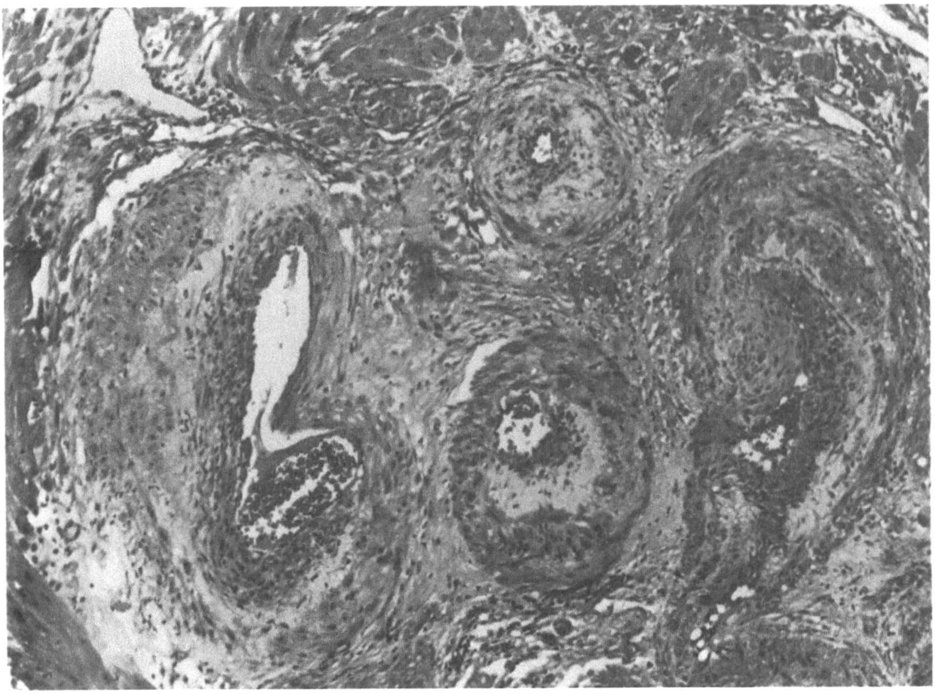

Fig. 7. Placental bed biopsy from a case of essential hypertension. Myometrial spiral arteries lacking physiological changes but showing hyperplastic arteriosclerosis with luminal stenoses. X 125

centa supplied by the artery in question (WILKIN, 1965; WALLENBURG, 1969; WIGGLESWORTH, 1969; BROSENS and RENAER, 1972). The hazards to the fetus in such cases are only too well known.

However the story does not end there. In reviewing our large collection of placental bed biopsies and caesarean hysterectomy specimens from normotensive and hypertensive women (BROSENS, ROBERTSON and DIXON, 1972) we noticed two other features associated with hypertension in pregnancy and, in particular, with pre-eclampsia. When we re-examined the cases of pre-eclampsia we found that the physiological changes, in contrast to normal pregnancy, involved only the decidual segments of the spiral arteries in the placental bed and did not extend retrogradely into the myometrial segments. Assessment of the myometrial zone of the placental bed revealed arteries affected by atherosis but spiral arteries free from atherosis were essentially normal in the strictly morphological sence (Fig. 12) unless there had been antecedent essential hypertension; this despite the presence of abundant trophoblast cells free in the surrounding myometrium.

Following on this observation we noted that acute atherosis almost always affected segments of arteries that had not undergone physiological changes, in effect the spiral arteries at the myometrial-decidual junc-

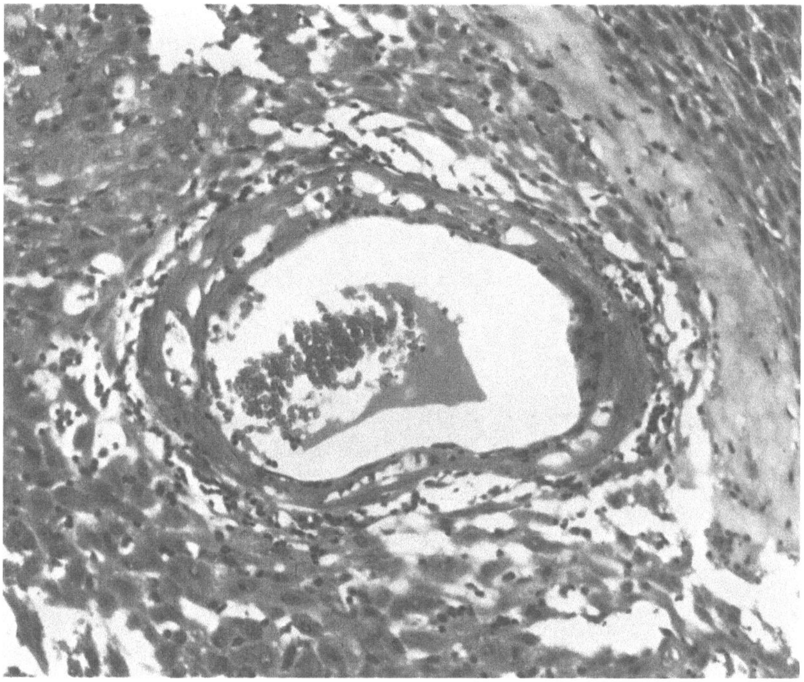

Fig. 8. Biopsy from decidua parietalis adjacent to the placental bed from a case of pre-eclampsia. Acute atherosis in decidual spiral artery with fibrinoid necrosis, intra-mural lipophages and infiltrate of small mononuclear cells around the damaged artery. X 200

tion of the placental bed, the basal arteries in the myometrium and their terminations in the decidua basalis, and the terminations of the spiral arteries in the decidua parietalis adjacent to, but not in, the basal plate (Fig. 13). The situation was similar where essential hypertension was complicated by pre-eclampsia except that, to make matters worse, the myometrial segments of the spiral arteries had already undergone hyperplastic arteriosclerotic changes. All the illustrations of hypertensive lesions in this presentation (Figs. 7, 8, 9, 10 and 11) come from arteries which show no physiological changes and all the photomicrographs published in the literature on this subject (HERTIG, 1945; ZEEK and ASSALI, 1950; DIXON and ROBERTSON, 1958, 1961; MARAIS, 1962; BROSENS, 1964; MAQUEO et al., 1964; WILKIN, 1965; ROBERTSON, BROSENS and DIXON, 1967; BENIRSCHKE and DRISCOLL, 1967; BROSENS, ROBERTSON and DIXON, 1972; KITZMILLER and BENIRSCHKE, 1973) confirm this to be so. We have carefully scrutinized all the published photomicrographs of decidual atherosis and they show small vessels that can only be terminations of the non-placental bed spiral arteries in the decidua parietalis or terminations of the basal arteries in the decidua basalis. Their small calibre and the absence of physiological changes clearly indicate that these vessels are not true utero-placental arteries and could not possibly supply the large volume of blood required by the placenta and fetus in the last trimester of pregnancy.

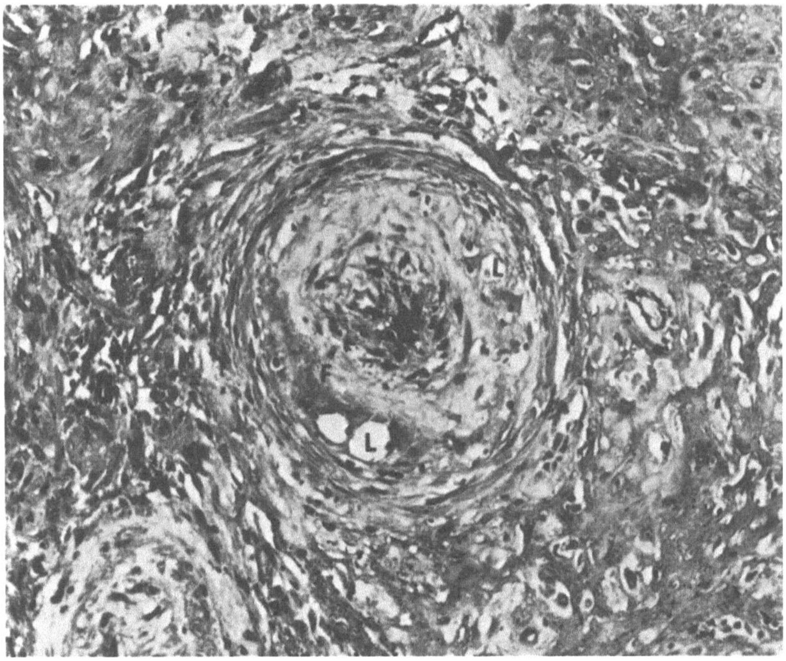

Fig. 9. Placental bed biopsy from a case of pre-eclampsia. Small spiral artery at myometrial-decidual junction without physiological changes. Intima is thickened by loose connective tissue, some fibrinoid necrosis (F) and vacuolated lipophages (L). X 250

Comments and Conclusions

It would therefore seem that in those women destined to develop pre-eclampsia later in pregnancy there is first of all an inadequate response of their spiral arteries to the normal, physiological processes of placentation with restriction of the vascular changes to the terminations of the spiral arteries in the decidua basalis. These findings do not, of course, by themselves explain the later onset of the clinical features of pre-eclampsia, the hypertension, albuminuria and oedema, but they do go a long way to explain why a small baby may be born to a woman who has shown the clinical features of pre-eclampsia for only a few days. They also correlate well with the observation that, in general, the infant of a woman with essential hypertension who subsequently develops pre-eclampsia is at an even greater risk.

It will be obvious that arising out of all this there are two important, related problems. The first is why the trophoblast in pre-eclamptic pregnancies is only partially successful in effecting the physiological changes in the spiral arteries and the second is the relation of this

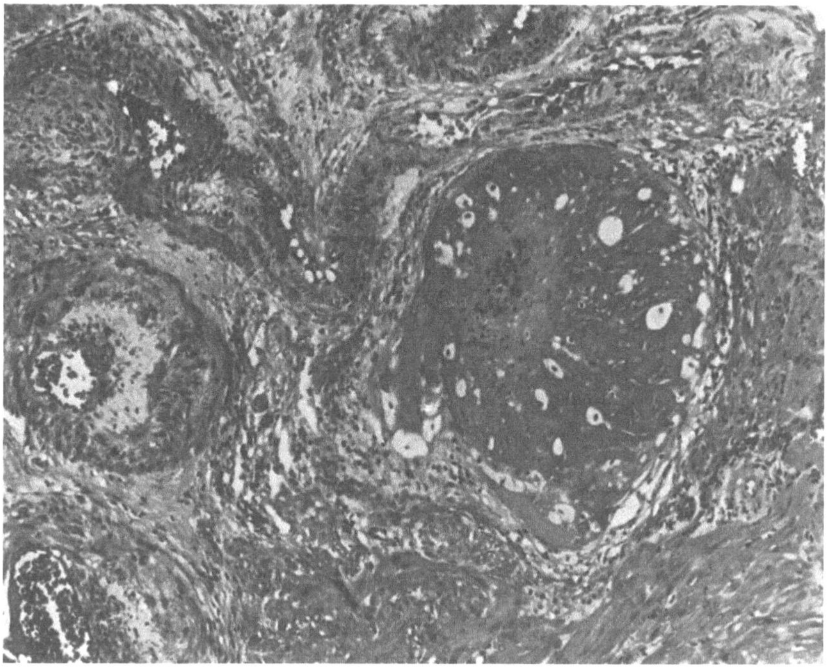

Fig. 10. Placental bed biopsy from a case of essential hypertension complicated by pre-eclampsia. No physiological changes in the myometrial spiral arteries which show hyperplastic arteriosclerosis (left) and acute atherosis with occlusion (right). X 125

inadequate vascular response to the clinical syndrome of pre-eclampsia. With regard to the first it may be that there is some intrinsic defect in the trophoblast itself but we think it more likely that the normal reaction of fetal with maternal tissues is in some way defective. It is tempting to postulate that the maternal tissues mount an immunological repulsion of the trophoblast in the vessels but, if so, why is the trophoblast in the surrounding myometrium immune? Following up the idea of an inappropriate immune response it would be attractive to regard the acute atherosis of pre-eclampsia as a delayed maternal hypersensitivity response to earlier fetal antigenic sensitization, and there is some recent evidence (KITZMILLER and BENIRSCHKE, 1973) that acute atherosis has an immunological component, a suggestion we made some time ago (ROBERTSON, BROSENS and DIXON, 1967). But here, too, there are snags amongst which are the facts that acute atherosis occurs in myometrial and decidual arteries remote from trophoblast, the presumptive source of the fetal antigens, and that acute atherosis affects only the arteries in the uterus and not arteries elsewhere.

One could argue equally strongly that the hypertensive lesions, both the hyperplastic and the necrotizing, can be explained in terms of haemodynamics. With the inadequate vascular response of early pregnancy there is maintenance of a high peripheral resistance in the placental bed, and

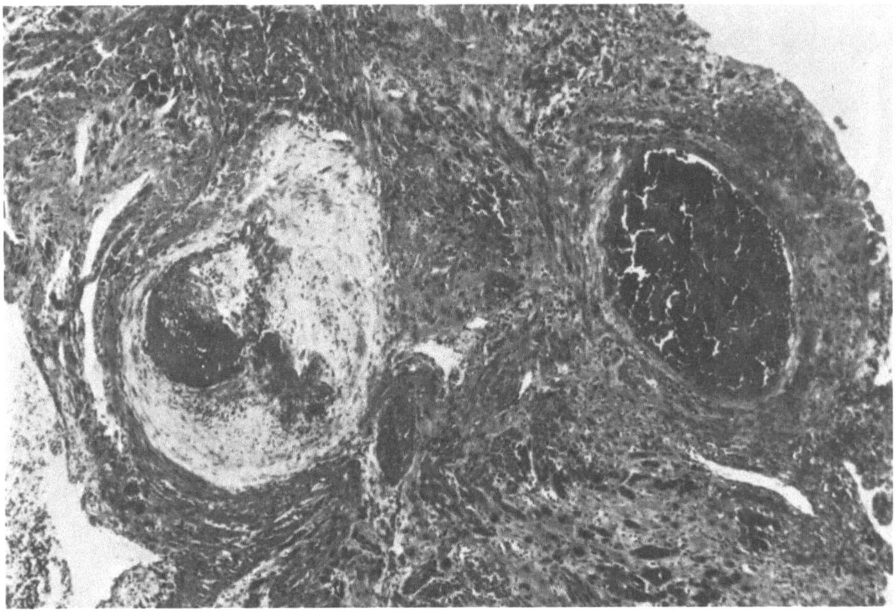

Fig. 11. Placental bed biopsy from a case of pre-eclampsia. Organising and recent thrombosis of spiral artery (left) with recent thrombus extending into the decidual segment (right) causing decidual infarction. X 60

essential hypertension can only increase it, so that hyperplastic arteriosclerosis may develop more quickly in an area where there is continuous adaptive and proliferative activity associated with the developing conceptus. The onset of the hypertension of pre-eclampsia is much more acute and probably the most vulnerable arterial segments are those at the myometrial-decidual junction and the terminations in the decidua parietalis. This is an analogous situation to that in malignant nephrosclerosis where the acute arterial lesions are thought to be due mainly to the rapid rise in blood pressure acting on unprotected small arteries, the afferent arterioles of the glomeruli at the extremity of the arterial tree. The terminal branches of the non-placental bed spiral arteries in the decidua vera or parietalis and the terminations of the basal arteries in the decidua basalis, although small, still retain their muscular coats and are therefore responsive to vasomotor influences. There is good evidence for believing that fibrinoid arterionecrosis in accelerated systemic hypertension is probably initiated by damage to smooth muscle by hyper-reaction to the altered haemodynamics of that condition and a similar situation may arise in the small decidual arteries in pre-eclampsia. On the other hand the decidual segments of the utero-placental arteries, having undergone physiological changes, have lost the bulk of their smooth muscle tissue, are already distended and incapable of reacting to vasomotor influences, normal or abnormal. Not so the myometrial segments of these spiral arteries which, unaffected by physiological changes, must bear the brunt of the rapid alterations in haemodynamics associated with pre-eclampsia.

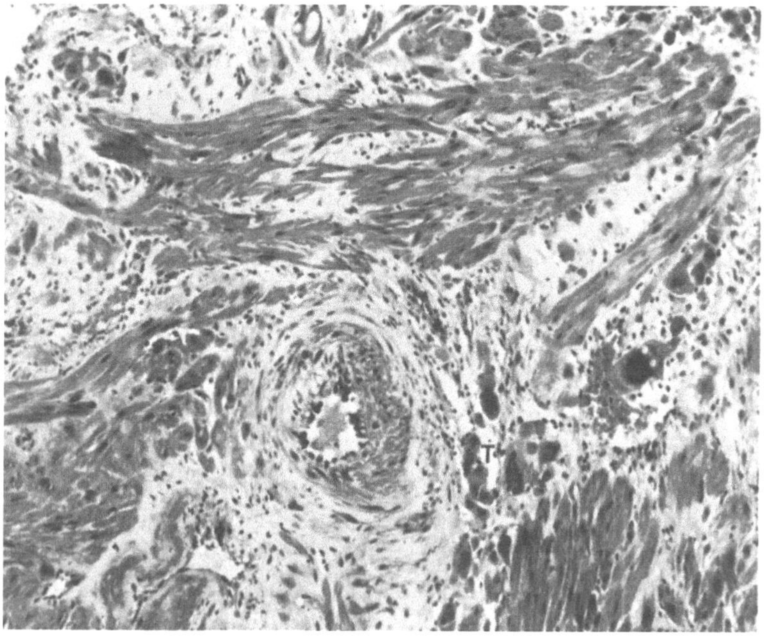

Fig. 12. Placental bed biopsy from a case of pre-eclampsia. Small spiral artery at myometrial-decidual junction; essentially normal artery with no physiological changes despite trophoblast (T) in surrounding myometrium. X 125

We can only offer our thoughts and speculations on these problems having no evidence other than morphological to support them but one conclusion from our findings would seem to be valid. If it is essential for normal haemochorial placentation that there be a marked lowering of the peripheral arterial resistance in the placental bed then anything that compromises the physiological changes in the spiral arteries must act to maintain a high peripheral resistance with consequent diminished perfusion of the intervillous space. The addition of pathological lesions in these same vessels can only worsen the situation and this seems to be what happens in the hypertensive states of pregnancy.

We wish we could report that we found similar defects in the physiological response of the placental bed vasculature in normotensive women with "small-for-dates" babies. We did find some cases with poorly developed physiological changes but others with an apparently normal response, at least as judged from placental bed biopsies. Morphometry applied to the fetal placenta (AHERNE and DUNNILL, 1966) has shown that, where the baby is small for the gestational age, the placenta is also small with considerable reduction in the total villous surface area, the mean volume of the intervillous space and the mean volume of the fetal capillaries. Since the fetal placenta is entirely dependant upon

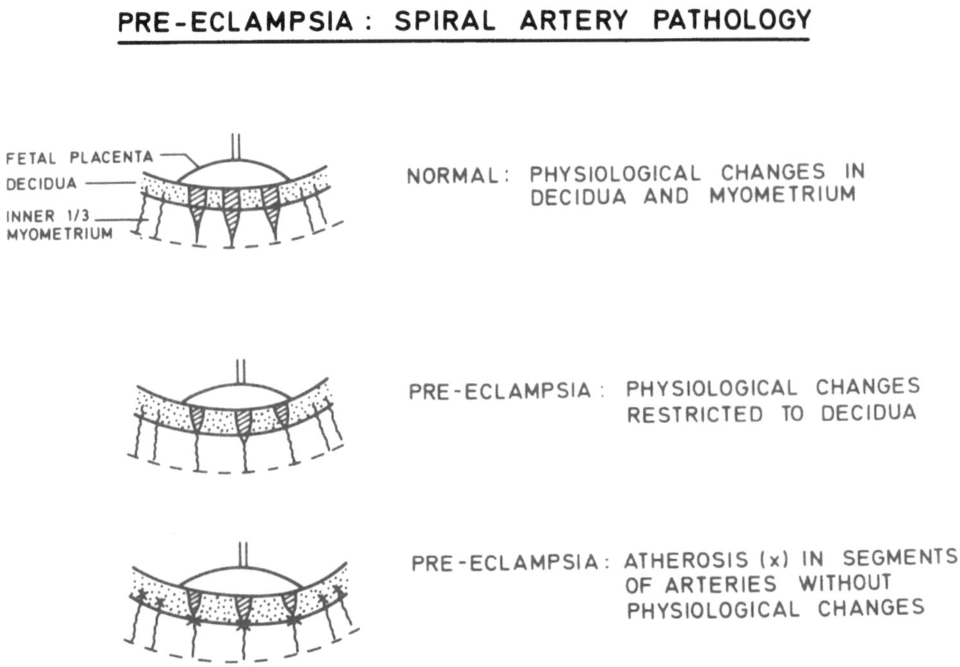

Fig. 13. Diagram summarising spiral artery pathology in pre-eclampsia. Note that the spiral arteries terminating in the decidua parietalis adjacent to the placenta do not undergo physiological changes but frequently show acute atherosis with the onset of pre-eclampsia

the maternal blood supply for its nutrition it would seem logical to apply morphometric methods to a study of the maternal blood supply in these cases to determine the number of spiral arteries opening into the intervillous space, the extent of the physiological changes and the degree of distension of the utero-placental arteries. Unhappily for the research worker but happily for the women concerned the essential material, the pregnant uterus, is seldom made available.

References

1. AHERNE, W., DUNNILL, M. S.: J. Path. Bact. 91, 123 (1966).
2. BENIRSCHKE, K., DRISCOLL, S. G.: The Pathology of the Human Placenta. p. 216. New York: Springer-Verlag 1967.
3. BOYD, J. D., HAMILTON, W. J.: J. Obstet. Gynaec. Brit. Commonw. 74, 161 (1967).
4. BROSENS, I.: J. Obstet. Gynaec. Brit. Commonw. 71, 222 (1964).
5. BROSENS, I., DIXON, H. G.: J. Obstet. Gynaec. Brit. Commonw. 73, 357 (1966).
6. BROSENS, I., RENAER, M.: J. Obstet. Gynaec. Brit. Commonw. 79, 794 (1972).
7. BROSENS, I., ROBERTSON, W. B., DIXON, H. G.: J. Path. Bact. 93, 569 (1967).

8. BROSENS, I., ROBERTSON, W. B., DIXON, H. G.: In Obstetrics and Gynecology Annual, Ed. R. M. Wynn, Appleton-Century-Crofts, New York, p. 177 (1972).
9. BROWNE, J. C. M., VEALL, N.: J. Obstet. Gynaec. Brit. Emp. 60, 141 (1953).
10. DIXON, H. G., BROWNE, J. C. M., DAVEY, D. A.: Lancet 2, 369 (1963).
11. DIXON, H. G., ROBERTSON, W. B.: J. Obstet. Gynaec. Brit. Emp. 65, 803 (1958).
12. DIXON, H. G., ROBERTSON, W. B.: Path. Microbiol. 24, 622 (1961).
13. GRUENWALD, P.: Anat. Rec. 173, 189 (1972),
14. HAMILTON, W. J., BOYD, J. D.: J. Anat. 94, 297 (1960).
15. HARRIS, J. W. S., RAMSEY, E. M.: Contrib. Embryol. Carneg. Inst. 38, 43 (1966).
16. HERTIG, A. T.: Clinics 4, 602 (1945).
17. KITZMILLER, J. L., BENIRSCHKE, K.: Am. J. Obstet. Gynec. 115, 248 (1973).
18. MAQUEO, M., CHAVEZ AZUELA, J., DOSAL DE LA VEGA, M.: Obstet. Gynec. 24, 350 (1964).
19. MARAIS, W.: J. Obstet. Gynaec. Brit. Commonw. 69, 234 (1962).
20. MOLL, W., KÜNZEL, W.: Pflügers Arch. 338, 125 (1972).
21. ROBERTSON, W. B., BROSENS, I., DIXON, H. G.: J. Path. Bact. 93, 581 (1967).
22. ROBERTSON, W. B., STRONG, J. P.: Lab. Invest. 18, 498 (1968).
23. WALLENBURG, H. C. S.: Arch. Gynäk. 208, 80 (1968).
24. WIGGLESWORTH, J. S.: J. Obstet. Gynaec. Brit. Commonw. 76, 979 (1969).
25. WILKIN, P.: Pathologie du Placenta, Masson, Paris (1965).
26. ZEEK, P. M., ASSALI, N. S.: Am. J. Clin. Path. 20, 1099 (1950).

Search for a Disturbance of Coagulation during Pregnancy in Cases of Intra-Uterine Growth Retardation

A. Benbassa, L. Kolodie, M. Mas, D. Villemin, C. Racinet, and Y. Malinas

It has been recognized for a long time that in cases of pre-eclampsia and eclampsia, occasionally intra-vascular coagulation may be present. (1, 2, 3, 10). The aetiology is unclear. It is not known whether it is primary or secondary to some vascular abnormality. However in 50 per cent of cases of intra-uterine growth retardation (I. U. G. R.) maternal reno-vascular pathology is found.

Placental insufficiency presumably originates from impaired placental blood supply and this leads to I. U. G. R. This impairment of the placental blood flow does not necessarily accompany any vascular or renal pathology, for some women with renal or vascular disease give birth to normal weight infants.

Recently (4) it has been suggested that a state of hypercoagulability could play a part in these cases of growth retardation and we wonder if hypercoagulability is present in pregnancies complicated by I.U.G.R. Nevertheless, such a hypothesis does not necessarily imply that this suggested hypercoagulability is responsible for the impairment of the placental blood flow. It could equally well be secondary to placental insufficiency.

In this study, we have attempted to answer the first question. We split 60 patients into three groups:
1. Group A (20) normal pregnancies
2. Group B (20) pregnancies with reno-vascular pathology (TA > 14/9) and children of normal weight.
3. Group C (20) pregnancies with reno-vascular pathology and I.U.G.R. (the birth weight being 10 % below the normal figures which have been established at the Grenoble Clinic of Obstetrics and Gynaecology).

Table 1

n = 20	KCCT (sec)	KCCT control group (sec)	Platelets	Fibrinogen 9/1	Thrombin clotting time (sec)
Group A normal pregnancy	34 (±3.37)	34 (±3.28)	184500 (±56000)	5 (±1.4)	1 (±1.45)
Group B R.Vasc. Path. + normal weight	32.6 (±3.10)	35 (±2.68)	177600 (±50000)	5.5 (±1.2)	2 (±2)
Group C R.Vasc. Path. + I.U.G.R	32.1 (±2)	35 (±3.87)	160000 (±40000)	4 (±1)	1.33 (±2)

We have excluded pre-eclampsia and eclampsia because of a limited number of cases during the period of study (1970 - 1972).

We performed the following tests:
1. Measurement of the Kaolin Cephalin Clotting Time (KCCT) using the technique of KOLODIE (5).
2. Fibrinogen measurement by the technique of FOSTER (6). A shortening of KCCT and an increase in fibrinogen are the classical tests for hypercaogulability (7).
3. Platelet counts, by CAEN'S method (8). A thrombocytopenia suggests the presence of a disseminated or localized intra-vascular coagulation.
4. Measurement of increase in thrombin clotting time according to the technique CAEN (8). Increase in thrombin clotting time permits a rough estimate of PDF (3). This however, cannot always be verified (9).

Results

1. KCCT. There is a significant difference ($p \leqslant 0.07$) between group C and the control group, which might indicate the existence of an hypercoagulability in these pathological pregnancies. There is no significant difference between groups B and C.

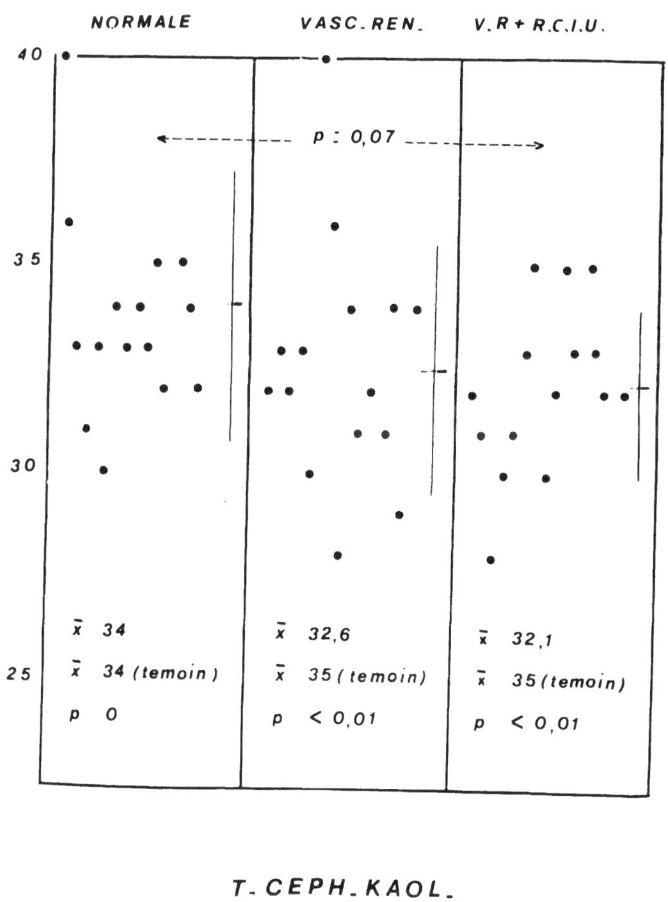

Fig. 1

2. Fibrinogen. There is a significant difference ($p \leqslant 0.01$) in fibrinogen titres in groups B and C. This difference is slight between groups A and C (Fig. 2).

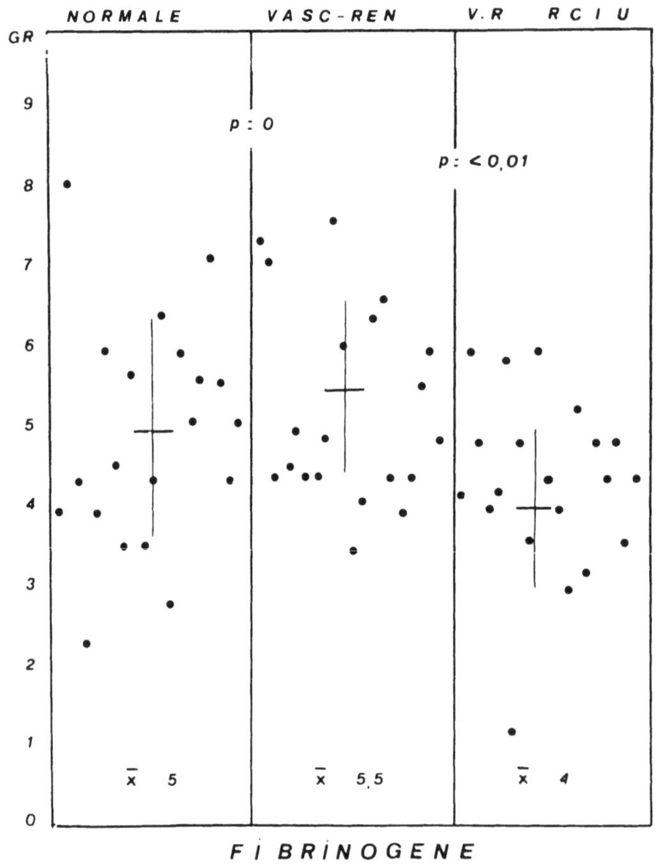

Fig. 2

3. Platelets. There is no significant difference between the platelet counts of groups B and C but a slight difference ($p \leq 0.12$) between groups A and C. There is often some thrombo-cytopenia in pregnancies with reno-vascular pathology and I. U. G. R. (group C) (Fig. 3).

4. Thrombin Clotting Time. The difference is not significant between the 3 groups. In normal pregnancies, the increase in Thrombin Clotting Time is always less than 5 seconds while it is more than 5 seconds in five cases with reno-vascular disease (Fig. 4).

We have a few tentative suggestions:
Reno-vascular pathology, with or without I. U. G. R., is accompanied by hypercoagulability as shown by the KCCT.

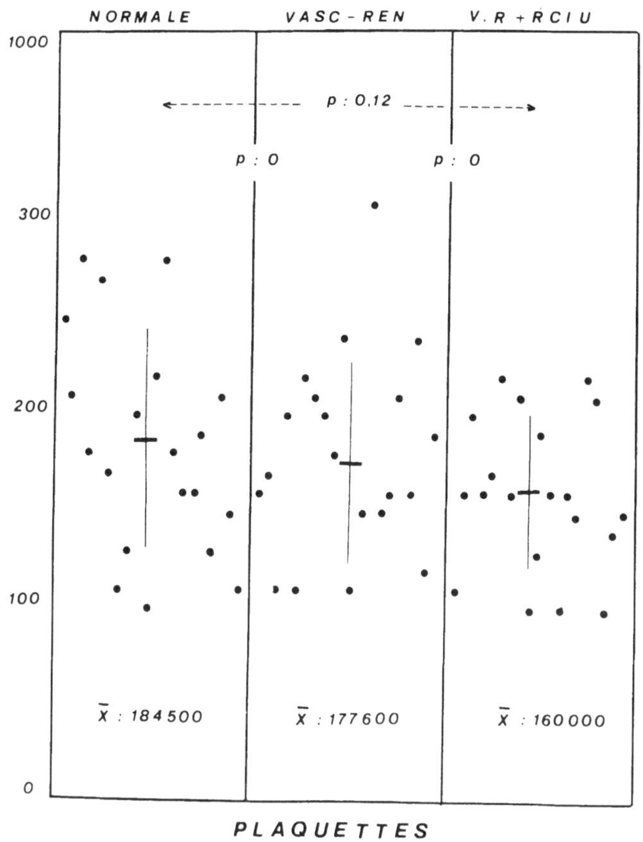

Fig. 3

The decrease in the platelet count is greater in group C than in group A which could favour the presence of intra-vascular coagulation.

The significantly reduced fibrinogen titres in group C as compared with group B are of interest.

Fibrinogen concentration represents a balance between the rate of hepatic synthesis and peripheral breakdown. In acute or sub-acute conditions, destruction is more rapid than synthesis leading to hypofibrinogenaemia.

In chronic conditions fibrin degeneration products, from fibrinolysis after intra-vascular coagulation, are followed by an increase in hepatic synthesis. Thus paradoxically a hyperfibrinogenaemia occurs. We are unable to explain our measured hypofibrinogenaemia.

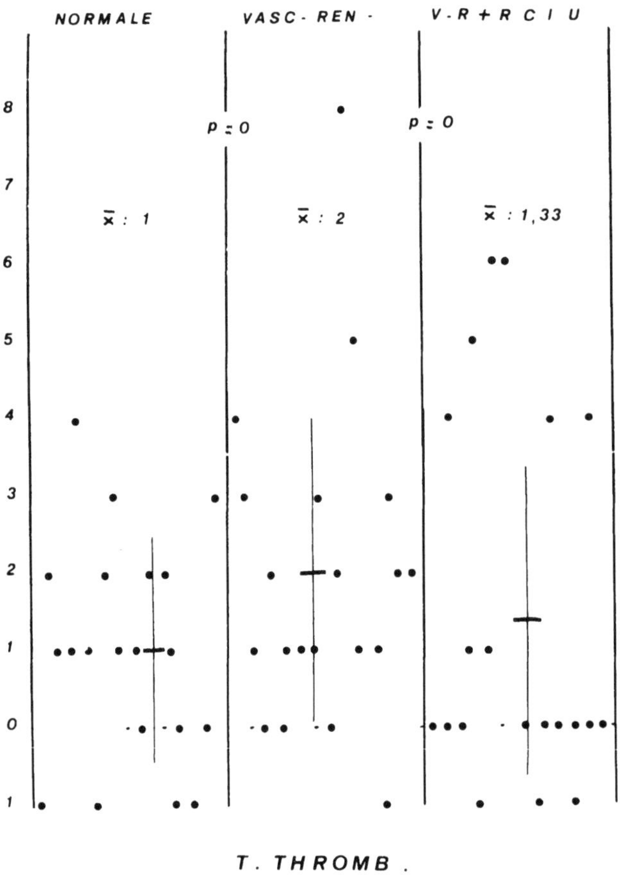

Fig. 4

References

1. HOWIE, P. W., PRENTICE, C. R. M., MC NICOL, G. P.: Coagulation, Fibrinolysis and platelet function in pré-éclampsia, essential hypertension and placental insufficiency. The Journal of Obstet. and Gynaec. Brit. Sclth. 78, 992 - 1003 (1971).
2. REID, D. E., FRIGOLETTO, F. D., TULLIS, J. L., HINMAN, J.: Hypercoagulable states in pregnancy. Amer. Journal. Obstet. Gynec. 111, 4, 493 - 504 (1971).
3. DAVIDSON, E. Z., PHILLIPS, L. L.: Coagulation studies in the hypertensive toxemias of pregnancy. Amer. J. Obstet. Gynec. 113, 7, 905 - 910 (1972).
4. FRIGOLETTO, F. D., TULLIS, J. L., REID, D. E., HINMAN, J.: Hypercoagulability in the dysmature syndrome. Amer. J. Obstet. Gynec. 111, 7, 867 - 873 (1971).
5. KOLODIE, L., BENSA, J., HOLLARD, D.: Le temps de Céphaline Kaolin - son intérêt pour le dépistage de l'hémophilie modérée. Grenoble Médico Chirurgical 8, 5 - 11 (1970).
6. FOSTER, J. B. T., DE NATALE, A., DOTTI, L. B.: Determination of plasma fibrinogen by means of centrifugation after heating. Amer. J. Clin. Path. 31, 42 - 45 (1959).

7. BONEN, B., CATHALA, B., JORDA, M. F., BIERME, R., LARENG, L.: Réanimation des maladies à haut risque hémorragique et thrombo-embolique. Surveillance biologique. Indications de l'héparinothérapie contrôlée. Nouv. Press. Méd. I, 29 - 32 (1972).
8. CAEN, J., LARRIEU, M. J., SAMAMA, M.: L'hémostase, méthodes d'exploration et diagnostic pratique. Expansion Edit. Paris 1968
9. KOLODIE, L., RACHAIL, M., SEIGNEURIN, D.: Dosage des PDF dans le sérum au cours des cirrhoses du foie. Etude critique de leur signification. Lyon Médical 229, 7, 671 - 678 (1973).
10. BONNAR, J., MC NICOL, G. P., DOUGLAS, A. S.: Coagulation and fibrinolytic systems in pre-eclampsia and eclampsia. Brit. Med. J. 2, 12 - 16 (1971).

Pathways of Glucose Metabolism in Human Placentae

P. Beaconsfield and J. Ginsburg

Rapidly growing embryonic cells utilise glucose at a much higher rate than mature adult non-proliferating tissues (1). The relative functioning of the two main routes for glucose metabolism - the pentose phosphate and glycolytic pathways - varies accordingly during development. Thus, glucose breakdown in pre-implantation ova is virtually exclusively through the pentose route (2) whilst glycolytic activity predominates after blastocyst formation (1, 2). Similarly, we found pentose shunt activity higher in early proliferating placentae before 16 weeks than at term, when it was only detectable after addition of an electron acceptor (3), with parallel changes in ribose formation, nucleic acid and protein turnover (4). Glycolytic activity was relatively increased at term (5). In early placentae from spontaneous abortion, pentose phosphate pathway activity was low (6).

In view of the primary importance of the pentose shunt for the maintenance of normal pregnancy and its possible role in placental insufficiency, we were surprised at the report (7), contrary to our own (3), and other studies (5), of very high pentose activity in term placentae (7) where cell replication had ceased. We therefore reinvestigated placental pentose activity and protein synthesis during human gestation and critically examined our experimental techniques.

Determination of the precise amount of glucose metabolised by the pentose route is extremely difficult. Consequently pentose shunt activity in different circumstances is conventionally assessed in relation to relative fractional recoveries of $^{14}CO_2$ after incubation with differentially labelled glucose (8).

On this basis, we found again higher pentose shunt activity before 12 weeks than at term, with corresponding variations in protein turnover, incorporation from both $U^{14}C$ glucose and $U^{14}C$ glycine being 2 - 3 times higher early in gestation than at term. However, in agreement with others (5) we now found pentose activity at term, a mean $C_1 : C_6$ ratio of 3.5 significantly less than that of 5.9 in early placentae, but not of the high order reported by SYBULSKI and TREMBLAY (7).

We further found CO_2 production less, particularly that from $^{14}C_1$ glucose, and hence pentose activity apparently reduced in placentae incubated after a two hour delay from delivery, compared with tissue incubated within half an hour. Increased tissue handling prior to incubation had similar influence. Pyruvate addition, as by SYBULSKI and TREMBLAY (7), lowered CO_2 production from $^{14}C_6$ glucose. The $C_1 : C_6$ ratio and hence <u>calculated</u> pentose shunt activity was increased, but this is an artefact induced by pyruvate, not an indication of tissue pentose activity.

Parallel ultra-structural examination revealed marked tissue changes after incubation, not apparent in placentae left in cold media and not incubated, or on examination by light microscopy. The major damage was to the syncitial trophoblast, with abnormal nuclear chromatin precipitation, damage to syncitial organites and cytoplasmic disintegration in the intervillous lake. The cytotrophoblast, stroma and foetal capillaries showed little change.

The discrepancy between our previous and present findings in respect of pentose activity at term can be explained by technical factors - the sensitivity of CO_2 production, particularly from $^{14}C_1$ glucose, to tissue handling and storage, whilst the depressant influence of pyruvate on $^{14}CO_2$ production from $^{14}C_6$ glucose accounts for the spurious high shunt reported at term. The effect of incubation on ultrastructure indicates further that biochemical responses after incubation may in part reflect reactions in damaged cells, and that electron-microscopical control is essential for the full evaluation of tissue biochemical sequence. Nevertheless the fact that, as in healing wounds, carcinomata and other proliferating tissues (9, 10), protein synthesis was consistently greater early in gestation than at term, confirms our previous conclusion of much higher pentose route activity in early foetal development than at term. The very low pentose activity in early abortions (6) is yet another illustration of the critical role of this pathway in cellular homeostasis and normal pregnancy. Insufficient attention has been paid to placental activity of this pathway and its possible relation to disorders of pregnancy.

References

1. TANIMURA, T., SHEPHARD, T. H.: Proc. Soc. Exp. Biol. Med. 135, 51 (1970).
2. FRINDHANDLER, L.: Exp. Cell Rs. 22, 303 (1961)
3. BEACONSFIELD, P., GINSBURG, J. JEACOCK, M. K.: Dev. Med. & Child. Neurol. 6, 469 (1964).
4. BEACONSFIELD, P., GINSBURG, J., KOSINSKI, Z.: Nature 205, 50 (1965).
5. SAKURAI, T., TAKAGI, H., HOSOYA, N.: Amer. J. Obstet. & Gynec. 105, 1044 (1969).
6. BEACONSFIELD, P., MORRIS, N. F.: Europ. Medica. 3, 3 (1967).
7. SYBULSKI, S., TREMBLAY, P. C.: Amer. J. Obstet. Gynec. 103, 1148 (1969).
8. BLOOM, B., STETTEN, DE W.: J. Amer. Chem. Soc. 75, 5446 (1953).
9. BEACONSFIELD, P.: Experentia 19, 437 (1963).
10. BEACONSFIELD, P., CARPI, A.: Nature 201, 825 (1964).

Experimental Investigations about Blood Flow and Oxygen-Consumption in Normal Pregnancy and Placental Dysfunction

A. Bolte

The circulation of the isolated uteri of 19 pregnant rabbits was maintened by aorta-aorta-anastomosis with non-pregnant donor animals after a gestation period of 22 - 34 days.

In Nembutal anesthesia the uteri were dissected free from surrounding tissue and the aorta and inferior vena cava isolated. An anastomosis between the abdominal aorta of a donor animal and the descending aorta supplying the uterus of pregnant test animal then was constructed (Fig. 1). With the exception of those vascular connections the preg-

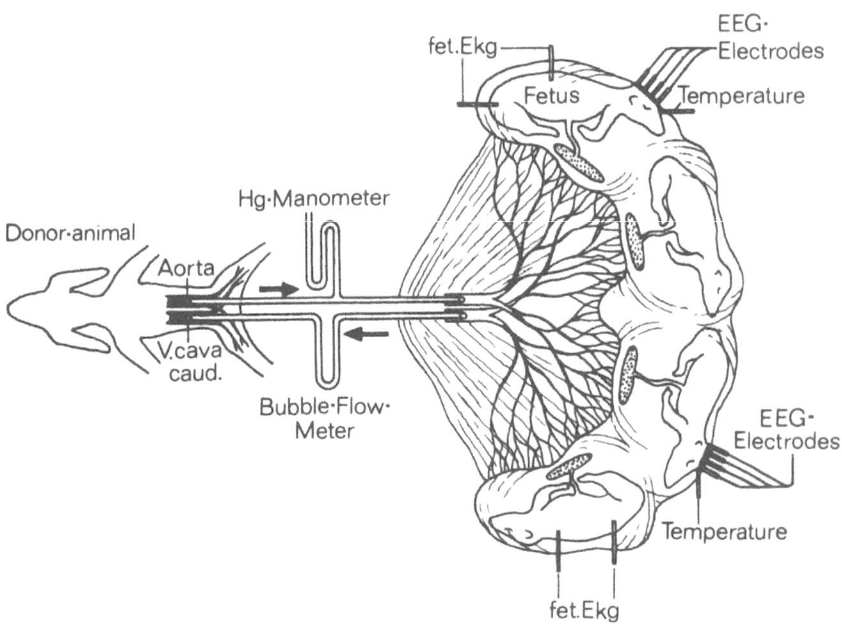

Fig. 1. Aorta-aorta-anastomosis between a pregnant uterus of a rabbit and a non-pregnant donor animal

nant uterus was completely isolated (BOLTE)+. The blood flow was measured by use of a bubble-flow-meter in the venous side of the uterine circulation. The O_2-consumption of the isolated uterus was

+BOLTE, A.: Bestimmung des fetalen Lebens nach Isolierung und Extrakorporierung des graviden Kaninchen-Uterus. Pflügers Arch. ges. Physiolog. 277, 577 (1963).

calculated under normothermic condition (36° C) by determination of the arterial-venous-difference of the O_2-saturation by means of VAN SLYKE analysis. The spontanous electrical activity of the fetal brain registered by use of intra-cortical needle electrodes served as an indicator for the survival time of the fetuses. In Fig. 2 the dependence of frequency and amplitude of the cortical activity from temperature is shown. The prolongation of the duration of the rabbits pregnancy from normally 31 to 34 days was achieved by progesteron.

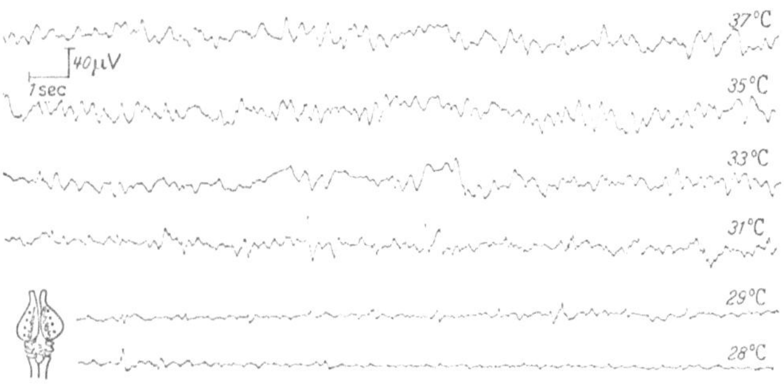

Fig. 2. Fetal cortical spontanous activity after isolation of a pregnant uterus (31st day of pregnancy) and perfusion by a donor animal. Frequency and amplitude of the cortical potentials are depending on temperature (bipolar leads 4 - 5)

Under the described conditions the fetal survival time in 14 isolated uteri ranged from 2 - 5 1/2 hours, fetal death accured in 5 experiments, 4 of them were over term.

Between the 22nd and 30th day of pregnancy (Figs. 3 and 4) the uterine blood flow increased from 7 to 15 ml/min/100 g pregnant uterus and the O_2-consumption from 1.0 to 2.1 - 2.4 ml/min/100 g pregnant uterus

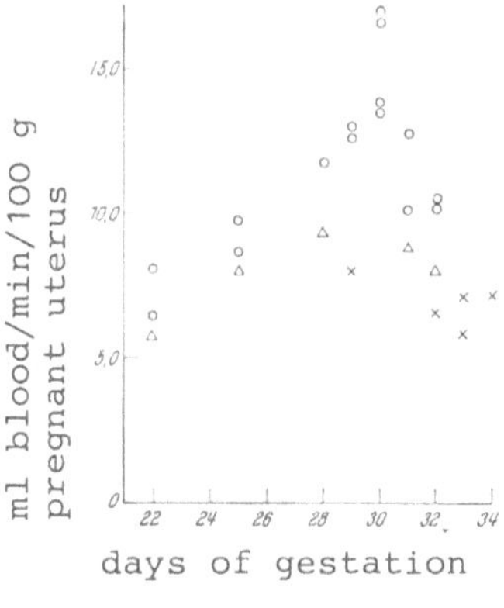

Fig. 3. Dependence of uterine blood flow on duration of pregnancy.
o blood flow when the fetuses survive the isolating operation,
Δ blood flow in non-surviving fetuses,
× blood flow when fetuses died preoperatively

measured at 36° C. The oxygen consumption which was found highest at term, was shown to decreased with prolongation of the gestation period to 1.8 - 2.0 ml/min/100 g, simultanously the uterine blood flow decreased to values about 10 ml/min/100 g on the 32nd day of gestation.

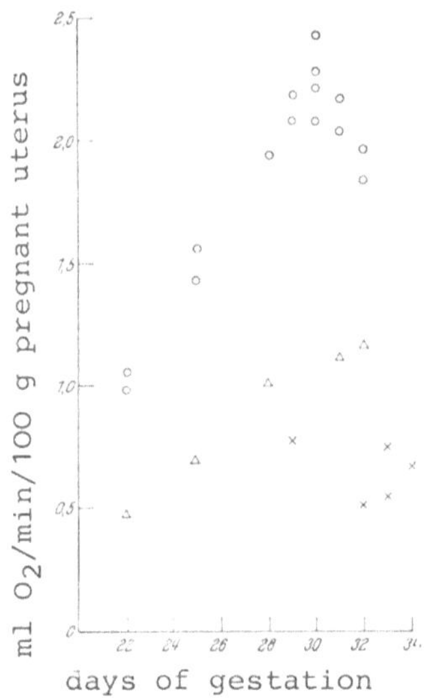

Fig. 4. Dependence of uterine oxygen consumption on duration of pregnancy. ○ *O_2-consumption, when the fetuses survive the isolating operation,* Δ *O_2-consumption in non surviving fetuses,* × *O_2-consumption when fetuses died preoperatively*

The increase of blood flow and oxygen consumption was thought to be due to an increase of fetal and placental metabolism between the 22nd and 30th day of gestation. Since the uterine blood flow and the O_2-consumption were found to decrease after term and fetal deaths were seen frequently in those cases we may assume that a placental dysfunction as well as a decrease of uterine blood flow are factors for the increased fetal death rate in cases with prolonged duration of pregnancy.

The Role of the Fetal Circulation in Placental Insufficiency

H. Fox

The term "placental insufficiency" refers to a clinical syndrome and is often thought of as being comparable to renal or pulmonary insufficiency. It has, however, become increasingly apparent that "placental insufficiency" is largely secondary to alterations in blood flow through the placenta and attention has been principally focussed on alterations in the maternal circulation.

It cannot be assumed, however, that uteroplacental ischaemia is the invariable cause of placental insufficiency. In prolonged pregnancy there is, in many cases, evidence of a decline in placental function but the maternal blood flow through the placenta is decreased only to a minor degree (1), almost certainly not to the extent that the reduction would severely impair placental function or fetal viability. In a personal study of fifty placentae from pregnancies extending to, or beyond, the forty-second week of gestation the principal abnormality noted was villous hypovascularity (2), the fetal vessels were, instead of being sinusoidally dilated, small and centrally situated; the degree and extent of villous hypovascularity increased progressively with increasing length of the gestational period beyond the fortieth week. The villi showed undue fibrosis and an excess of syncitial knots but these changes were secondary to the reduced villous blood flow. The trophoblast itself showed no evidence of any degenerative or "ageing" change and this has been confirmed at the ultrastructural level in an electronoptical study of ten placentae from prolonged pregnancy (3). Similar findings were noted in ten out of twenty placentae from cases of low birth weight of unknown aetiology; in four of the remaining placentae there was a generalised failure of villous maturation with, as a defining feature of immaturity, failure of the villous vessels to become dilated.

These findings suggest that in many cases of placental insufficiency the basic abnormality is an inadequate fetal perfusion of the villi. In the absence of an adequate fetal circulation through the villi the vasculo-syncytial membranes will either regress or fail to develop. These membranes, which are seen as attenuated, anuclear areas of trophoblast directly overlying dilated fetal capillaries, are the site of optimal oxygen transfer across the placenta and a deficiency of such membranes is very often associated with fetal hypoxia (4). It is obvious, however, that these membranes will not develop if there is a primary failure of villous blood flow and will regress if there is a secondary failure of villous perfusion. Thus a reduced fetal blood flow through the placenta will inevitably lead to inadequate fetal oxygenation and this may well be accentuated by the reduction in the villous "pulse" which probably assids the flow of maternal blood through the intervillous space, thus causing an elevation of intervillous space pressure and a mild reduction in maternal utero-placental blood flow.

It is thus apparent that in many cases of placental insufficiency attempts at therapy should be aimed primarily, not towards the maternal circulation, but towards improving the fetal villous perfusion. There is no real evidence that the vascular failure is due to any primary defect within the extra-placental circulation and hence attention must be directed to the factor, or factors, within the placenta that lead to underperfusion.

References

1. DIXON, H. G., BROWNE, J. C. Mc, DAVEY, D. A.: Lancet 2, 369 - 373 (1963).
2. FOX, H.: In the Foeto-Placental Unit ed. A. Pecile and C. Finzi. Excerpta Medica, Amsterdam, pp. 3 - 7 (1969).
3. FOX, H., JETLEY, U.: (in preparation).
4. FOX, H.: In Fetal Evaluation during Pregnancy and Labor. ed. P. G. Crosignani and G. Pardi. Academic Press, New York. pp. 5 - 10 (1971).

Effect of an Adrenergic ß-Mimetic Compound (Ritodrine Hydrochloride) on the Feto-Placental Unit in Chronic Fetal Distress

A. Scommegna, W. P. Dmowski, and J. Bieniarz

Chronic fetal distress in high risk pregnancy is one of the major unresolved problems in obstetrics, responsible for high perinatal mortality and morbidity. No treatment so far has been able to improve materno-fetal interchanges in these pregnancies, so that their usual management consists of bed rest and early delivery when a hostile intra-uterine environment becomes more dangerous for the fetus than prematurity for the newborn.

The rate of placental blood flow is the determinant factor of materno-fetal interchanges. Placental perfusion could be augmented by increasing cardiac output and thus regional blood flow. While studying uterine and cardiovascular effects of an adrenergic β-mimetic compound, ritodrine hydrochloride[1], in the treatment of premature labor, we observed a rise in systolic pressure, pulse pressure and acceleration of heart rate suggesting increased cardiac output (1). If this assumption could be proved by direct methods, then ritodrine treatment could conceivably increase placental perfusion and form a new modality in the treatment of chronic fetal distress.

The aims of this study were: 1. to test the postulated cardiovascular effects of ritodrine on blood pressures and cardiac output; and 2. to investigate the action of ritodrine administration on the fetus in chronic distress.

In five women in premature labor, arterial pressure and heart rates were recorded by direct electronic methods. Cardiac output was measured by a dye dilution technic. A catheter was inserted through the antecubital vein into the superior vena cava and 5 mg of indocyanine green[2] was injected. Arterial blood was concomitantly drawn with a Harvard pump from an indwelling catheter and photometric analysis was performed by a Gilford densitometer . Dye curves were recorded and the output signals were fed to a Lexington cardiac output computer[4] that provided an immediate integration curve read-out. This method has several advantages: there is no need for cumbersome calculations; there is no significant blood loss; oxygen saturation has no effect on the output curves; and the indicator is very rapidly cleared from the blood by the liver, thus permitting repeated measurements without problems of rising baseline.

Peripheral resistance was calculated by dividing the mean blood pressure by cardiac output and was expressed in peripheral resistance units:

$$PRU \quad \frac{136 \times 950 \text{ dynes}}{\text{cm } 3}$$

---

[1] = N.V. Philips-Duphar, Weesp, The Netherlands

[2] = Cardio-Green Flyson, Wetscot & Dunning, Inc., Baltimore, Maryland 21201

[3] = Gilford Instrument Labs., Inc., Oberlin, Ohio

[4] = Model COC-5, Lexington Instruments Corp., 241 Crescent Street, Waltham, Massachusetts 02154

All recordings and measurements were carried out in supine position. The mean of all factors under study, measured between uterine contractions were calculated for a 30 minute control period and compared with the respective means during 10-minute intervals of uniform ritodrine infusion. The infusion started at 100 μg/min and was increased by 40 μg at 10 minute intervals until complete uterine relaxation or unacceptable side effects occured. After 12 hours of infusion treatment continued by oral administration of 20 mg ritodrine every 6 hours. The significance of the difference between the average mean value obtained during the control period in all patients and the respective average obtained after a 30 minute ritodrine infusion was assessed for each factor under study using the t test for paired values, each patient acting as her own control.

During ritodrine infusion in a primigravida at 32 weeks, a remarkable increase in systolic and pulse pressure accompanied by acceleration in maternal heart rate coincided with a rise in cardiac output from 5.0 liters/min to 6.1 liters/min at 10 minutes of infusion, to 6.8 liters/min at 30 minutes, and to 7.5 liters/min at 40 minutes. Note the remarkable rise in pulse pressure and in cardiac output to 150 % of control (Fig. 1).

In a 33 week primipara, a transient hypotension during ritodrine infusion recovered spontaneously in spite of an inhibition in uterine contractility. The cardiac output increased from 3.8 liters/min to 5.5 liters/min, 145 % of control (Fig. 2).

In a 33 week pregnant primipara, ritodrine infusion accelerated maternal heart rate, relaxed the uterus, increased systolic pressure and cardiac output from 5.0 liters/min to 6.0 liters/min, 120 % of control at 20 minutes of infusion. Fetal heart rate remained unchanged (Fig. 3).

Further increase in ritodrine infusion during the next 20 minutes accelerated maternal heart rate even more, increased systolic and pulse pressure with a concomitant decrease in diastolic pressure. Cardiac output increased to 8.7 liters/min, 174 % of control at 40 minutes of infusion (Fig. 4).

During the next 20 minutes of infusion, maternal heart rate remained stable, but blood pressure and cardiac output decreased, remaining still above the preinfusion values. Fetal heart rate increased slightly (Fig. 5).

This graph (Fig. 6) and the corresponding Table 1, summarize the effect of ritodrine on arterial blood pressure in five women in supine position expressed as average ± standard error of the preinfusion control value. Diastolic pressure decreased progressively by 10 % while the systolic pressure increased during 40 minutes 12 % above control value. A significant rise in pulse pressure resulted, and levelled off eventually because of a slight decrease in systolic pressure.

Average cardiac output and related hemodynamic factors ± S. E. are shown in Fig. 7 (compare with Table 2) obtained in 10 minute intervals during ritodrine treatment in 5 women in premature labor. The decrease in peripheral resistance represented by the descent in diastolic pressure in the preceding figure is compensated by a rise in stroke volume during first ten minutes and later by acceleration in heart rate between the 10th and 40th minute of infusion. These inotropic and chronotropic effects of ritodrine result in a rise in cardiac output, 57 % over the control value.

These significant changes compensate for the decreased diastolic pressure by a concomitant rise in systolic and pulse pressure and

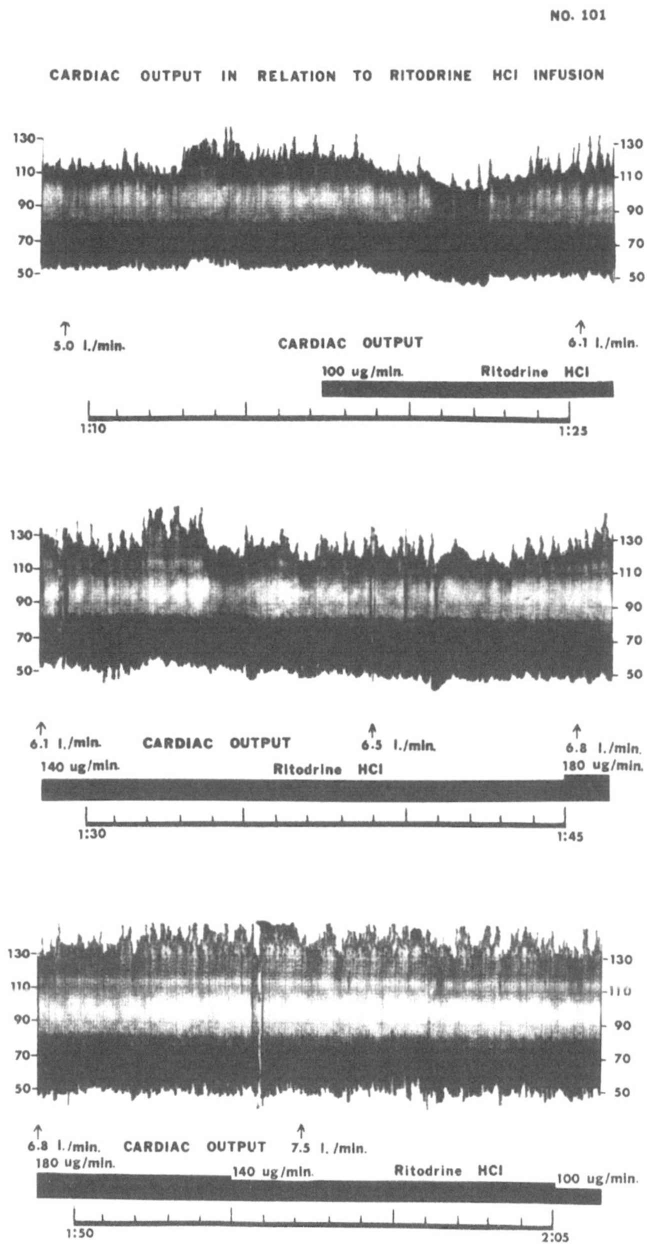

Fig. 1

result in a remarkably stable mean arterial pressure. This is in contrast to the marked hypotension observed during treatment with other β-mimetic drugs, all of which cause relaxation of smooth muscles including those of resistance vessels. Compensatory mechanisms resulting in elevated cardiac output and assuring circulatory homeostasis are

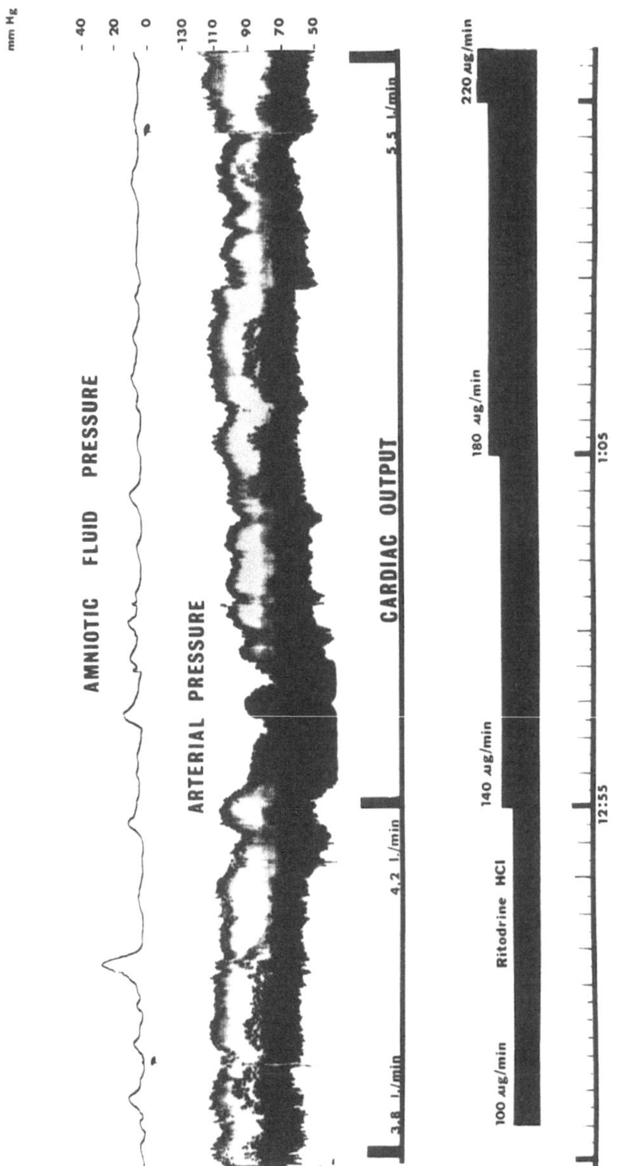
NO. 100
mm Hg
AMNIOTIC FLUID PRESSURE
ARTERIAL PRESSURE
CARDIAC OUTPUT
3.8 l./min
4.2 l./min
5.5 l./min
Ritodrine HCl
100 µg/min
140 µg/min
180 µg/min
220 µg/min
12:55
1:05
40
20
0
130
110
90
70
50

Fig. 2

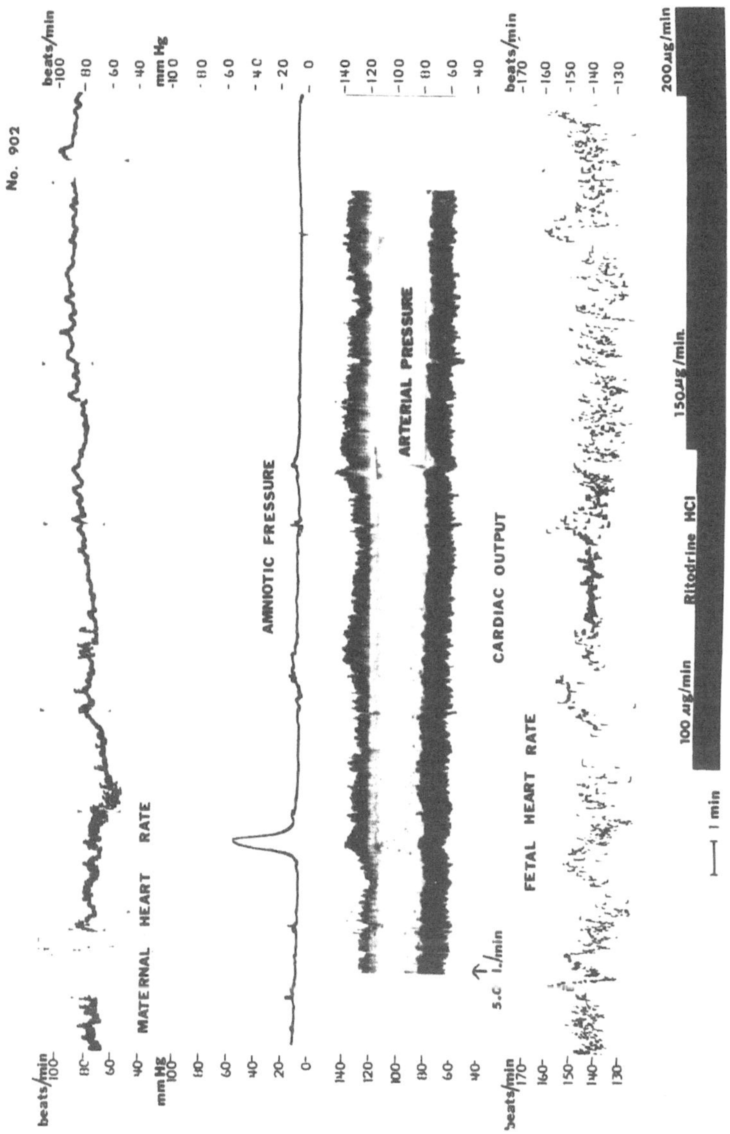
No. 902
beats/min
mm Hg
MATERNAL HEART RATE
AMNIOTIC PRESSURE
ARTERIAL PRESSURE
CARDIAC OUTPUT
5.0 l./min
FETAL HEART RATE
Ritodrine HCl
100 µg/min
150 µg/min
200 µg/min
1 min

Fig. 3

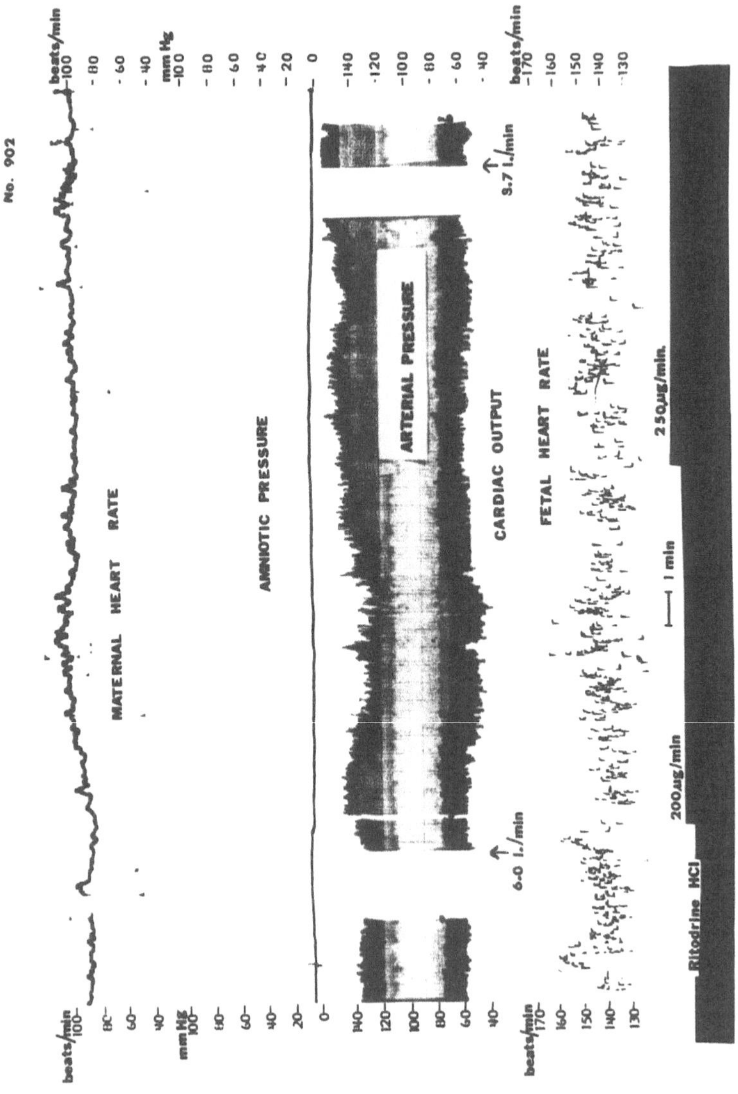

No. 902
beats/min
mm Hg
MATERNAL HEART RATE
AMNIOTIC PRESSURE
ARTERIAL PRESSURE
CARDIAC OUTPUT
FETAL HEART RATE
6.0 l./min
9.7 l./min
1 min
Ritodrine HCl
200 µg/min
250 µg/min

Fig. 4

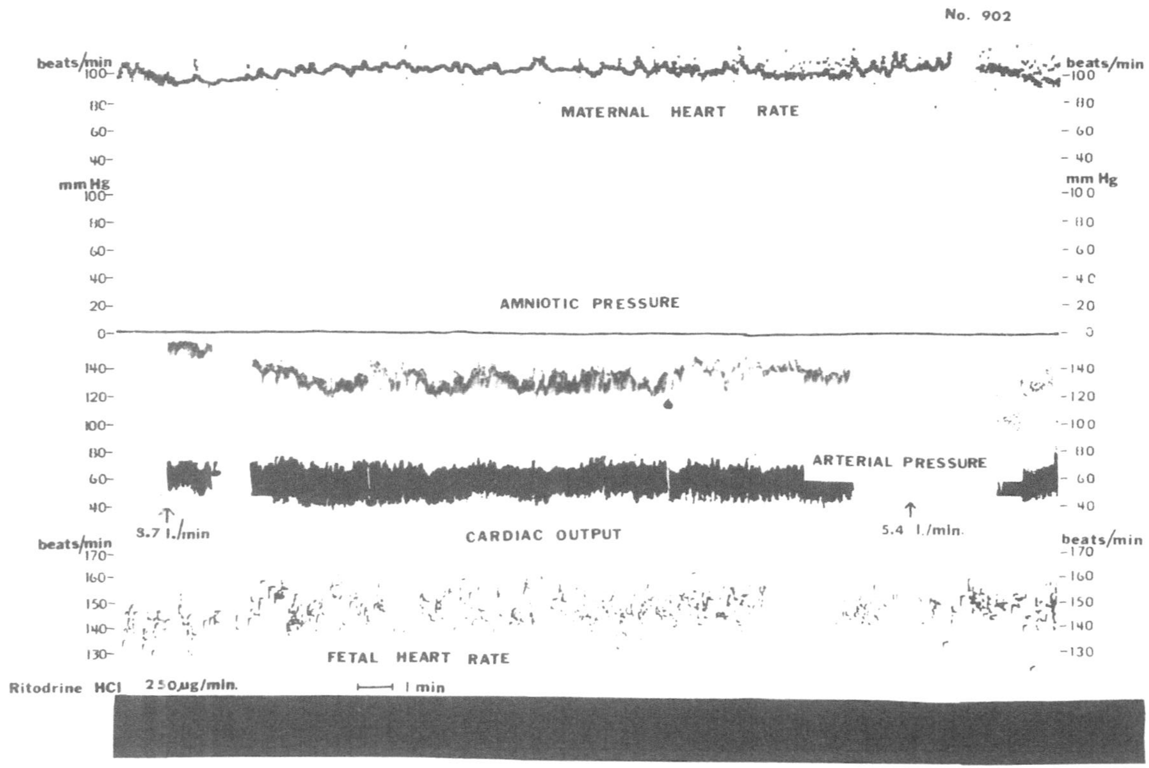
No. 902
beats/min
MATERNAL HEART RATE
mm Hg
AMNIOTIC PRESSURE
ARTERIAL PRESSURE
3.7 l./min
5.4 l./min.
CARDIAC OUTPUT
beats/min
FETAL HEART RATE
Ritodrine HCl 250 µg/min.
1 min

Fig. 5

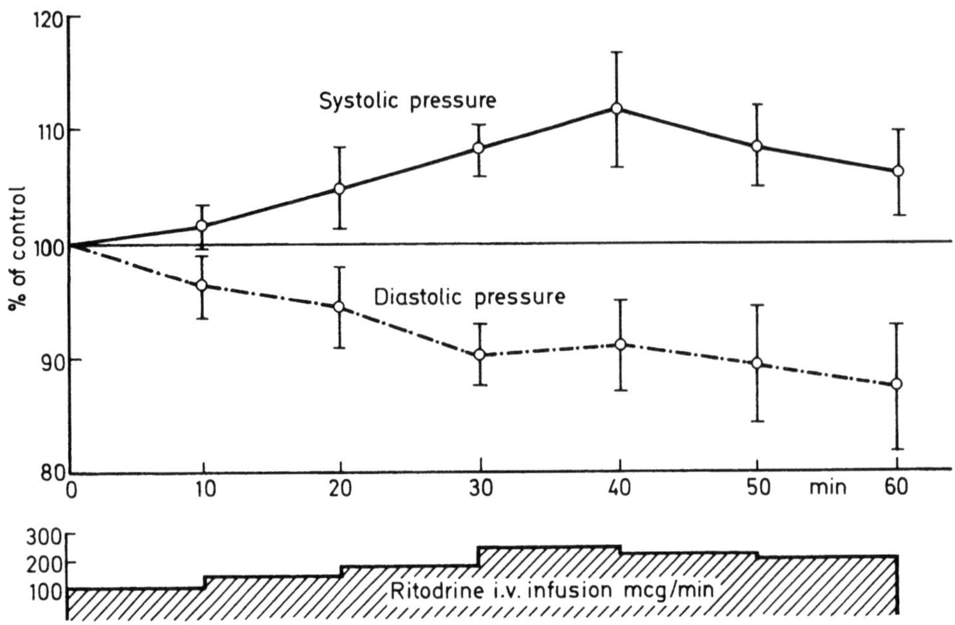

Fig. 6

Table 1. Arterial pressure values (M ± S. D.) during ritodrine treatment in 5 women in premature labor

Blood pressure	Control period	Minutes of infusion 10	20	30	40	50	60
Systolic	113±6	115±11	118±13	123±11	127±17	125±11	121±13
Diastolic	61±4	59± 5	57± 4	55± 5	56± 4	55± 6	53± 5
Pulse	52±6	55±10	61±12	67±11+	71±16+	68±15+	68±16+
Mean	74±4	78± 7	79± 8	78± 7	79± 8	77± 4	76± 6
Ritodrine hydrochloride i.v. mcg/min	0	100	142	176	218	208	203

+p <0.05

evidently specific for ritodrine and missing with other β-mimetic compounds. They cannot therefore be attributed exclusively to the inotropic and chronotropic effects common to all β-mimetic adrenergic drugs. The consistent rise in cardiac output indicates that an increase in venous return must coexist because the heart cannot expell more blood than it receives from the venous side. An elevated venous return at time when the driving force of uterine contractions abates could be explained by an increase in venous tone which maintains filling pressure and cardiac output. Examples of a similar dissociation in the responses of capacitance vessels concomitant with relaxation of resistance vessels are known and have been reported under various circumstances (3).

Having confirmed the effect of ritodrine on cardiac output, we undertook preliminary observations on the ritodrine effect in 4 women with chronic fetal distress and intra-uterine growth retardation. The condition of the fetus was assessed by the following indices: feto-placental and trophoblastic activity by urinary estriol (E_3) excretion measured by a gas chromatography technic (4), plasma level of unconjugated estriol (5), and chorionic somatomammotropin (HCSM)by radioimmunoassays (6), as well as progesterone by the competitive protein binding assay (7).Fetal oxygen reserve was evaluated by the oxytocin challange test (8) and fetal growth by ultrasonic measurement of the biparietal diameter (9).The dangers of intra-uterine demise were weighed against those of prematurity by amniotic fluid sampling, determination of lecithin sphingomyelin (L/S)ratio (10), creatinine level (11) and percent of orange cells in the sediment (12).

Fig. 8 shows the results obtained in a gravida 7 para 6 diabetic Class B, hospitalized in the 33rd week because of intra-uterine growth retardation and history of fetal demise in the 35th week of her last pregnancy. Ritodrine treatment coincided with an increase in urinary E_3 excretion, while plasma E_3 and progesterone levels significantly decreased, and HCSM slightly increased.

The oxytocin challange test initially positive, became negative and the biparietal diameter increased to become larger than compatible with dates. Amniotic fluid studies indicated rapid maturation of fetal lungs. In these conditions, falling insulin requirements during the 36th week of gestation, and the history of fetal loss in a previous pregnancy were considered sufficient indications for induction of labor. The newborn, 2360 gms with Apgar 9/10 developed well.

H. L., 17 years old gravida 1 para 0 was hospitalized at the 32nd week of pregnancy because of pre-eclampsia with a nephrotic syndrome, small for date baby and low estriol excretion. During ritodrine infusion, the estriol excretion rose to near normal values and the plasma E_3 as well as HCSM increased transiently (Fig. 9).

The oxytocin challange test initially positive became repeatedly negative. Fetal growth indicated by the biparietal diameter became compatible with dates. At the end of the 34th week of pregnancy vaginal bleeding, uterine tenderness and falling estriol levels raised the suspicion of abruptio placentae, confirmed during a LSCS at the 35th week. The newborn 2220 gms with Apgar score 6/8 survived without problems.

L. E., a 34 year old gravida 2 para 2 with chronic hypertension was hospitalized at the 31st week because of history of intra-uterine fetal demise at the 32nd week of previous pregnancy and falling urine estriol in the present pregnancy. Unlike the previous patients, ritodrine treatment did not influence the low urinary E_3 excretion. Plasma E_3 levels decreased markedly, plasma progesterone decreased slightly and HCSM remained stable. Signs of severe superimposed pre-eclampsia gradually developed during the 2nd week of hospitalization. When meconium stained amniotic fluid was obtained and E_3 values decreased further, it was decided to induce labor at the 33rd week rather than to risk a repeated fetal loss, although L/S ratio indicated still poor prognosis for the newborn (Fig. 10).

A small for date 1460 g baby developed a severe respiratory distress syndrome and died in 48 hours.

L. T., a primigravida was hospitalized at the 30th week of pregnancy because of pre-eclampsia with a nephrotic syndrome and small for date baby. Treated conservatively by bed rest and high protein diet, pregnancy was continued until the 32nd week when E_3 urinary and plasma estriol levels, as well as HCSM clearly declined. Although the increase in the biparietal diameter indicated fetal growth the oxytocin challange test, originally negative became positive. This patient, agreed only at this late date to ritodrine treatment. Infusion was accompanied by a tendency to increase of plasma E_3 and HCSM, however the latter remained at very low level, while urinary E_3 excretion declined even more as did plasma progesterone. The oxytocin challange test was repeatedly positive. In spite of low L/S ratio it was decided to deliver the patient by cesarean section in view of intolerance to uterine contractions. The 1980 g newborn did surprisingly well in the premature nursery (Fig. 11).

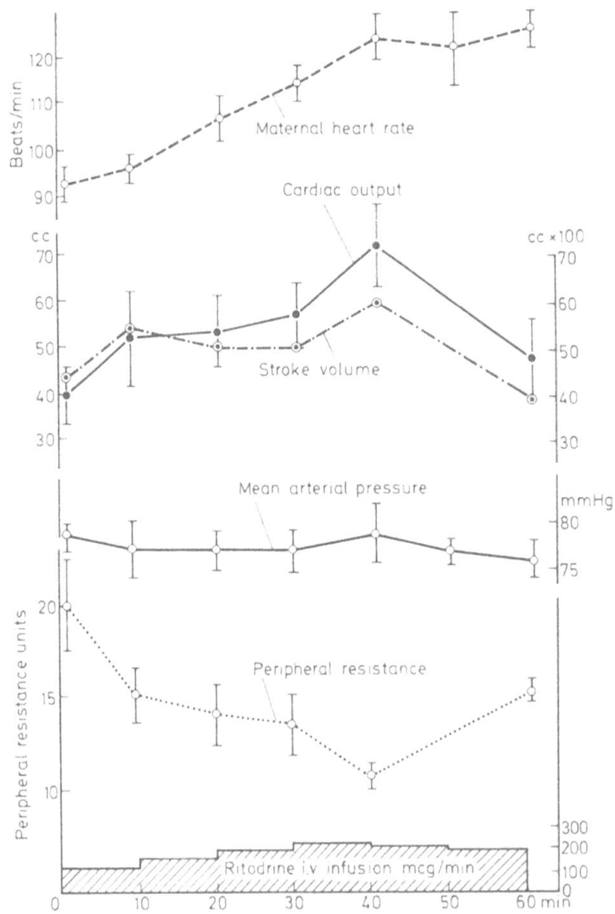

Fig. 7

Table 2. Cardiac output and related hemodynamic factors (M ± S. D.) during ritodrine treatment in 5 women in premature labor

	Control period	10	20	30	40	50	60
Maternal heart rate beats/min	92 ± 9	95 ± 9	107 ±12^{++}	114 ± $^{++}$	122 ±13^{++}	121±18^{++}	125 ±10^{+}
Cardiac output l/min	3.92± 1.28	5.15±	5.20± 1.67	5.70± 1.29^{+}	7.23± 1.55^{+}		4.75± 1.23
Stroke volume ml/min	42.5 ±10.47	54.2 ± 4.35	48.6 ±12.4	50.0 ±10.44	59.3 ± 7.59		38.0 ± 5.75
Peripheral resistance PRU Units	20.05± 5.7	15.1 ± 3.0^{+}	14.9 ± 3.6^{++}	13.7 ± 2.0^{++}	10.97± 1.44^{++}		16.93± 1.18^{+}
Fetal heart rate beats/min	157 ±13	153 ±16	155 ±13	155 +13	157 ±12	160±12	155 ±11
Ritodrine hydrochloride i.v. µg	0	100	142	176	218	208	203

$^{+}p < 0.05$
$^{++}p < 0.01$

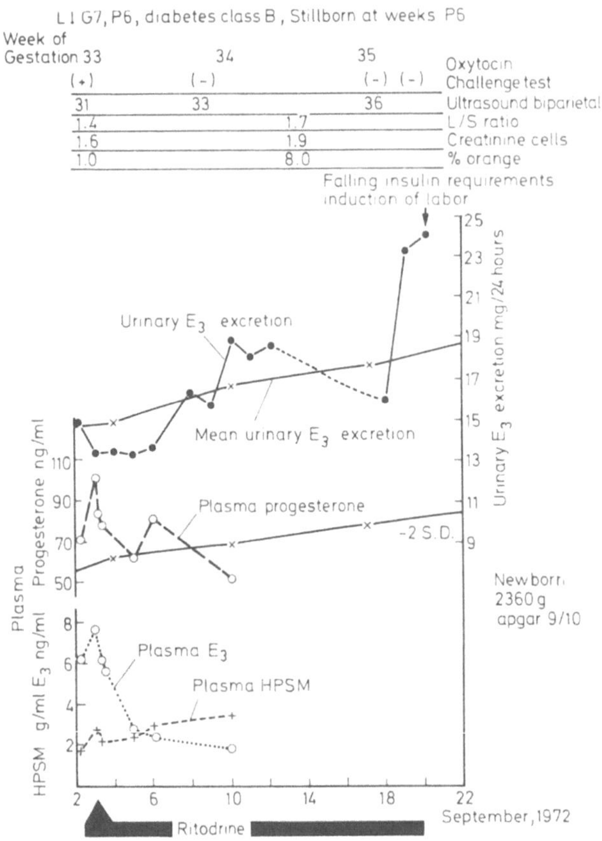

Fig. 8

Discussion

The administration of adrenergic β-mimetic compounds for the purpose of increasing utero-placental blood flow is not a new concept. BROTANEK and HODR (13) in 1966 administered isoxsuprine to women with toxaemia and measured uterine blood flow by a thermistor probe applied to the uterine cervix. An increase in uterine blood flow was registered. Except for measurements of fetal heart rate no other objective index of fetal well being was monitored. However, on discontinuation of the isoxsuprine infusion, the fetus reacted with violent and frequent movements in about half of the cases treated.

In our patients, administration of ritodrine at no time caused any untoward effects on the fetus. Clear cut beneficial effects however, were less clearly demonstrable.

Estriol has been claimed to be an accurate index of the feto-placental status. In 3 patients, intravenous administration of ritodrine caused a temporary increase in plasma estriol. This increase was short lived and soon the plasma values returned to preinfusion levels or even below, in spite of continued oral administration of ritodrine. In one patient with chronic hypertension, the control estriol sample prior to ritodrine administration was lost, but subsequent values were clearly decreasing.

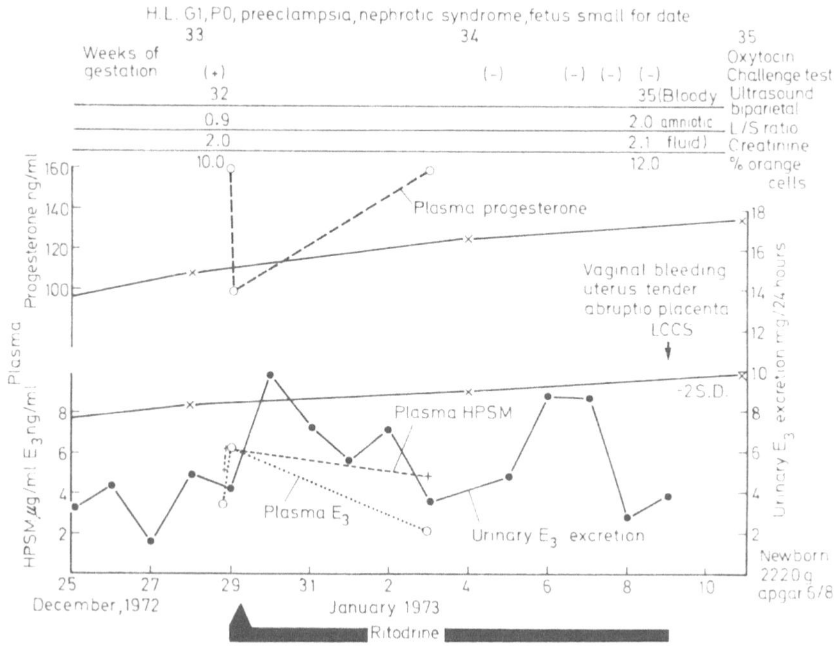

Fig. 9

Urinary estriol also did not show a clear rise except in the diabetic patient in whom the values were normal prior to ritodrine treatment and continued to increase with progression of pregnancy.

Plasma progesterone and placental somatomammotropin, thought to represent mainly placental activity and perhaps more closely related with placental blood flow, showed a clear trend, mostly downward with the progression of pregnancy, in spite of ritodrine administration.

Our data do not indicate a clear beneficial effect of ritodrine in chronic fetal distress, as shown by changes in some endocrine indices of feto-placental activity. The increased cardiac output after ritodrine administration is perhaps not sustained as evidenced by the tendency of the cardiac output to return towards preinfusion level at as early as 1 hour of ritodrine administration (Fig. 7). This would explain the short lived initial rise in plasma estriol.

Alternatively, pathologic alterations in the placental vascular bed caused by the pre-existing disease may impede placental circulation and reduce this regional blood flow in spite of increased maternal cardiac output. Whether administration of ritodrine in chronic fetal distress would improve feto-placental exchange if given earlier in the course of the disease, prior to the time when placental vascular changes have irrevocably affected placental flow, remains to be proven.

Summary

A study by direct electronic methods of recording in 5 women in premature labor has proved that ritodrine, in contrast to other β-mimetic inhibitors of uterine contractility which tend to cause marked hypo-

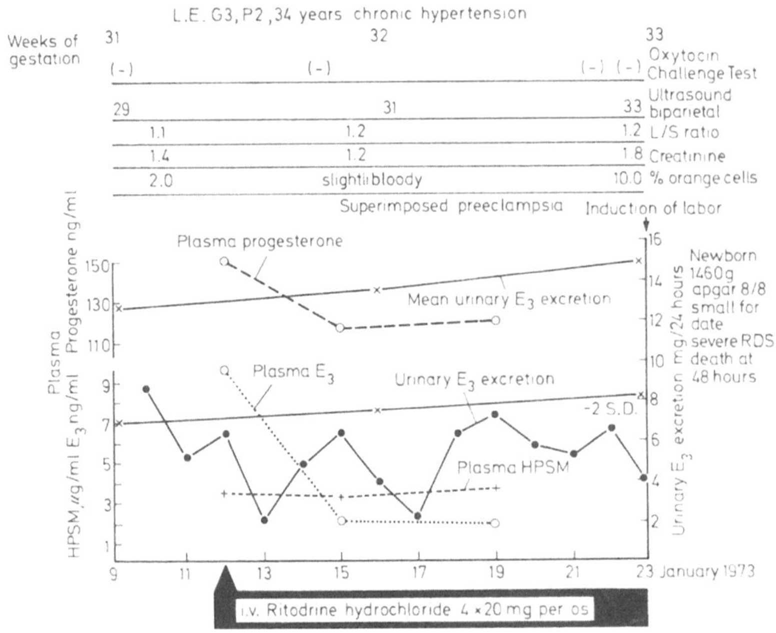
L.E. G3, P2, 34 years chronic hypertension
Weeks of gestation
31
32
33
(-)
(-)
(-) (-)
Oxytocin Challenge Test
29
31
33
Ultrasound biparietal
1.1
1.2
1.2
L/S ratio
1.4
1.2
1.8
Creatinine
2.0
slightli bloody
10.0
% orange cells
Superimposed preeclampsia
Induction of labor
Plasma progesterone
Mean urinary E3 excretion
Newborn 1460g apgar 8/8 small for date severe RDS death at 48 hours
Plasma E3
Urinary E3 excretion
-2 S.D.
Plasma HPSM
Plasma Progesterone ng/ml
HPSM,μg/ml E3 ng/ml
Urinary E3 excretion mg/24 hours
9
11
13
15
17
19
21
23 January 1973
i.v. Ritodrine hydrochloride 4 × 20 mg per os

Fig. 10

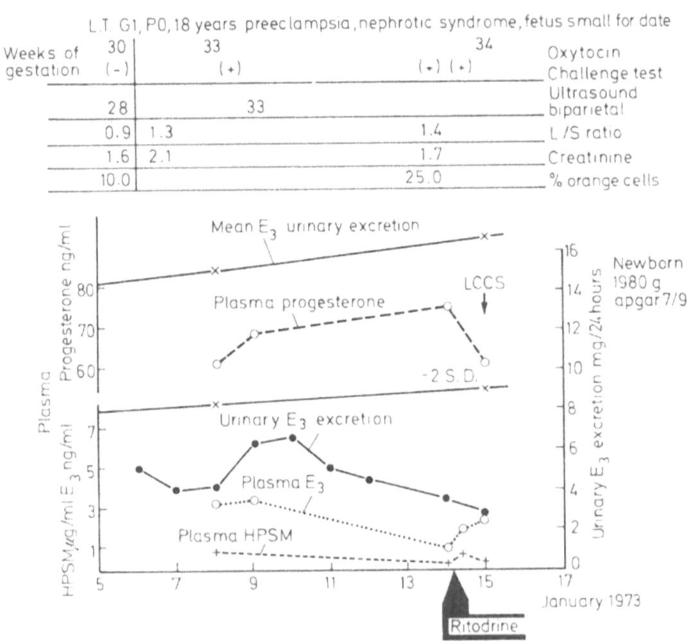
L.T. G1, P0, 18 years preeclampsia, nephrotic syndrome, fetus small for date
Weeks of gestation
30
33
34
(-)
(+)
(+) (+)
Oxytocin Challenge test
28
33
Ultrasound biparietal
0.9
1.3
1.4
L/S ratio
1.6
2.1
1.7
Creatinine
10.0
25.0
% orange cells
Mean E3 urinary excretion
Newborn 1980 g apgar 7/9
LCCS
Plasma progesterone
-2 S.D.
Urinary E3 excretion
Plasma E3
Plasma HPSM
Plasma Progesterone ng/ml
HPSM,μg/ml E3 ng/ml
Urinary E3 excretion mg/24 hours
5
7
9
11
13
15
17
January 1973
Ritodrine

Fig. 11

tension, decreased only the diastolic pressure, while systolic pressure and pulse pressure increased. These changes accompanied by tachycardia, suggested an increase in cardiac output during ritodrine treatment, confirmed by an indicator dilution technic: a rise in cardiac output was found, 56 % over the control value. This remarkable rise has been attributed to adrenergic inotropic and chronotropic effects of ritodrine. These effects along with a postulated increased venous tone and decreased compliance of capacitance vessels compensate for the relaxation of resistance vessels, providing for adequate venous return at a period of abating uterine contractility.

A novel concept has been explored: the use of ritodrine induced hyperkinetic circulation and accelerated placental perfusion to improve materno-fetal interchanges in chronic fetal distress with intra-uterine growth retardation. A series of hormonal and metabolic indices has been used to test the effectiveness of this approach. Preliminary results are reported and discussed.

References

1. BIENIARZ, J., MOTEW, M., SCOMMEGNA, A.: Obstet. Gynec. 40, 65 (1972).
2. FOX, T. J., BROOKER, L. G. S., HESELTINE, B.: Proc. Mayo-Clin. 32, 18 (1957).
3. EPSTEIN, T. E., STAUPFER, M., BEISER, G. D.: Circulation 37, 524 (1968).
4. SCOMMEGNA, A., CHATTORAJ, S. C.: Amer. J. Obstet. Gynec. 99, 1087 (1967).
5. SCOMMEGNA, A., KULKARNI, B.: Plasma unconjugated estriol determination in pregnancy by solvent partition and radioimmunoassay. (In preparation).
6. SPELLACY, W. N., TECH, E. L., BUHI, W. C.: Amer. J. Obstet. Gynec. 109, 588 (1971).
7. SCOMMEGNA, A., BURD, L., BIENIARZ, J.: Amer. J. Obstet. Gynec. 113, 60 (1972).
8. POSE, S. V., CASTILLO, J. B., MORA-ROJAS, E. D.: Pan. Americ. Health Organization 185, 96 (1969).
9. DONALD, M.: Proc. Roy. Soc. Med. 64, 991 (1971).
10. GLUCK, L., KULOVICH, M. V., BORER, R. C. Jr.: Amer. J. Obstet. Gynec. 109, 440 (1971).
11. PITKIN, R. M., ZWIREK, S. J.: Amer. J. Obstet. Gynec. 98, 1135 (1967).
12. BROSENS, J., GORDON, H.: J. Obstet. Gynaec. Brit. Comm. 73, 88 (1966).
13. BROTANEK, V., HODR, J.: The effect of isoxsuprine on utero-placental circulation. IN Hodr, J. and Stembera, Z. Jr. (eds): Intra-uterine Dangers to the Fetus. Excerpta Medica Foundation, Amsterdam, 1967, pp. 424 - 427.

The Effect of a Beta-Mimetic (Ritodrine) on the Uterine Circulation during Normal and Pathological (Chronic Fetal Distress) Pregnancies. Therapeutic Implications

J. P. Brettes, A. Chavas, A. Constantinesco, M. Irrmann, R. Renaud, and R. Gandar

With the objective of assessing changes in the uterine circulation induced by a beta-mimetic agent (ritodrine) and attempting to recognise the possible role of this substance in the treatment of chronic fetal distress, we have conducted a double-blind cross-over study in a series of normal and pathological (chronic fetal distress) pregnancies.

To measure changes in the circulation we used the technique of anemometric thermometry described by BROTANEK. A number of parameters were simultaneously recorded: maternal heart rate, arterial blood pressure and fetal heart rate.

Of 29 cases studied between the 31st and 40th week of pregnancy the results were suitable for analysis in 26: 16 normal and 10 pathological pregnancies (Table 1).

The combined results of both groups (Table 2) show a significant difference between ritodrine and placebo as far as changes in cervical blood flow are concerned. There is a general trend, that, as compared with placebo, ritodrine was more often associated with an increase in uterine blood flow.

In the normal cases (Table 3), the cervical blood flow increased in two patients with ritodrine and in three with placebo. It remained unchanged in 7 patients after ritodrine and in 10 patients with placebo. There was no significant difference between the changes in cervical circulation with ritodrine or with placebo.

By contrast, in the pathological cases (Table 4) in 7 of 10 studies with ritodrine there was an increase in the cervical blood flow, while with placebo the cervical blood flow remained unchanged in 9 out of the 10 cases. Statistical analysis shows a significant difference between these two groups.

Uterine blood flow was statistically significantly increased only in the pathological pregnancy group when treated with ritodrine. However, at the dose employed (maximum 150 μg/min) the fetal heart rate was not significantly altered in either of the two series.

This study confirms our earlier results in a smaller series. Only in the pathological cases did this beta-mimetic cause a significant increase in the uterine blood flow, but it is in this group where there were changes in the general cardiovascular haemodynamics of the mother. It is logical to connect the changes in the uterine circulation with ritodrine to this change in the systemic maternal circulation.

The use of the beta-mimetic with the aim of improving the utero-placental circulation raises new therapeutic possibilities which are of primary interest for the treatment of chronic fetal distress during the third trimester of pregnancy.

Table 1. Pathologic cases - clinical summary

	Parity	Abnormality of pregnancy	Duration of pregnancy at time of test (week)	Duration of pregnancy at delivery	Weight/ length	Apgar
P 1	1	clinically small for dates severe tobacco abuse	38	39	1980/46	4 - 8
P 2	0	severe P. E. T.+ pyelitis at 26 weeks	35	37	2400/45	9 -10
P 3	0	clinically small for dates	32	41	2800/46	6 -10
P 4	2	recurrent P. E. T.	35	36	2500/46	9 -10
P 5	0	P. E. T. at the end of pregnancy	39	40	2900/49	10 -10
P 6	0	moderate P. E. T. in late 3rd trimester	37	39	3400/51	10 -10
P 7	0	hypertension during pregnancy	31	-	-	-
P 8	0	severe, recurrent urinary infection	37	38	3000/50	8 -10
P 9	1	moderately severe intra-uterine growth retardation. Small for dates infant in previous pregnancy	31	-	-	-
P10	0	moderate P. E. T. at the end of the 3rd trimester	37	40	3300/50	7 -10

+P. E. T. = pre-eclamptic toxaemia

Table 2. Effect of ritodrine and placebo on cervical blood-flow - all cases combined - significant difference [$p < 0.05$]+

Cervical blood-flow	Increased	Unchanged	Decreased	Not interpretable
Ritodrine	9	10	3	4
Placebo	4	19	0	3
Total	13	29	3	7

+$p > 0.05$, Chi^2 test, one-sided, with Yates correction

However, because of the varied aetiology of such cases, the decision concerning treatment would depend upon the results of a study of uterine blood flow during administration of ritodrine. Such an investigation would allow one to determine those cases where the uterine blood flow was already decreased and then to assess the local vascular changes under the effect of treatment.

Table 3. Effect of ritodrine and placebo on cervial blood-flow - normal cases. Difference not significant.

Cervical blood-flow	Increased	Unchanged	Decreased	Not interpretable
Ritodrine	2	7	3	4
Placebo	3	10	0	3

Table 4. Effect of ritodrine and placebo on cervical blood-flow - pathologic cases. Significant difference [$p < 0.05$]+

Cervical blood-flow	Increased	Unchanged	Decreased
Ritodrine	7	3	0
Placebo	1	9	0

+$p = 0.01$, Chi^2 test, one-sided, with Yates correction

The Effects of Beta-Mimetic Treatment (Ritodrine) during Pregnancy on Carbohydrate Metabolism and Hepatic Function of the Newborn Infant

H. Freysz, D. Willard, H. Berland, J. Messer, G. Tissier, R. Renaud, and R. Gandar

We set up a study to determine whether Ritodrine had any adverse effects on the carbohydrate metabolism and hepatic function of newborn children.

In the adult, beta-mimetics have been shown to increase free insulin (IMURA, PORTE), plasma glucagon (LECLERC MEYER) and to inhibit the secretion of growth hormone. We decided to investigate these three indices.

Full details of the complete study will not be given. The study involved an intravenous glucose tolerance test on the first and fourth days of life and many other tests shown in the tables.

We shall base our conclusions on the following tables.

These include results from 21 children whose mothers had received Ritodrine for a mean duration of 45 days (range ante-partam 10 - 98 days) in comparison with a test group of infants of comparable weights (Table 1).

Table 1

	Normal for dates at term	Small for dates at term	Small for dates: premature
Treated group	12	5	4

Table 2 shows that the blood glucose levels between 0 and 60 minutes after injection are similar on the first day of life for the two groups.

Table 2

	Blood glucose (gr. per 1)			
	fasting	1 minute	30 minutes	60 minutes
Treated group	0.53 ± 0.16	3.45 ± 0.63	2.26 ± 0.40	1.72 ± 0.38
Test group	0.52 ± 0.16	3.93 ± 0.62	2.04 ± 0.30	1.52 ± 0.34

Table 3 shows plasma insulin levels before glucose loading insulin levels after glucose loading are so wide that it is impossible to draw firm conclusions. There does not seem however to be any obvious discrepancy between the two groups.

Table 3

	Plasma insulin (micro-units per ml)			
	fasting	1 minute	30 minutes	60 minutes
Treated group	13.6 ± 6.7	25.0 ± 24.1	26.5 ± 14.3	42.2 ± 22.3
Test group	12.7 ± 7.6	23.7 ± 21.1	31.3 ± 22.7	41.1 ± 28.2

The range of growth hormone (Table 4) is also too great for analysis, but again no considerable discrepancy between the two groups is apparent.

Table 4

	Serum growth hormone (nanogrammes per ml)			
	fasting	1 minute	30 minutes	60 minutes
Treated group	16 ± 9.3	12.6 ± 7.9	23.7 ± 18.5	44.4 ± 32
Test group	10.5 ± 7.5	8.3 ± 5.9	18.1 ± 17.4	29.5 ± 14.7

Table 5 shows plasma glucagon levels (this is the only determination which could not be made in our laboratory; the concentrations were kindly measured by Dr. BLOOM of London).

It is noticeable that values for the two groups are almost identical after glucose loading.

Table 5

	Plasma glucagon (picogrammes per ml)			
	fasting	1 minute	30 minutes	60 minutes
Treated group	160 ± 74	202 ± 42	171 ± 44	155 ± 44
Test group	183 ± 42	196 ± 39	191 ± 16	174 ± 33

Blood sugar levels induced on the 4th day of life are shown in Tables 6, 7, 8 and 9. The concentrations measured are similar to those found on the first day of life.

Table 6

	Blood glucose (gr per l)			
	fasting	1 minute	30 minutes	60 minutes
Treated group	0.53 ± 0.20	3.65 ± 0.72	1.88 ± 0.37	1.22 ± 0.35
Test group	0.74 ± 0.24	3.88 ± 0.77	2.04 ± 0.26	1.46 ± 0.29

Table 7

	Serum insulin levels (micro units per ml)			
	fasting	1 minute	30 minutes	60 minutes
Treated group	8.0 ± 5.6	50.5 ± 50.1	30.4 ± 28.4	29.9 ± 23
Test group	9.6 ± 4.5	22.3 ± 15.3	28.9 ± 15.1	27.8 ± 16

Table 8

	Serum growth hormone (nanogrammes per ml)			
	fasting	1 minute	30 minutes	60 minutes
Treated group	17.0 ± 10.2	15.6 ± 11.0	14.3 ± 7.9	21.3 ± 8.8
Test group	17.1 ± 11.8	16.7 ± 12.2	19.7 ± 11.0	24.3 ± 11.3

Table 9

	Plasma Glucagon (picogrammes per ml)			
	fasting	1 minute	30 minutes	60 minutes
Treated group	172 ± 81	165 ± 40	157 ± 35	138 ± 27
Test group	148 ± 53	159 ± 54	127 ± 74	128 ± 52

Table 10 shows that liver function tests were not different between the control and experimental group.

Table 10

	Treated group	Test group
Bilirubin (mg/100 ml)	3.0 ± 1.5	2.5 ± 1.8
Transaminases SGOT (i.u./l)	30.1 ± 17.1	31.5 ± 18.6
SGPT (i.u./l)	12.2 ± 9.1	24.4 ± 15.7
Alkaline phosphatase (i.u./l)	63.5 ± 13.8	67.2 ± 14.1
Serum lactate dehydrogenase (i.u./l)	609 ± 255	612 ± 258
Prothrombin (%)	72.5 ± 18.0	77.5 ± 22.9

Our work suggests that Ritodrine can be administered for a prolonged period to pregnant women without obvious detrimental effects on the hepatic function and glucose metabolism of the newborn child.

The Influence of a Beta-Mimetic on Placental Function-Tests

H. Fröhlich, W. Gruber, and K. Baumgarten

Many methods have been described to recognize a fetal distress and/or evaluate the placental function. In contrast to this our therapeutic possibilities to influence the well-being of the fet in utero or a placental insufficiency are but few. All the substancies applied up to now could neither improve the nutritive nor the respiratory function of the placenta. The infusion of glucose and protein into the amniotic cavity failed as well as the application of ATP, vasodilators or buffers to the mother to be.

At the 2nd European Congress for Perinatal Medicine in London GAMISSANS, co-worker of ESTEBAN-ALTIRRIBA reported that beta-mimetic substances given to the mother during delivery prevent or reduce a fetal acidosis. SIVASAMBOO found that babies born in mothers who were treated with such a substance during pregnancy because of threatened premature labour had a higher average birth-weight than those out of a control group. In the meantime it could be proved that this fact is not due to an influence on the glucose metabolism neither of the mother nor of the fet.

According to the quoted findings it seems possible that the application of beta-mimetics improves the placental function - probably by increasing the uterine blood flow (GAMISSANS, COSMI). To find out if this thesis were true we treated - in a preliminary study - 7 pregnant women who were admitted to our clinic because of toxaemia with PREPAR. After 3 days bedrest those mothers to be got 40 mg of the substance per day over 6 days. Before, during and after the treatment the amount of urinary estriol was measured by means of a thin layer chromatographic technique.

Fig. 1 shows the normal values and the 2 sigma border lines. The disturbance of placental function in our cases is expressed by the excretion curves being close to the lower border line. The values found during treatment are shown in red.

If the average estriol excretion before treatment started is 100 % one can see that during application of the remedy the amount of urinary steroid increases in all but one case. The 2 control cases show a distinct decrease (Fig. 2).

If the substance is given to prevent threatened premature labour that means to suppress uterine contractions before term the increase of estriol takes some days, - evidently until the uterus is at rest (Fig.3).

Of course, a preliminary study would not allow us to draw any conclusions that beta-mimetics do improve the placental function indeed. In our opinion these findings indicate that further investigations based on more cases are necessary.

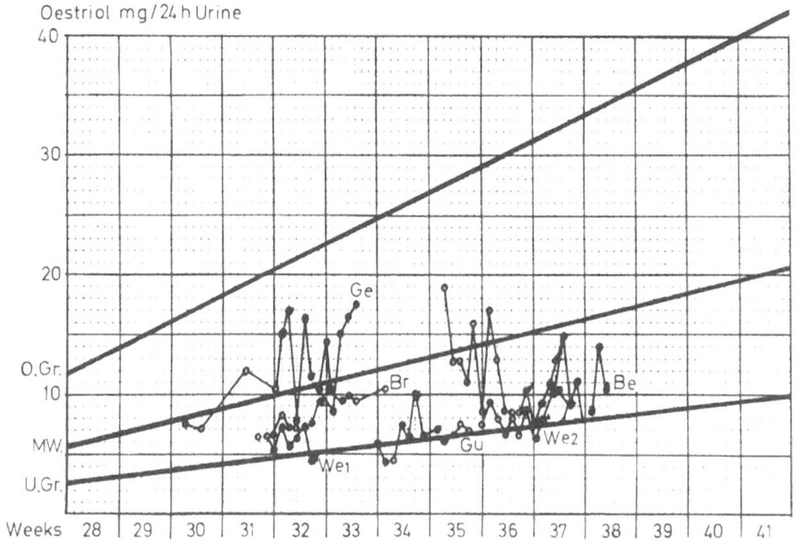
Oestriol mg/24 h Urine
40
30
20
O.Gr.
10
MW.
U.Gr.
Ge
Br
Be
We1
Gu
We2
Weeks
28
29
30
31
32
33
34
35
36
37
38
39
40
41

Fig. 1

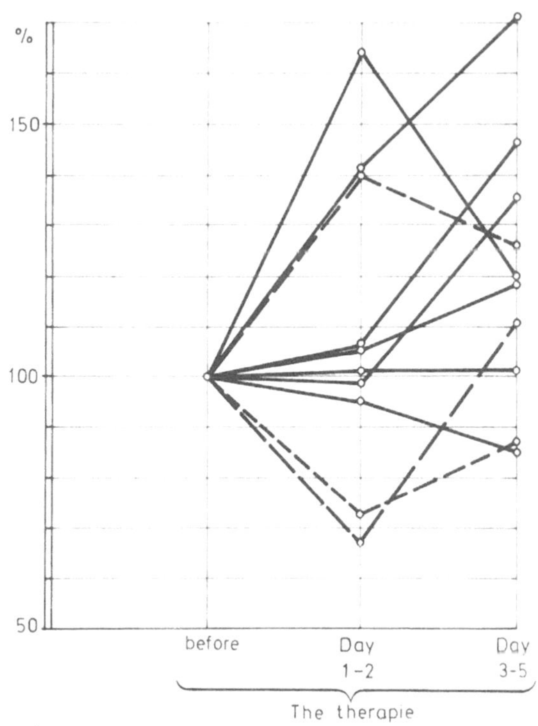
%
150
100
50
before
Day
1-2
Day
3-5
The therapie

Fig. 2

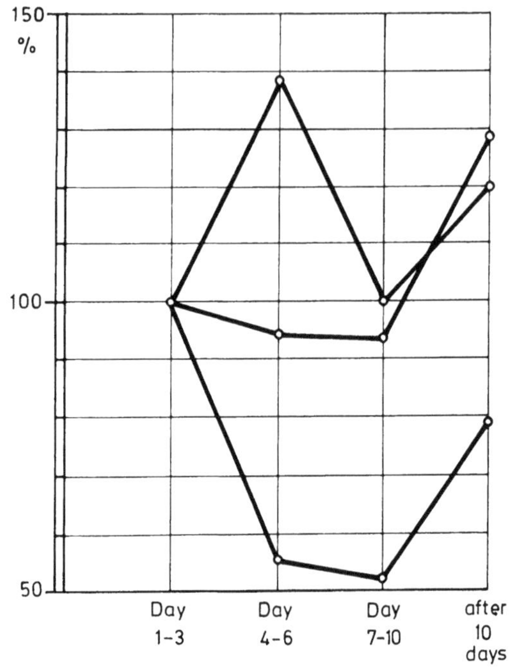

Fig. 3

Adrenergic ß-Mimetic-Compounds and Utero-Placental Blood Supply in Risk Pregnancies

H. Janisch, S. Leodolter, and E. Reinold

By means of the radio isotope placental blood flow technique developed by them (2), JANISCH et al. were able to demonstrate that in risk pregnancies - predominantly patients with EPH gestosis - a significantly reduced blood supply in the utero-placental unit is to be expected (3). The causes are likely to be multifactorial in nature, primarily morphological changes affecting the capillaries (6) and functional disorders such as increased tonus at rest of the uterine musculature as compared to normal pregnancies and arteriolar spasms. Placental insufficiency is the result of all these changes.

Since isoprotenerol derivatives, in addition to their cardiac action, also exert a relaxing effect on the smooth muscle fibers (4), these neuropharmaca, the socalled β-sympathicomimetics have been introduced to all special fields of modern medicine. Within the scope of obstetrics they are primarily administered as tocolytics (5). Because we felt that the functional element is of importance in deficient placental blood supply, we tried to expand the scope of indications for the use of β-adrenergic substances and test their action on the blood supply of the utero-placental unit in risk pregnancies (1).

22 patients with EPH gestosis and insufficient blood supply had been diagnosed by means of our technique for recording the placental blood flow; they were divided in 2 groups to whom long-term infusion therapy with β-adrenergic substances was administered. The 10 patients in group A received 50 mg of RITODRINE, the patients in group B 0.08 mg of Th 1165 a - administered in twice daily for a period of 14 days by means of slow intravenous continuous drip. After this long-term therapy the recording of the placental blood flow was repeated. This report covers these results.

In the recording of the placental blood flow by means of radio isotopes the following parameters are taken into consideration: the shape of the curve itself; type 1 conforms to an undisturbed pregnancy, it is characterized by a rapid rise and an early apex, corresponding to an unimpaired flow of the radio-pharmacon into the utero-placental unit. On the other hand, type 3, which must be termed pathological, manifests a considerable delay in the rise and manifests a mere gradual ascent up to the peak of the curve. Type 2 represents a transitional type. By applying FICK'S principle, approximate values for the flow volume (expressed in cc/min/100 g tissue) were obtained as an additional parameter (2).

The therapy leads to a significant rise of the blood flow values in patients of group A (RITODRINE). From an initial level of 97 cc an increase to 147 cc/min/100 g tissue was achieved. The time (in seconds) required to reach the curve's peak was but slightly reduced. This value, just like the one for the average flow type that improved from 2.0 prior to therapy to a value of 1.63, did not differ significantly from the initial values.

Table 1. Results of placental blood flow recordings prior to (1st) and after (2nd) therapie with 2 x 50 mg/d RITODRINE r (group A) and 2 x 0.08 mg/d Th 1165 a (group B).

	group A				group B			
	1st		2nd		1st		2nd	
n	10		10		12		12	
ml	98	± 9	147	± 10++	88	± 8	135	± 10++
sec	117	± 10	106	± 9	167	± 14	93	± 10+++
type	2.0	± 0.2	1.6	± 0.2	2.5	± 0.1	1.85	± 0.1+

Significance: +++ ....$p < 0.001$
++ ....$p < 0.005$
+ ....$p \leq 0.01$

The results in pregnant women of group B following the administration of β-mimetics confirmed a significant improvement in the utero-placental blood supply; this was reflected in all the parameters recorded. The time (in seconds) for the peak to be reached was reduced from an initial average of 167 sec to barely 93 sec, the volume in cc rose by approximately 50 % from a 88 cc to 135 cc and the average flow type dropped from an initial recording of 2.93 to 1.85.

Since these two groups of patients had differing initial values prior to therapy, we cannot assign a specific value to the results achieved with the two substances.

However, our findings lead us to conclude that following intravenous long-term therapy with both these β-adrenergic substances, considerable improvement in the utero-placental blood supply is obtained in cases where the blood flow had been reduced previously. This is due, on the one hand, to a lowering of the uterine tonus at rest plus vascular dilatation, and to the increase in the cardiac minute volume occasioned by the β-mimetic substances on the other. Undoubtedly, this improvement in the placental blood supply has a positive influence on the fetus in utero even though no definitive judgment may as yet be passed about this.

Long-term treatment with uterotonolytics during pregnancy provides a new possibility for improving deficient placental blood supply as it occurs, for example, in gestosis.

References

JANISCH, H., LEODOLTER, S., REINOLD, E.: Der Effekt von Ritodrin auf die Plazentadurchströmung. Internat. Symposium "Behandlung fetaler Gefahrenzustände" Baden / Wien 1972.

JANISCH, H., LEODOLTER, S.: Plazentainsuffizienz und Funktionsdiagnostik mit Radioisotopen. Z. Geburtsh. Perinat. 177/1, 11 (1973)

JANISCH, H., LEODOLTER, S.: Ergebnisse der Plazentadurchströmungsmessung bei Risikoschwangerschaften. Z. Geburtsh. Perinat., im Druck.

KONZETT, H.: Neue broncholytisch hochwirksame Körper der Adrenalinreihe. Arch. exp. Path. Pharmak. 197, 27 (1940).

MOSLER, K. H.: Tocolysis. Bibl. gynaec., Fasc. 42, Basel - New York: S. Karger 1966.

ROBERTSON, W. B.: The pathology of feto-placental insufficiency in hypertensive pregnancy. Simposio "Terapia dell insufficienza feto-placentare durante la gravidanza". Parma - 1973.

Early Trials in the Treatment of Placental Insufficiency with Ritodrine

J. Melchior and N. Bernard

Whilst neonatal therapeutics is advancing rapidly, fetal therapy is in its early stages and there are as yet very few studies on the treatment of the fetus.

Administration to the mother of beta-adrenergic agents may be used to improve uterine haemodynamic conditions and to treat placental insufficiency which is a cause of fetal growth retardation. This report describes the results of an experimental and clinical study of the effects of a beta-adrenergic agent (Ritodrine).

In the dog, or pregnant sheep, an intravenous infusion of Ritodrine is followed by a marked increase in cardiac output with a simultaneous increase in heart rate. During prolonged administration of the drug the heart rate remains unchanged, but arterial flow has not been measured. It is possible that the mother becomes accustomed to the drug, and that blood flow returns to control values. We have started a study to clarify this point.

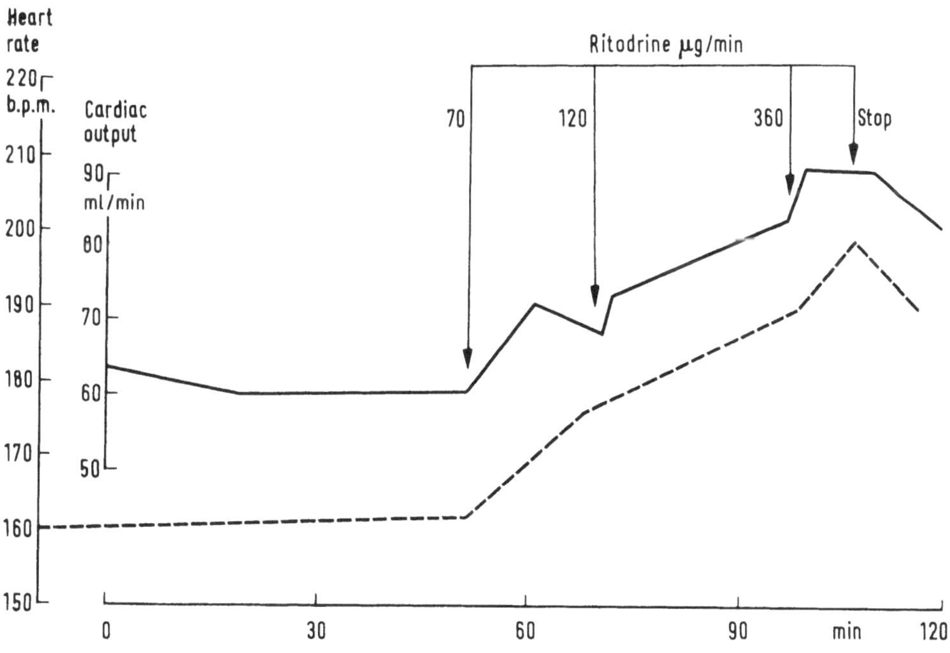

Fig. 1. Heart rate and renal artery blood flow increased by an intravenous infusion in a dog

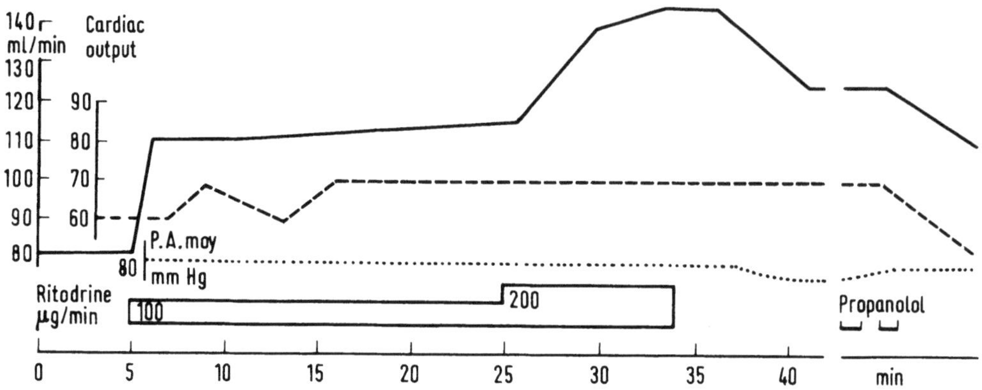

Fig. 2. Recording of heart rate, carotid artery blood flow and the mean arterial blood pressure during an intravenous infusion in a sheep

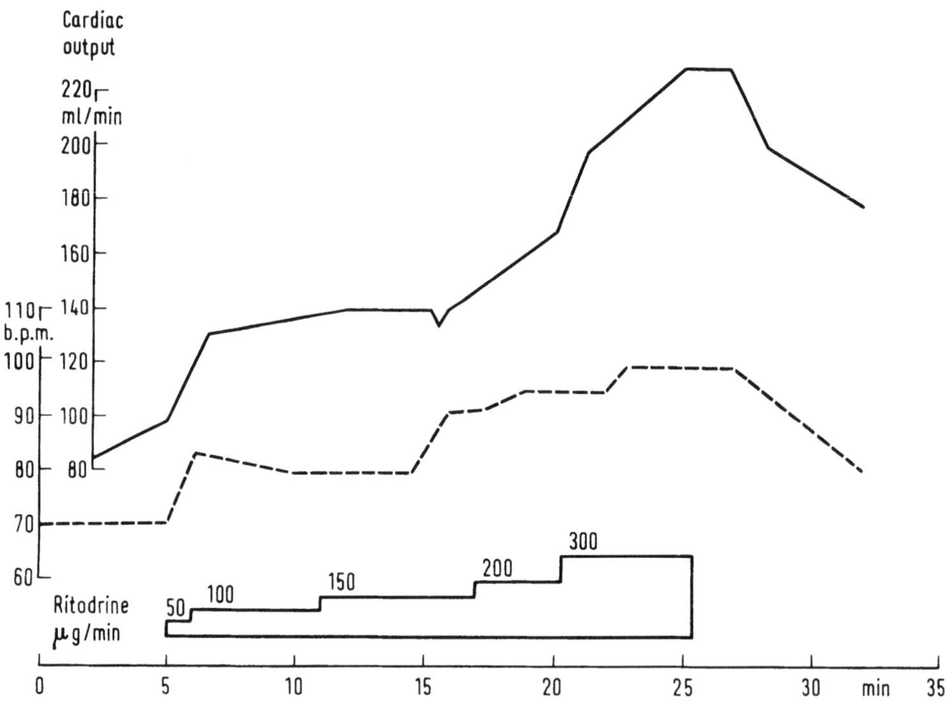

Fig. 3. Increase in heart rate and blood flow in the hypogastric artery during an intravenous infusion of Ritodrine in a non-pregnant patient

In patients undergoing a gynecological operation, uterine blood flow has been measured by an electromagnetic flowmeter with a probe placed over a uterine artery. Two observations have become clear:

1. In the treatment of threatened labour, with Ritodrine 100 to 400 micrograms per minute, uterine blood flow is considerably increased, and may reach levels twice control values. The effect is observed immediately after the infusion has begun, and stops as quickly after the end of the infusion.
2. Variations in flow rate do not always follow those of the heart rate and in some anesthetized women, flow increases, although heart rate remains unchanged.

To assess the benefits of prolonged administration of the drug to mothers carrying a low weight fetus, we have selected from our series of threatened premature labour treated with Ritodrine, the cases of low birth weight infants. The fig. shows that the birth weight of infants born of mothers treated for more than 3 weeks is nearer the normal values than those of mothers who were treated for a shorter time. There is a clear difference between the two groups. Moreover, when we

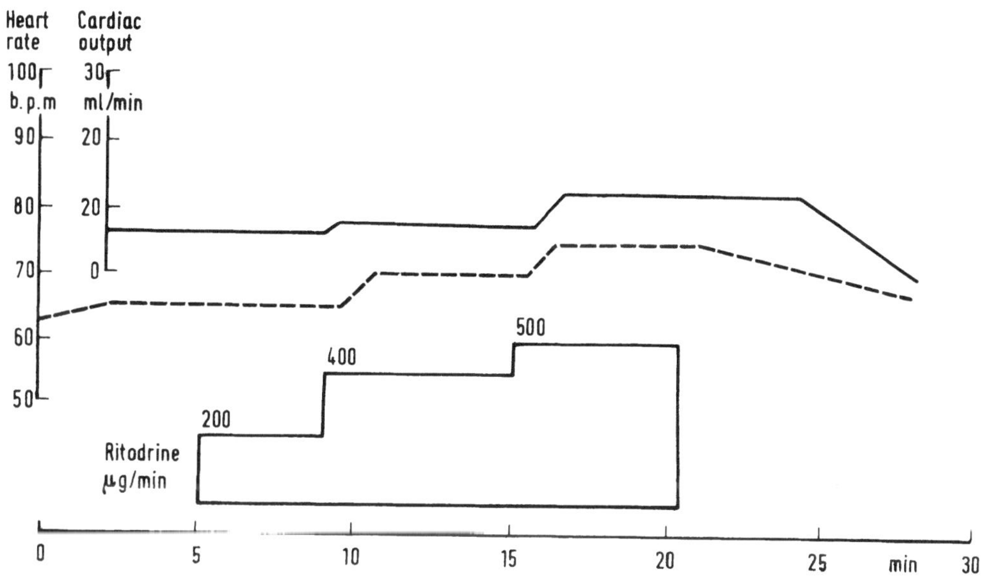

Fig. 4. Increase in the uterine arterial flow and heart rate in a non-pregnant patient

compare the results obtained in cases of prolonged treatment with a similar group of untreated mothers delivering low birth weight infants of the same gestational age born in our department, we notice that the weight of the infants born of treated mothers, is higher than in the group of untreated mothers. Further, the duration of pregnancy is prolonged as shown by the fact that 6 children out of 11 were born after 38 weeks, 3 were born between 36 and 38 weeks, only 2 before 36 weeks.

These are our initial conclusions regarding the treatment of placental insufficiency with Ritodrine. More important a prospective study has been commenced in our department. Its purpose is to determine the benefits using a double blind technique.

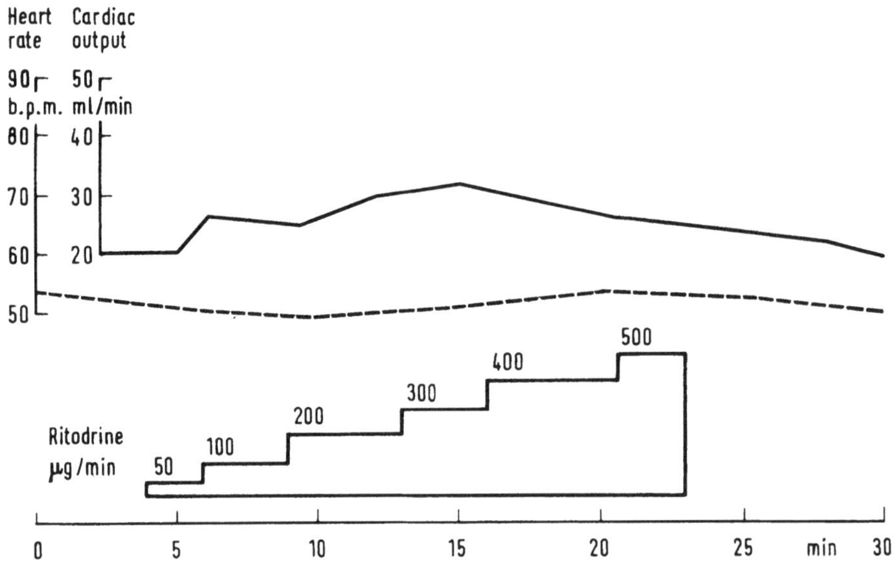

Fig. 5. Increase in the uterine arterial flow without increase in heart rate in a non-pregnant patient

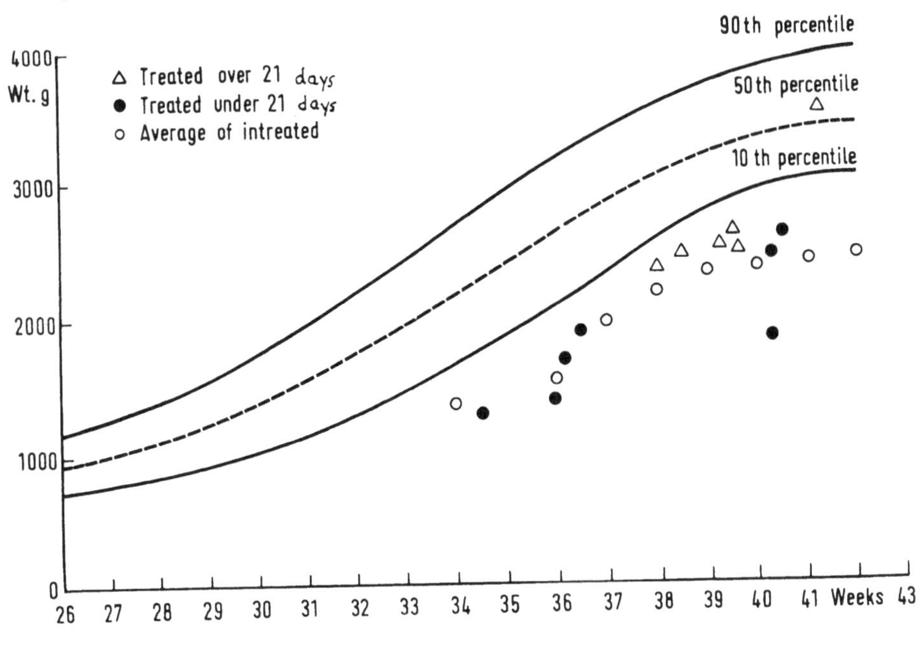

Fig. 6. Distribution of infant weights in treated and non-treated cases of fetal growth-retardation in relation to normal figures

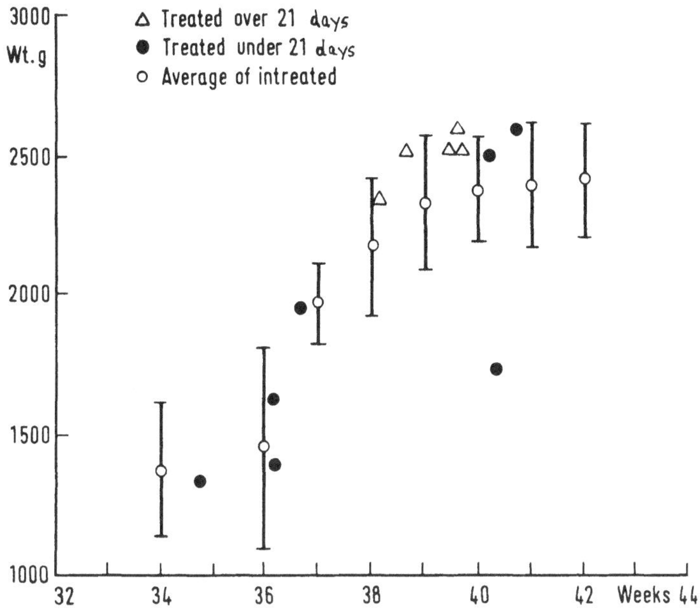

Fig. 7. Mean and distribution of the weights of non-treated cases of fetal growth-retardation and cases treated with Ritodrine

The Effect of Ritodrine on Infant Weight

M. J. Flynn

A number of authors have referred to the possible use of β-mimetic agents, in particular ritodrine hydrochloride (Pre-par ®) for the treatment of intra-uterine growth retardation. This summary describes the background upon which these proposals are based.

Early in the development of this drug for the planned indication field of premature labor, studies were performed in animals to assess the effect on the offspring of prolonged administration to the mother in high doses during pregnancy. No adverse effects on the offspring were seen but surprisingly the mean pup weight in one of the studies in rats was found to be significantly higher in the ritodrine treatment groups than in the controls (Fig. 1). After correction for litter size

Controls	3.55 grams
Ritodrine - oral administration	
10 mg / kg / day	3.64 grams
100 mg / kg / day	3.90 grams +
Ritodrine - intravenous administration	
1 mg / kg / day	3.68 grams
3 mg / kg / day	3.86 grams +
9 mg / kg / day	3.89 grams +

+Mean pup weight significantly greater than controls, $p < 0.01$ (WILCOXON Test).

Fig. 1. Mean pup weight after administration of ritodrine to pregnant rats from day 6 to day 15 of gestation

and subdivision into dosage groups this effect was found to be dose related (Fig. 2).

Before this finding was known however it had already been found in human pregnancy from a controlled trial with ritodrine and librium ® in premature labor (1) that after subdivision of the patients according to duration of gestation at the time of delivery the mean weight of all infants born after 33 weeks was higher in the ritodrine group than in the librium ® group. Despite the small numbers this difference was significant at 39 weeks (Fig. 3).

The possible reasons for the result are shown in Fig. 4.

Litter size	Treatment group mean pup weight (g)			
	Control	1 mg/kg	3mg/kg	9mg/kg
8	3.74	--	3.89	--
9	--	3.59	3.47	4.07
10	3.46	3.82	3.66	3.79
11	3 34	3 72	3 95	--
12	3.61	3.67	3.92	3.97
13	3.54	3.82	3.77	3.65
14	--	--	3 75	3 94

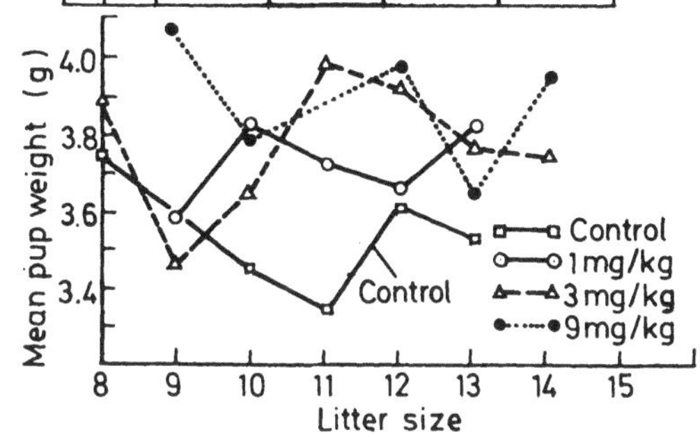

Fig. 2. Mean pup weight / litter size in control and treatment groups after intravenous administration of ritodrine to pregnant rats. (Based on data taken from report 3198/70/10, K. Palmer and D. D. Cozens Huntingdon Research Centre England)

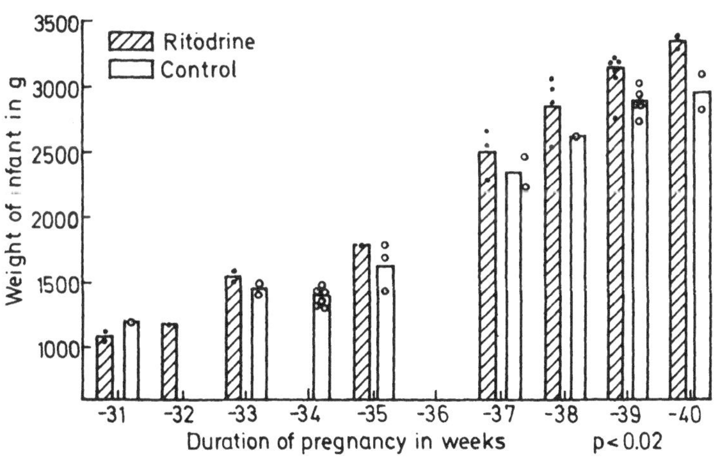

Fig. 3. A comparison by weight and duration of gestation of Ritodrine & control group from a controlled trial in premature labour

Fig. 5 shows a similar analysis from a double-blind study performed in a different centre to assess the effect of oral ritodrine or placebo in the treatment of mild, threatened premature labor. Once again at certain durations of gestation the babies in the active drug group

1. Librium caused small babies ?
2. Ritodrine caused large babies ?
3. The selection of patients had by accident caused the difference ?
4. The statistics are wrong ?

Fig. 4. Possible reasons for difference in infant weight in ritodrine and librium groups from a controlled trial in premature labor

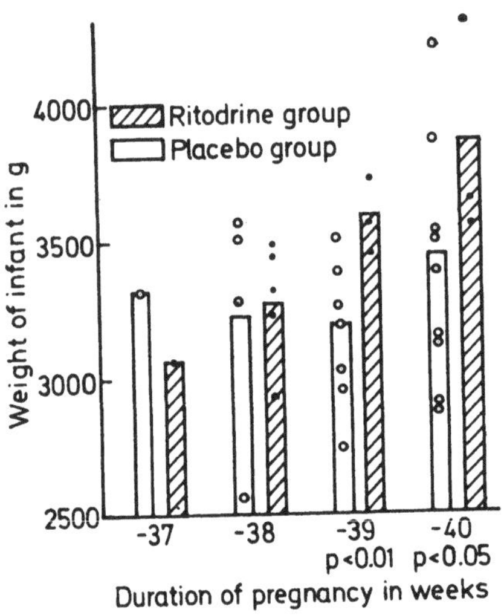

Fig. 5. A comparison by infant weight and durating of gestation of ritodrine and placebo groups from a controlled trial in premature labour

were significantly heavier than in the placebo group. There was a tendency to increased length of the infants but the difference was not significant (Fig. 6).

SEIDL et al. compared the weights and lengths, categorized for gestational age at time of delivery, of 110 infants of ritodrine treated mothers and 239 controls. They could detect no effect of the ritodrine treatment on mean infant weight (2). They did however draw attention to the fact that when treatment was started after 34 weeks of gestation the incidence of infants weighing less than 3000 grams at term in their own study and in a multicentre study reported by THIERY et al. (3) was higher than when treatment was started earlier in the pregnancy (Fig.7). This apparent effect of ritodrine could however be due to factors related to the different reasons for premature labor at 35 and 36 weeks of gestation than at 28 - 33 weeks of gestation.

A number of mechanisms were considered as being possibly causal to the effect on infant weight. These are shown in Figs. 8, 9 and 10.

The studies by DE SWIET (4), JANISCH et al. (6) and BRETTES et al. (5) raised the possibility of a possible use for ritodrine in certain cases of intra-uterine growth retardation. It was however first con-

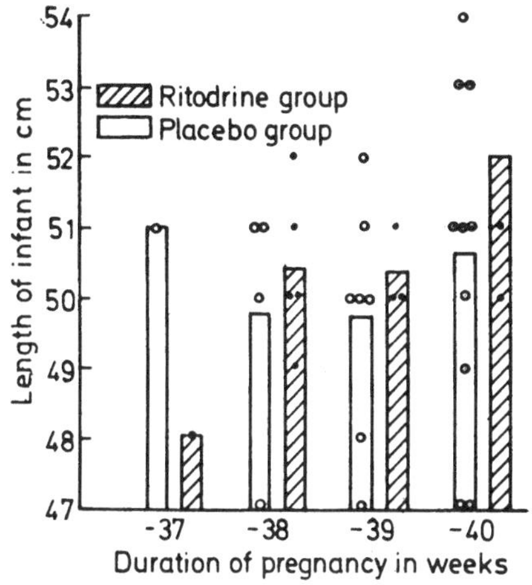

Fig. 6. A comparison by infant length and duration of gestation of ritodrine and placebo groups from a controlled trial in premature labour

Onset of treatment (weeks)		30	31	32	33	34	35	36
SEIDL et al.	Total No. of infants % <3000 grams	43 21 %	12 33 %	9 22 %	10 37 %	8 38 %	13 38 %	13 69 %
THIERY et al.	Total No. of infants % <3000 grams	22 32 %		2	5 20 %		9 78 %	10 60 %

SEIDL et al. 1972

Fig. 7. Relationship between time of onset of treatment with ritodrine and number of infants born after 36 weeks with a birthweight below 3000 grams

Possible causal factors for effect of ritodrine on infant weight
1. Increase of uterine or placental blood flow ?
2. Metabolic effect involving metabolism of glucose ?

Fig. 8. Possible causal factors for effect of ritodrine on infant weight

1. DE SWIET (1970)	Pregnant rabbits, microsphere technique - increased placental flow (4)
2. BRETTES et al. (1972)	"Uterine blood flow", thermistor probe technique. (double-blind study)------- increased uterine blood flow in patients with "placental-insufficiency" (5)
3. JANISCH et al. (1972)	"Placental blood flow" - pertechnetate bolus.------- increased placental blood flow (6)

Fig. 9. Studies with ritodrine on uterine or placental blood flow

Non-pregnant patients: oral treatment, no effect on glucose tolerance curve or fasting blood glucose	MRAVUNAC (1972) (7)
Pregnant patients: intra-venous infusion, increase of maternal and fetal glucose levels	GAMISSANS et al. (8) GRUBER et al. (9)
Pregnant patients: intra-venous infusion----- increased maternal glucose and insulin responses to a glucose load	URBAN et al. (10) BERGSTEIN et al. (11)
Pregnant patients: long term administration--- return of glucose tolerance curve to normal	BERGSTEIN (12)
Pregnant patients: no abnormality of fasting blood glucose during long-term administration	Several authors

Fig. 10. Metabolic studies with ritodrine -----carbohydrate metabolism

sidered worthwhile to perform animal studies in experimentally induced intra-uterine growth retardation.

After consideration of a number of possible animal models one was selected which is attributed to GARMASHEVA, 1968 (13). GARMASHEVA reported that cooling of pregnant rats on day 4 of pregnancy resulted in significant growth retardation of the fetuses. In a large series of experiments MORSINK and DE WACHTER found that in their hands the maximum effect on pup weight was obtained by cooling to 20° C for 3 hours on day 8 of pregnancy (14). Figs. 11 and 12. Fig. 12 shows that 56 % of the offspring of the cooled rats were small for dates, that is, they were below the 10th percentile of the normal population.

MORSINK and DE WACHTER (1973)		
Pregnant rats cooled to 18 - 22° C for 3 hours on day 8 of pregnancy. Caesarian section on day 18.		
Controls (n = 114)	Mean weight = 749 mg	Difference = 16 %
Cooled rats (n = 68)	Mean weight = 629 mg	

$p < 0.01$

Fig. 11. Induction of intra-uterine growth retardation in rats by cooling

MORSINK and DE WACHTER (1973)		
Controls	No of pups smaller than 600 mg = 1.75 % = 2/114	$p < 0.01$
Cooled rats	No of pups smaller than 600 mg = 36.5 % = 25/ 68	
Controls	No of pups smaller than 650 mg = 10 % = 11/114	$p < 0.01$
Cooled rats	No of pups smaller than 650 mg = 56 % = 38/ 68	

Fig. 12. Induction of intra-uterine growth retardation in rats by cooling

A series of further studies by the same investigators showed that the growth inhibiting effect of cooling could be significantly counteracted by administration of ritodrine from pregnancy day 7 to 20 (15). Without ritodrine 61 % of the offspring of the cooled rats were growth retarded as compared with 30 % in the group of cooled rats which received ritodrine.

Fig. 13 shows a final comparison of the weight distribution of cooled rats and control rats, with or without ritodrine administration, while fig. 14 demonstrates that ritodrine administration resulted in heavier

MORSINK and DE WACHTER (1972)

	mean pup weight on day 21	number of pups < 3000 mg
Not cooled - no ritodrine	3350 mg	12/111 = 11 %
not cooled - ritodrine	3420 mg	3/ 62 = 6 %
cooled - no ritodrine	2960 mg	54/ 89 = 61 %
cooled - ritodrine	3150 mg	18/ 59 = 30 % $p<0.01$

Fig. 13. Effect of ritodrine on intra-uterine growth retardation in rats induced by cooling

pups not by producing giant rats but by decreasing the incidence of growth retarded ones.

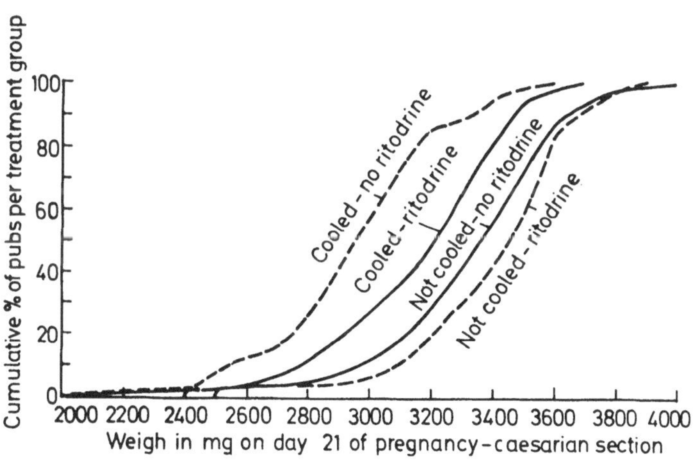

Fig. 14. Effect of ritodrine on intra-uterine growth retardation induced by cooling in rats

These animal and human studies are felt to indicate the careful investigation of ritodrine for the treatment or prophylaxis of intrauterine growth retardation. Such studies can only be conclusive if they involve careful selection of patients, randomised allocation to drug or control group, with identical handling of the two groups in other respects, due care to evaluation of group comparability before treatment and finally assessment of the success or failure of management only on the basis of direct criteria - namely the relative weight, condition and subsequent development of the infants from each group.

References

1. SIVASAMBO, R.: Premature Labor. Paper presented at an international symposium on the "treatment of fetal risks". Baden (Austria) 11 - 13 May 1972. In Press.
2. SEIDL, A., BAUMGARTEN, K., EISNER, R., FRÖHLICH, H., GRUBER, W., URBAN, G.: Auswirkung der Ritodrine-Behandlung auf das Kindesgewicht. Paper presented at the international symposium on "Treatment of fetal risks" Baden (Austria) 11 - 13 May 1972. In Press.
3. THIERY, M., BAUMGARTEN, K., BROSENS, I., ESTEBAN-ALTIRRIBA, J., GAMISSANS, O., YO-LE-SIAN, A., FLYNN, M., VAN STRIK, R.: A multicentre trial with ritodrine in the treatment of premature labor in patients with intact membranes . Paper presented at an international symposium on the "Treatment of fetal risks". Baden (Austria) May 11 - 13, 1972. In Press.
4. DE SWIET, M.: Personal communication to Philips-Duphar B. V. 1970.
5. BRETTES, J. P., CHAVAS, A., CONSTANTINESCO, A., IRRMAN, M., RENAUD, R., GANDAR, R.: L'action d'un beta mimétique (ritodrine) sur la circulation utérine au cours de grossesses normales et pathologiques (souffrances foetales cliniques). Paper presented at an international symposium on the "treatment of fetal risks." Baden (Austria) May 11 - 13, 1972. In Press.
6. JANISCH, H., LEODOLTER, S., REINOLD, E.: "Der Effekt von ritodrine auf die Plazentadurchblutung". Paper presented at an international symposium on the treatment of fetal risks, Baden (Austria) 11 - 13 May, 1972. In Press.
7. MRAVUNAC, B., FLYNN, M.: A double blind investigation into the effects of ritodrine on blood chemistry. Paper presented at an international symposium on the "Treatment of fetal risks", Baden (Austria) 11 - 13 May 1972. In Press.
8. GAMISSANS, O., CARRERAS, M., DURAN, P., CARARACH, J., CALAF, J., ABRIL, V., ESTBAN-ALTIRRIBA, J.: The treatment of fetal acidosis with β-mimetic drugs, studies on acid base balance, blood glucose levels and uterine motility. International symposium on the "Treatment of fetal risks", Baden (Austria) May 11 - 13, 1972. In Press.
9. GRUBER, W., BAUMGARTEN, K., BAUMUNG, H., FRÖHLICH, H., SEIDL, A., URBAN, G.: Der Einfluß kurzzeitiger Infusion von Ritodrine auf Blutzucker, Insulin und somatotoropes Hormon. International symposium on the "Treatment of fetal risks". Baden (Austria) May 11 - 13, 1972. In Press.
10. URBAN, G., BAUMGARTEN, K., BAUMUNG, H., BECK, A., FRÖHLICH, H., GRUBER, W., SEIDL, A.: Die Beeinflussung des Glukosetoleranztestes bei normalen Schwangerschaften mit Ritodrine und Th 1165 a. International Symposium on the treatment of fetal risks, Baden (Austria) May 11 - 13, 1972. In Press.
11. BERGSTEIN, N. A. M., STOLTE, L. A. M., FLYNN, M. J., V. DOORN, G. A.: An investigation into the effects of β-mimetic agents on the response to intravenous glucose loads. International symposium on the "Treatment of fetal risks". Baden (Austria) 11 - 13 May, 1972. In Press.
12. BERGSTEIN - Personal communication, 1973.
13. GARMESHEVA, N. L.: The influence of experimental chronic impairment of utero placental circulation upon the embryo. Wissenschaftliche Zeitschrift der Friedrich-Schiller-Universität Jena.

Mathematisch-Naturwissenschaftliche Reihe. Heft 1 Jahrgang 17. 1968. Herausgeber: Der Rektor
14. MORSINK, L., DE WACHTER, M.: Ontwikkeling methode voor het verkrijgen van hypotrophie van feut en placenta bij de rat. Report No. 56648/44/73, Dept. of Pharmacology, January 1973. Philips-Duphar B. V. The Netherlands.
15. MORSINK, L., DE WACHTER, M.: Invloed ritodrine na orale toediening op hypotrophie van de rattefeut. Report No. 56648/39/72, Dept. of Pharmacology, Philips-Duphar B. V. The Netherlands.

Oestrogen Excretion in a Group of 90 Pregnant Women Treated with Ritodrine

E. Moneta, C. Romanini, and E. Menini

We have treated a group of 90 pregnant women showing signs of threatened premature labour with a new beta-mimetic drug, Ritodrine. This drug has been used according to the therapeutic schedule shown in Table 1.

Table 1. Therapeutic schedules using ritodrine

1. Initial treatment	
a) intravenous increasing dose from 50 to 200 mcg/min	
b) intravenous constant dose:	150 or 200 mcg/min
2. Maintenance treatment	
a) oral:	4 x 10 mg daily
b) intramuscular:	4 x 10 mg daily

In all cases the treatment was begun between the 28th and the 37th weeks of pregnancy. Ritodrine was given for different periods of time as shown in Table 2. Table 3 illustrates the main clinical features of the patients studied: age, parity and previous pathological events.

During the whole period of treatment several parameters were frequently determined in order to assess the condition of the mother and the fetus together with the benefits and side-effects of the drug.

Table 2. Duration of treatment with ritodrine in the patients studied

Intravenous		Oral		Intramuscular	
duration	No. of patients	duration	No. of patients	duration	No. of patients
over 25 days	1 (29)	over 100 days	1 (103)	14 days	1
20 - 25 days	1 (20)	90-100 days	1 (91)	10 days	1
10 - 19 days	-	71- 90 days	1	9 days	1
5 - 9 days	12	61- 70 days	2	7 days	1
1 - 4 days	43	51- 60 days	-	5 days	4
		41- 50 days	6		
		31- 40 days	5		
		26- 30 days	4		
		21- 25 days	7		
		16- 20 days	10		
		11- 15 days	20		
		1- 10 days	16		

Table 4 shows the measurements made during treatment. Other measurements were also made as and when indicated by the clinical pictures.

Table 3. Age, parity, and maternal pathology of the patients studied

Age	No. of patients
less than 20	1
from 21 to 29	55
from 30 to 34	21
from 35 to 40	12
over 41	1
Parity	
0	46
1 - 2	38
3	1
4 and over	5
Previous premature deliveries	
1	23
2	2
3	1
Main maternal pathology	
Prediabetes	6
Hepatitis	6
Cervical incompetence	3
Nephropathy	2
Placental insufficiency	1
Ulcerative colitis	1
Severe anaemia	1
Epilepsy	1

In other communications (1, 2) we have reported on the use of Ritodrine at appropriate dosage in premature labour and on the relatively modest side-effects of the drug.

Table 4. Scheme of maternal and fetal measurements during ritodrine treatment

1. Cardiotocography
   - a - during intravenous infusion: during the whole period of infusion, and at least 30 min after cessation.
   - b - during maintencance treatment: at least 60 min every 2-5 days.
2. Arterial pressure and maternal heart rate
   - a - during intravenous infusion: every 15 - 30 min.
   - b - during maintenance treatment: at least once or twice a day.
   - c - in presence of subjective symptoms: every 5 - 15 min.
3. Total oestrogen excretion/ 24 hrs
   - a - every 1 - 4 days during the whole period of treatment (intravenous, intramuscular or oral)
4. Other maternal parameters
   - a - on admission: E. C. G.; general blood chemistry, and in particular electrolytes and blood glucose.
   - b - every 7 days: E. C. G.; electrolytes and blood glucose.
   - c - in presence of subjective symptoms: E. C. G. and electrolytes.

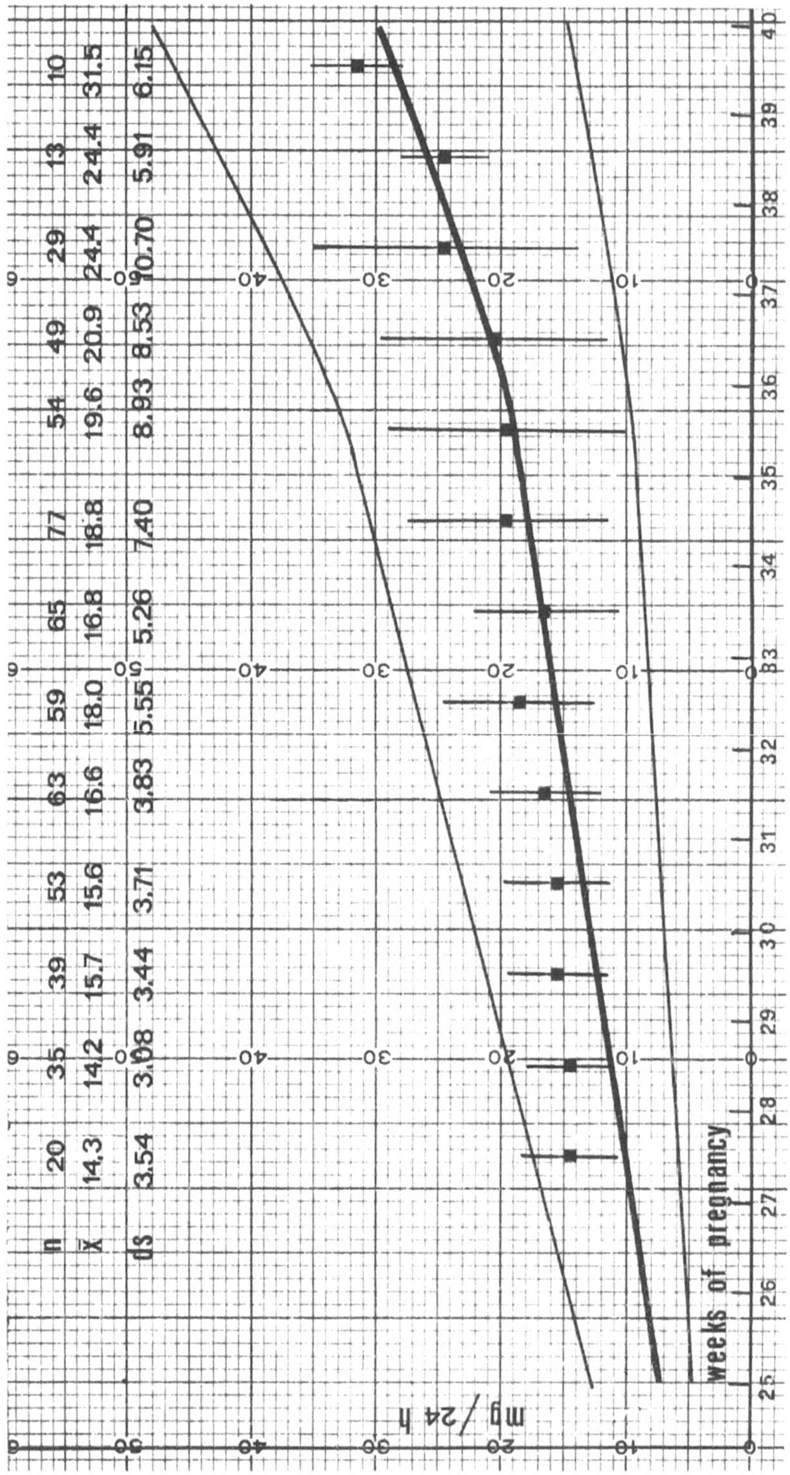

Fig. 1. Total urinary oestrogens (mean for each week ± S. D.)

Fig. 1 shows the results of serial determinations of urinary oestrogens (24 hours collections) and it is of interest to note that in all cases they are within the limits of a normal statistical variation (3).

The data presented, resulting from 556 determinations, clearly shows the lack of serious effects of the drug on the fetus, even after long treatment. We believe that this observation is valuable with respect to the increasing use of beta-mimetic drugs in prolonged treatment of premature labour.

We also believe that our figures, which include patients not only with threatened premature labour but also with other conditions, demonstrate the innocuity of the drug.

References

MONETA, E., ROMANINI, C., OLIVA, G. C., PLOTTI, G.: International Symp. on treatment of fetal risks, Baden, 1972.

ROMANINI, C., MONETA, E., OLIVA, G. C.: Annali di Ostetricia, Cinecologia e Medicina Perinatale, 1973 (in press).

MENINI, E., BOMPIANI, A.: Technicon Symposia, Roma, 1969.

The Influence of Some Preparations on the Feto-Placental Insufficiency

J. Sieroszewski, T. Pajszczyk-Kieszkiewicz, and J. Kieszkiewicz

The concentration of steroid hormones excreted in the urine during pregnancy is some measure of the viability of the feto-placental unit. A positive correlation exists between steroid excretion and feto-placental function. Oestriol measurements are of particular importance.

Uterine blood supply is important in leading to the formation of oestriol. We decided to investigate the influence of preparations improving uterine perfusion and so the excretion of oestriol in urine of pregnant women in various months of pregnancy.

We examined 290 pregnant women, in the obstetrical clinic of our Institute, who delivered prematurely. We found intra-uterine dystrophy in 10 % of them.

Table 1 shows the number of women separated into months of pregnancy and the drugs used.

Table 1

Treatment	Period of pregnancy in months				
	V	VI	VII	VIII	Total
Isoxuprine - Duvadilan/ (Duphar)	50	94	79	19	242
Euphyllinum (Polfa)	8	14	16	12	50
Total	58	108	95	31	292

Duvadilan (Duphar) was given to patients with hypertonic uterine activity in doses of 30 - 80 mg/24 hours orally or 20 - 40 mg in 5 % glucose solution intravenously over a few hours. Duvadilan was never used during delivery and/ or accompanying haemorrhage. Euphyllinum (Polfa) was used in similar cases - twice daily in suppositories 0.36 mg each.

In most cases Duvadilan has been used for 2 - 3 months. Euphyllinum was given for a shorter time.

Studies on effectiveness of the preparations were based on regression of uterine over-contractility and on measurement of urinary oestriol. With treatment, we succeeded in decreasing the percentage of premature deliveries to 2.2 % among the treated women, compared with 10.5 % in the control group.

Oestriol in 24 hours urine was estimated by the ITTRICH method. Table 2 presents mean values of oestriol in various months of pregnancy before and after treatment. The mean excretion values of oestriol before and

Table 2

Kind of investigation	Period of pregnancy / months V	VI	VII	VIII
Oestriol value before treatment/ mg/24 hours	5.8/ 3.6-12.3	10.9/ 6.8-13.7	12.3/ 8.0-20.5	18.3/ 11.4-30.0
Number of estimations	58	108	95	31
Oestriol value in time of treatment/ mg/24 hours	6.7/ 3.8-14.5	15.2/ 12.3-23.1	18.9/ 11.3-27.6	28.6/ 24.0-39.4
Number of estimations	50	94	79	19
p	$p<0.05$	$0.001<p<0.05$	$0.001<p<0.05$	$0.001<p<0.05$

after treatment were calculated from 4 - 6 estimations from 24 hour urine. The urinary excretion of oestriol, after using both medicines, rose.

It is worth noting that long-term (some months) treatment of cases of dystrophy with Duvadilan apparently causes a significant increase in birth weight of fetuses compared with the untreated cases.

Table 3

Investigation	Length of pregnancy (months) V	VI	VII	VIII
Oestriol excretion before treatment mg/24 hours	5.8/ 3.6 - 12.3	10.9/ 6.8 - 13.7	12.3/ 8.0 - 20.5	18.3/ 11.4 - 30.0
Number of estimations	58	108	95	31
Oestriol excretion at time of treatment mg/24 hours	6.3/ 4.1 - 13.2	14.6/ 11.8-21.7	18.1/ 12.0 - 26.9	25.3/ 18.1 - 29.6
Number of estimations	8	14	16	12
p	$p<0.05$	$p<0.05$	$0.001<p<0.05$	$0.001<p<0.05$

Conclusion

1. Preparations improving the perfusion of uterus cause:
   a) Increase in urinary excretion of oestriol.
   b) Decrease of premature deliveries.
2. Improvement in uterus perfusion led to an increase in the birth weight of ten dystrophic fetuses.

Effects of a Beta-Adrenergic Agent on the Angiographically Visualized Uteroplacental Circulation in the Rhesus Monkey

H. C. S. Wallenburg, J. Mazer, and D. L. Hutchinson

Introduction. Recent studies (1, 2) suggest that administration of a beta-adrenergic receptor stimulating catecholamine to the mother may increase uteroplacental blood flow and thus could be useful for intra-uterine treatment of fetal asphyxia and acidosis. This effect is attributed to decompression of uteroplacental vasculature due to inhibition of myometrial activity. The objective of the present study has been to investigate by means of a radioangiographic technique the possible intrinsic effects of a potent and specific beta-adrenergic compound (metaproterenol, Alupent®) on uteroplacental vasculature and circulation in the absence of myometrial activity under standardized conditions in the pregnant rhesus monkey.

Material and methods. Thirteen experiments have been performed in seven lightly anesthetized pregnant rhesus monkeys. Aortic, intra-amniotic and central venous pressures as well as a maternal E. K. G. were continuously written. Serial placental radioangiography was performed following the procedure described by RAMSEY et al. (3). Each experiment consisted of two angiographies made during uterine relaxation at a 20 minutes interval; the first angiography served as a control, the drugs to be studied were infused prior to the second angiography. In the two sets of angiograms from each experiment the arterial entries ("spurts") into the intervillous space were compared. The times of appearance of the first spurts (Initial Spurt Appearance Time, I.S.A.T.), of the maximum number of spurts (Maximum Spurt Appearance Time, M.S.A.T.) as well as the rate of appearance from the first spurt until the maximum number (Spurt Appearance Rate, S. A. R.) were determined. The following experiments were performed:

1. Control experiments (n = 4), without infusion of drugs.
2. Metaproterenol experiments (n = 6) in which metaproterenol (Alupent®) was infused intravenously (.7 or 1.0 μg/kg/min) prior to the second angiography.
3. Propranolol followed by metaproterenol experiments (n = 3) in which propranolol - a specific beta-receptor blocker - was infused (3.1 - 5.0 μg/kg/min) followed by metaproterenol, (.7 - 1.0 μg/kg/min) prior to the second angiography.

Results. In the control series the spurt appearance times did not differ between the first and the second series of angiograms.

Metaproterenol in the dosage used appeared to have no effects on aortic, central venous or intra-amniotic pressures, or maternal heart rate. Following infusion of metaproterenol, I. S. A. T. and M. S. A. T. were shortened, while S. A. R. was increased (Fig. 1).

These effects were not observed when metaproterenol was preceded by propranolol.

Comment and conclusions. The angiographic parameters I. S. A. T., M. S. A. T. and S. A. R. measured under standardized conditions are indices of uteroplacental circulation time (U. C. T.). In the present experimental model U. C. T. is inversely proportional to flow; the

A

B

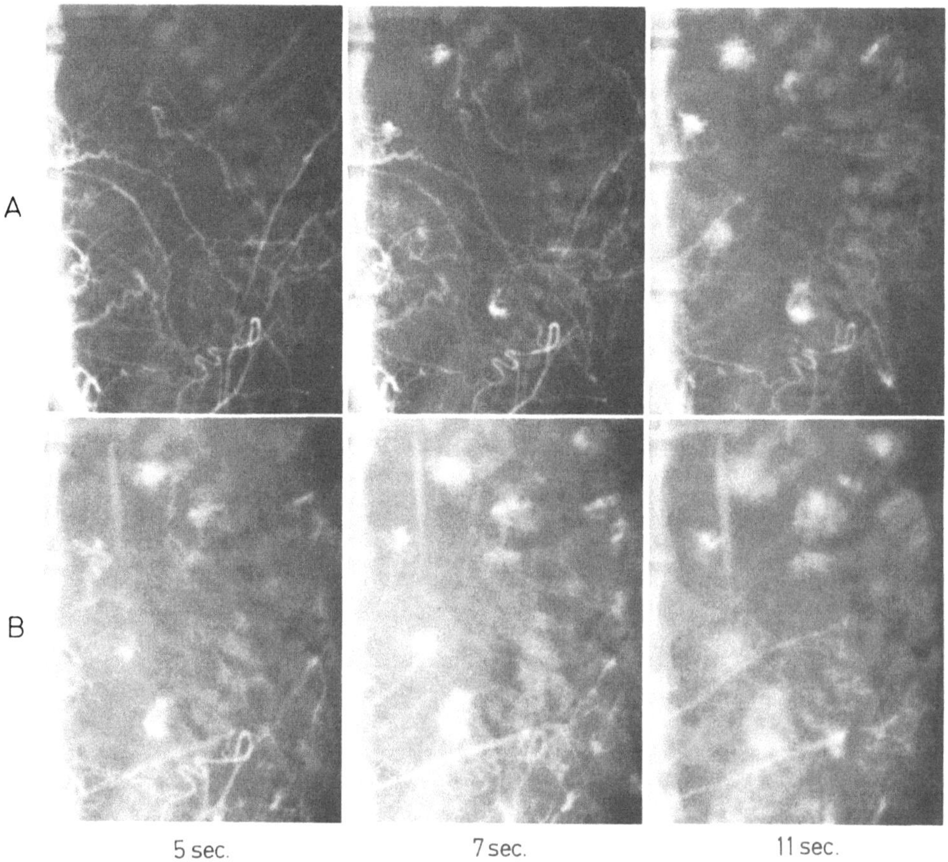

Fig. 1. Identical areas taken from anteroposterior placental angiograms made at 5, 7 and 11 seconds, respectively, following injection of contrast medium.
Top row: control angiography.
Bottom row: second angiography, following intravenous infusion of metaproterenol, .7 µg/kg/min.
The intervillous spurts appear sooner and faster than in the control series

vessel radius is the only variable that influences both U. C. T. and uteroplacental flow. Thus, in this model administration of metaproterenol to the mother appears to shorten U. C. T. and to increase uteroplacental blood flow, on the basis of intrinsic vasodilatation. The observation that this effect can be blocked by propranolol indicates that it is due to stimulation of beta-adrenergic receptors. Since human uterine arteries have been shown to possess beta-receptors (4) administration of a beta-receptor stimulating agent like metaproterenol in a dosage, small enough to prevent general cardiovascular effects might, in analogy with the results obtained in the rhesus monkey, lead to uterine vasodilatation resulting in an increased uteroplacental flow. It might thus be used for intra-uterine treatment of impaired fetal condition, particularly when uterine vasospasm seems to be involved, like in pre-eclampsia.

References

1. CONDORELLI, S., TONELLI, F., COSMI, E. V.: Acta Anaesth. 21, 707 (1970).
2. CALDEYRO-BARCIA, R., MAGAÑA, J. M., CASTILLO, J. B., POSEIRO, J. J., MENDEZ-BAUER, C., POSE, S. V., ESCARCENA, L., CASACUBERTA, C., BUSTOS, J. R., GIUSSI, G.: Arch. Ginec. Obstet. 24, 15 (1969).
3. RAMSEY, E. M., CORNER JR., G. W., DONNER, M. W.: Am. J. Obstet. Gynec. 86, 213 (1963).
4. BELL, C.: J. Obstet. Gynaec. Brit. Cwlth. 76, 1123 (1969).

Orciprenaline in the Treatment of Premature Labour

L. Zichella and L. Marzetti

Beta-receptor stimulation inhibite uterine activity and seems to increase utero-placental flow. The presence or absence of beta-adrenergic receptors in the uterine vessels have never been clearly proved, but clinical and experimental studies have shown that beta-stimulators increase uterine blood flow and decrease the resistance of uterine vessels. This paper reports the results we obtained with orciprenaline in the treatment of premature labour.

In 72 cases of premature labour between weeks 20 - 35 of pregnancy orciprenaline was administered by intravenous infusion at a rate of 10 - 20 γ per min (2.5 mg in 500 ml of 5 % dextrose). After the first 30 minutes, a lower rate was given (5 γ per min) to a maximum of 2.5 mg. If uterine contractions recurred, the infusion was repeated up to four times daily for a maximum of 20 days. Oral medication with isoxuprine 20 mg every eight hours was used when uterine contractions ceased. Orciprenaline infusion was reduced when the maternal heart rate exceeded 120 - 130 beats per minute.

We assessed the results of treatment from patients using the following criteria: cervical condition, intact or ruptured membranes and fetal weight.

The patients were divided into five groups, according to their condition at the beginning of treatment:

1. Uterine activity with closed or effaced cervix.
2. Uterine activity with cervical delatation of 3 - 4 cm and intact membranes.
3. Ruptured membranes without uterine contractions.
4. Ruptured membranes with uterine contractions.
5. Cervical dilatation of 3 - 4 cm in patients who had undergone cerclage.

Table 1.

Group	No.	Cervical dilatation cm	Membranes	Uterine activity	Gestational age weeks	Delivery postponement days
I	42	0	Intact	+	27 - 35	> 10
II	12	3	Intact	+	28 - 34	1 - 2
III	9	0	Ruptured	-	30 - 34	5 - 15
IV	5	0	Ruptured	+	26 - 34	1 - 3
V	4	3 - 4	Intact	±	20 - 24	10 - 14

Orciprenaline inhibits uterine contraction of early premature labour as well as advanced labour with 3 - 4 cm of cervical dilatation using 20 γ per min, even when the membranes are ruptured.

The inhibiting dose is related to the frequency of the uterine contractions. However, in the first group it was possible to obtain a long extension of the pregnancy (10 - 70 days). In the others, uterine activity resumed soon after the discontinuing of the infusion. In the fifth group (patients with cervical incompetence, 20th - 24th week), even after cerclage and inhibition of uterine activity, it was not possible to postpone premature labour for more than 10 - 15 days. After this time membranes were always ruptured, probably because of infection.

Maternal blood pressure changes were not significant; at higher doses there was tachycardia and occasionally balpitations. The drug dose was then reduced. Even after many days treatment, increase in urinary oestriol was not significant during and after the therapy.

When uterine activity resumes rapidly after discontinuing the infusion, this means that there is a strong stimulus to labour which will be difficult to arrest. Successful treatment, therefore, depends on the ability to abolish uterine activity for many days. However, the suppression of uterine contractions and the postponement of labour give minimal clinical advantages if it is not possible to achieve a gestational age with a good index of fetal maturity.

References

1. BROTANEK, V., HODR, J.: The effect of isoxsuprine on uteroplacental circulation. Intra-uterine dangers of the fetus. Excerpta Medica, Foundation ED., Amsterdam,424, 1967.
2. GREISS, F. C. Jr.: The uterine vascular bed. Effect of adrenergic stimulation. Obstet. Gynec., 21, 295 (1963).
3. KLOCK, F. K., KUNZEL, W., JUNGE, D.: The uterine flow and the uterine resistance of the vessels in highly pregnant sheep under influence of beta-stimulators. Third European Congress of Perinatal Medicine, 1972.
4. MARZETTI, L., ZICHELLA, L.: Treatment of premature labour with orciprenaline. Comun. International Symposium on the Treatment of Fetal Risks, 11/5/1972: Baden - Vienna.
5. RENAUD, R., BOOG, G., BRETTES, J. P. et al.: Souffrance foetale. Aspects thérapeutiques. XXII Congrès Nat. Anesth. Réanim, p. 958, 1972. Paris, Librairie Arnette.

Betamimetic Drugs and the Feto-Placental Function

G. Zinelli, E. Vadora, D. Debiasi, and F. Coppola

Starting out from the assumption that the betamimetic drugs, apart from having a relaxing effect upon the uterine musculature, can also regulate the variations of the utero-placental circulation, their use was suggested for therapy in foeto-placental insufficiency.

From among the very numerous cases coming regularly to the clinic for treatment with these substances, we selected 12 pregnant patients with low urinary estrogen levels to whom quite a different drug was administered designated LU 52, which from the pharmacological point of view corresponds to 4-hydro-alfa-1-2-4-hydroxyphenyl-ethylamino-benzyl-alcohol hydrochloride, or Ritodrine hydrochloride, for the purpose of evaluating the effect of this substance within all the parameters of the foeto-placental function.

Administration was almost exclusively intravenous in doses of 25 mg in 500 ml of 5 % glucose solution with a feed rate of 20 drops a minute, equal to 0.05 mg for the first 10 - 15 minutes, and of 40 drops a minute, equal to 0.10 mg thereafter. In all cases the treatment was continued with doses of 40 mg a day administered orally.

In all the patients we evaluated some biochemical and blood constants (azotaemia, glycaemia, transaminasis, bilirubinaemia, serum and urine electrolytes, peripheral haematic crasis) without noticing any significant variations even after prolonged treatment lasting several days. The ECG showed no important changes: in one case, in which the trace was recorded only during the infusion, there was noted a sinusal arhythmia with tachycardia and phase changes of the repolarisation: on ending administration, however, it returned to normal.

In all cases after the 30th week of pregnancy a cardiotocographic check was carried out and in some cases internal tocography also.

The most frequently occurring side effects on the part of the mother were tachycardia, mild arterial hypertension, tremors, heart palpitations, but not such as to cause treatment to be suspended, although the drip feed rate was reduced. On the part of the foetus mild tachycardia was noticed during infusion.

As parameters for the foetal-placental functioning we have used total urinary estrogens, pregnenolone and pregnanediol, and plasmatic HCS (Fig. 1). For the measurement of total urinary estrogens we used the spectrophotometric method of ROURKE, MARSHALL and SHELLEY.

For the measurement of urinary pregnenolone and pregnanediol the SCOMMEGNA and CHATTORAJ method of gas chromatography was used. For plasmatic HCS the radioimmunological method using the ethanol precipitation of LETCHWORTH et al.

In so far as total estrogens are concerned (Fig. 2), in the group of patients treated it was not possible to pick out a typical behaviour. The curve for total estrogen excretion does not appear to be signi-

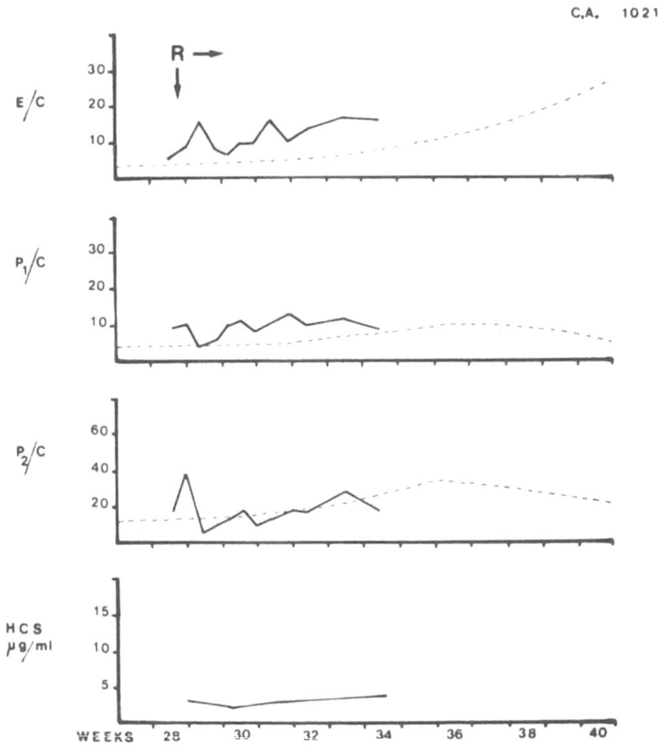

Fig. 1. Essential foeto-placental insufficiency treated with LU 52 (ritodrine hydrocloride)

ficantly influenced by treatment with Ritodrine. Observed variations are within individual daily fluctuations. The figure for estrogen gain calculated from all the percentage variations in the basic values gave a mean percentage value of + 37.75 % ± 66.56. This figure indicates a wide fluctuation with a tendency to increase. On the other hand it is not possible to determine whether this increase is due to therapy or is the physiological increase resulting from the advancing state of pregnancy.

Total Estrogen % gain	Pregnanolon % gain	Pregnanediol % gain	H. C. S. % gain
37.75 ± 66.56	42.86 ± 100.54	13.13 ± 88.41	15.17 ± 25.41

Fig. 2. Hormonal gain after treatment with LU 52 (ritodrine hydrocloride) (Mean values and standard deviation)

The behaviour of pregnenolone is similar to that for total estrogens with a mean percentage increase of 42.86 % ± 100.54. This figure shows, as does that for estrogens, a tendency to increase. Again, in this parameter, it is not possible to separate the part due to therapy from that due to the physiological progress of the pregnancy.

With pregnanediol the mean percentage increase had a value of 13.13 $\pm$ 88.41. With HCS we noted a mean increase of 15.17 % $\pm$ 25.41.

Study of the correlation coefficients between the behaviour of the various metabolic functions (total estrogens, pregnenolone, pregnanediol) shows a direct analogy in behaviour.

Et	vs	P_1	r = 0.815	P 0.001
Et	vs	P_2	r = 0.982	P 0.001
P_1	vs	P_2	r = 0.957	P 0.001

Analysis of the parameters studied does not permit definite conclusions to be drawn on the action of RITODRINE on foeto-placental function. We can only point to analogy in behaviour between the total estrogens (indicative of foeto-placental function) and pregnenolone but would point out that it is suggested by some that this is partially of foetal origin. With pregnanediol and HCS, indicative only of placental functioning, the increase is, on the other hand, considerably lower in comparison with that of the above parameters.

Mrs. D. BOLZONI and Mr. R. SPALLANZANI, Laboratory Technicians at the Obstetric and Gynaecological Clinic of the University of Parma, collaborated actively in the hormonal analyses.

Betamimetics and Placental Insufficiency Due to Uterine Hypoplasia

G. Gardey, J. J. Serrano, and J. L. Viala

The action mechanism of the betamimetics has been researched by ROBINSON, BUCHER and SUTHERLAND at the level of the cardiovascular system; intracellular adenyl-cyclase is activated. This enzyme catalyses ATP into AMPc, increased membrane potential hence increasing the threshold of excitability and inhibiting contractions. Similar effects occur in the uterus.

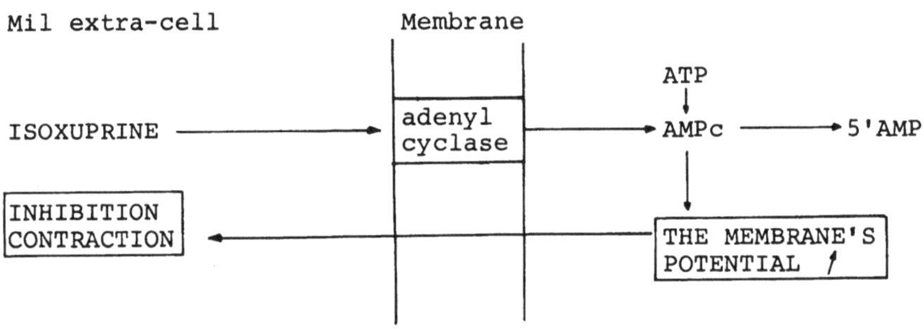

Fig. 1

The pharmacological study of the product used (isoxuprine) shows peripheral vasodilatation and an increase in arterial flow in the uterus because this organ has many beta receptors.

The uterine muscle relaxes, there is vasodilatation and increase in blood flow. The best clinical illustration of these pharmacological properties is the treatment of threatened premature delivery induced by uterine hypoplasia. The myo-relaxant effect is sufficient in such cases to arrest the contractions of an onset of labour, and continuation of treatment permits an appreciable increase in the volume of the uterus.

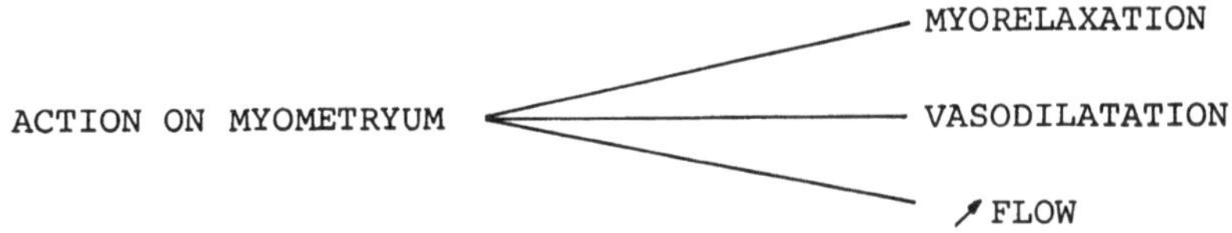

Fig. 2

We think that the myo-relaxant effect does not in itself explain this increase in uterine volume; probably the increase in blood flow plays as important a role.

It is very likely that the vascular system is underdeveloped and ischaemia is present. Thus chronic placental insufficiency occurs.

Uterine hypoplasia = Uterine vascular hypoplasia

during pregnancy

↘ placental flow

↓

chronic foetal distress

Fig. 3

The betamimetics act by both relaxation of the uterine muscle fibre and an increase in the blood flow, the final effect being growth of the uterus.

Similarly, improvement in placental nutrition allows growth and an increase in feto-placental exchange.

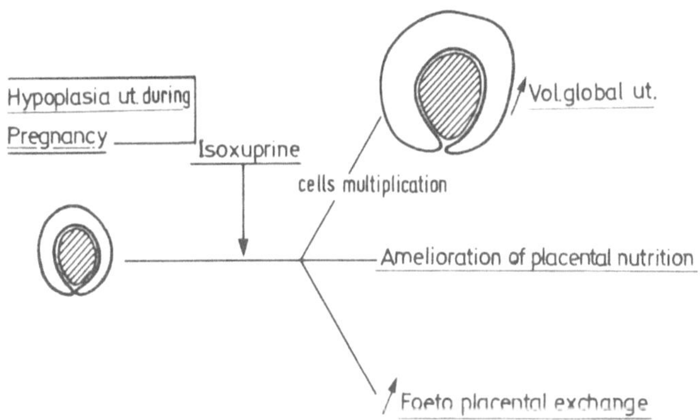

Fig. 4

We suggest that betamimetics should not be confined solely to threatened labour. Perhaps treatment should cover the entire pregnancy, and if possible, should precede it by eight to twelve weeks in order to prepare the uterine muscle for its development during pregnancy.

Since 1970, we have submitted to this treatment a certain number of women whose obstetrical histories are marked by recurring spontaneous abortions due to uterine hypoplasia. Isoxuprine is taken orally continuously until the eighth month, and if needed, for short periods, parenterally. The commencement of treatment is often at the same time as the first threatened abortion; progesterone and sometimes a cerclage are used in association with isoxuprine.

Here is an observation which supports our tentative suggestions: Mrs. D. between 1967 and 1971 had nine miscarriages between the sixth and tenth week of pregnancy, despite various hormone treatments and cerclage.

THE β MIMETICS DRUGS AS ISOXUPRINE

WILL BE GIVEN DURING THE ALL PREGNANCY

FOR UTERINE HYPOPLASIA

Fig. 5

	OESTROGENE	PROGESTERONE	CERCLAGE	β MIMETIQUE	RESULTS
1967	?	?			Abort.
1967	?	?			Abort.
1968	?	+			Abort.
1968	+	+			Abort.
1968	+	+			Abort.
1969	+	+			Abort.
1970	+	+			Abort.
1970	+	+			Abort.
1971	+	+	+		Abort.
1971		+	+	+	♂ 3080 g

Fig. 6

In 1971, the patient became pregnant again. At six weeks we began treatment with isoxuprine, 4 tablets daily, together with a weekly injection of progesterone and a cerclage procedure. The treatment was continued until the eighth month. In the 38th week, a boy of 3,080 kg was delivered.

Since 1970, some ten similar cases have been successfully treated. The results may be in doubt, as success has never been obtained by the administration of isoxuprine alone.

The facts seem to confirm our opinion of the effectiveness of isoxuprine on the utero-placental effects of uterine hypoplasia. We have seen an increase in plasma human placental lactogen levels in a number of pregnant women treated with isoxuprine. This could only be explained by an improvement in the utero-placental circulation.

We wanted to test these observations by animal experimentation - based on the hypothesis that poor vascular supply is critical in the genesis of uterine hypoplasia. We induced uterine hypoplasia by impairment of the blood supply and subsequently treated the animals with isoxuprine. We also attempted to measure the effect of isoxuprine on the capacity for gestation of the uteruses in experimental hypoplasia. We are using rats and hope to complete 200 experiments.

Hemi-uterine hypoplasia has been induced by interrupting the blood supply to half of the uterus in pre-pubertal rats - (under 3 weeks of age). The ovary on the side of the arterial interruption is not affected nor is the contralateral uterine cornu.

The animals operated on have been divided into two groups: the first group is treated with isoxuprine for six weeks in a dose proportionally twice as great as that given to patients. The control group is treated with distilled water.

Compared with the average weight of a uterus in a normal rat, that of a rat operated on as described above is reduced by 10 %. That of a rat operated on and treated is increased by 18 %. We also looked for any

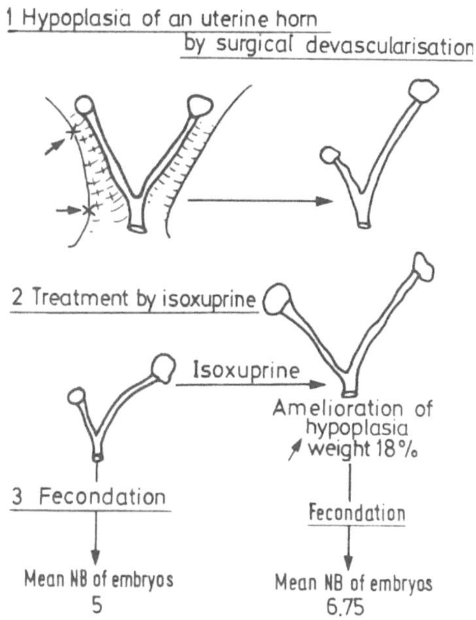

Fig. 7

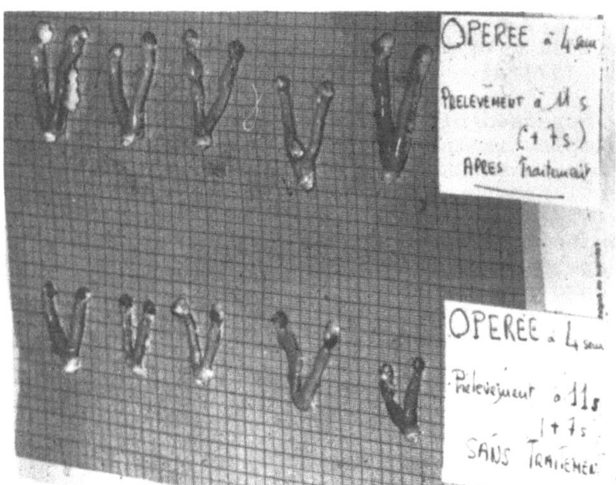

Fig. 8

effect of this drug on the capacity for gestation of the rats operated upon. An untreated hypoplasic gravid cornu contains on average 5 embryos; after six weeks of treatment, a hypoplasic gravid cornu contains on average 6.75 embryos, near the average normal figure.

These early results of experiments still in progress are encouraging, but to extrapolate to the ward must be done with care.

Placental Function and Xanthinol-Nicotinate

H. van Kessel

Introduction

The functional state of an organ or a tissue is obviously closely related to its capillary blood flow. This capillary blood flow is dependent upon the arterial blood pressure, the number of the capillaries and their functional and anatomical state.

In normal pregnancy, the growing uterus with its placenta constitutes an organ which needs an intensive perfusion with blood in order to facilitate the necessary exchange between mother and fetus of blood gases, nutrients and end products of metabolism. The uterine blood flow increases with increased vascularisation and increase of total blood volume. The placental perfusion is effected by the spiral arteries, which transverse the myometrium, penetrate the basal plate and eject arterial blood into the centre of the overlying cotyledon (FREEZE 1968). From the centre of the cotyledon, according to FREEZE's concept, the blood flows towards the periphery of the cotyledon and is finally collected in the venous return system. The functional state of the villi depends on this blood supply and deterioration in the supply causes insufficiency of the villi as a place for exchange, and leads to infarction (WALLENBURG et al. 1971 a).

Other organs, also, have an increased blood flow in normal pregnancy. The renal blood flow, for example, is increased and this results in an increased glomerular filtration, which explains the low values found for plasma creatinine in normal pregnancy.

In the course of normal pregnancy the spiral arteries undergo degenerative changes to a degree depending on their localisation in the placental bed and on the duration of pregnancy+.

These changes could be described as atheromatotic and arteriolosclerotic changes of the vessel wall, leading to obstruction and sometimes even to thrombotic processes. Hypertension may increase the progressive degeneration of the spiral arteries (BROSENS 1964).

Also in toxaemia of pregnancy there is an evident, progressive degeneration of the spiral arteries, leading in many cases to placental insufficiency and infarction (WALLENBURG 1969).

In toxaemia of pregnancy, the kidney too shows specific pathological alterations. The glomerular capillaries are constricted and their endothelial cells affected; a fibrinoid deposit can be seen on the basal membrane. These changes are accompanied by a decreased glomerular filtration rate and an increased permeability for plasma proteins. Even slightly elevated values for plasma creatinine and the development of a proteinuria are signs of the onset of toxaemia of pregnancy. The processes in kidney and placenta are closely interrelated.

+An excellent survey on this subject is given in WALLENBURG's thesis (1971 b).

Xanthinol-nicotinate is one of the drugs which are used to improve capillary blood flow, specifically in those regions where the capillaries are partly obstructed because of pathological processes. It is said that this substance, when it reaches the capillaries, is split into the base xanthinol and the nicotinate. The xanthinol is supposed to interact with the endothelial cells and to promote the uptake of the nicotinate. Pathological swelling of the endothelial cells should then diminish, the capillaries widen and the blood flow increase.

These facts, supported by clinical and experimental evidence, prompted the use of this drug also in toxaemia of pregnancy. It was hoped that the salutary effect on the capillaries would be accompanied by an increased uterine blood flow, inhibition of spiral artery degeneration and amelioration of placental function. Likewise, a favourable effect on the glomerular blood flow was expected with widening of the capillary lumen and inhibition of the capillary spasm, resulting in an increase of glomerular filtration.

MARZETTI and BENAGIANO (1964) used a therapy with Complamin (tradename for xanthinol-nicotinate) in nephrogenic toxaemia. They reported favourable results, and they ascribed this to the fibrinolytic activity of the drug in the capillaries of the glomeruli and the increased renal blood flow.

The more direct effect of Complamin on the placental function was studied by BERGSTEIN and VAN KESSEL (1968). To a small group of women, treated for suspected placental insufficiency, Complamin was given orally in a dosage of 2.000 mg per day. The urinary output of oestrogens and pregnanediol and the plasma heat-stable alkaline phosphate was measured before, during and after one week's treatment. Two non-toxaemix women, also treated with Complamin, served as controls. In these normal pregnant women no effect of the medication on the chosen parameters was seen. From the results obtained in the patient group we obtained the impression, but not more than that, that, especially in the women with raised values of plasma creatinine, the values for the chosen parameters for placental function increased more than might have been expected without treatment.

In a later study BERGSTEIN (1971) reported similar results: a striking increase in the excretion of oestrogens when Complamin was given to women with initially low urinary oestrogens. It must be noted, however, that there was no control group of women with suspected placental insufficiency. Therefore a double-blind trial was undertaken.

Materials

For a certain period of time, patients with a suspected placental insufficiency and with a duration of pregnancy of over 30 weeks, were selected from the visitors of several antenatal clinics. These patients were treated in the usual way with rest and dietary sodium restriction. In addition to this, each patient received a medication of 4 tablets a day until delivery. Each patient took the tablets from a coded bottle which contained either Complamin tablets (Complamin-retard, 500 mg of Complamin per tablet) or a placebo. Before this medication and weekly thereafter, assays were made of several parameters for placental function. At the end of the trial, when data were collected on 30 patients, the code of the bottles was broken. The Complamin group consisted of 13 patients and the placebo group of 17 patients. The values obtained from the patients who had received Complamin were compared with those of patients who had received the placebo. As parameters for placental function we chose the excretion of pregnanediol, of total oestrogen excretion and the weight of the newborns. The pregnanediol excretion was chosen as a parameter for pure placental activity, namely the secretion of progesterone. The excretion of oestrogens as a parameter of the combined foeto-placental hormone-producing activity. The birth-weight had to reflect the effective placental function as regards the supply to the foetus.

Methods

The pregnanediol was assayed by means of automated gas chromatography of toluene extracts of hydrolysed urine specimens (VAN KESSEL 1971). The oestrogens were assayed with a fully automated continuous flow system, based on ITTRICH's method (VAN KESSEL et al. 1969).

Results

The effect of Complamin on the excretion of pregnanediol

The values for the excretion of pregnanediol are given in Table 1 and Fig. 1. All the values collected for this excretion from each woman during the weeks of treatment until delivery, were expressed as a percentage of the value of the pregnanediol excretion, obtained immediately before the start of the treatment.

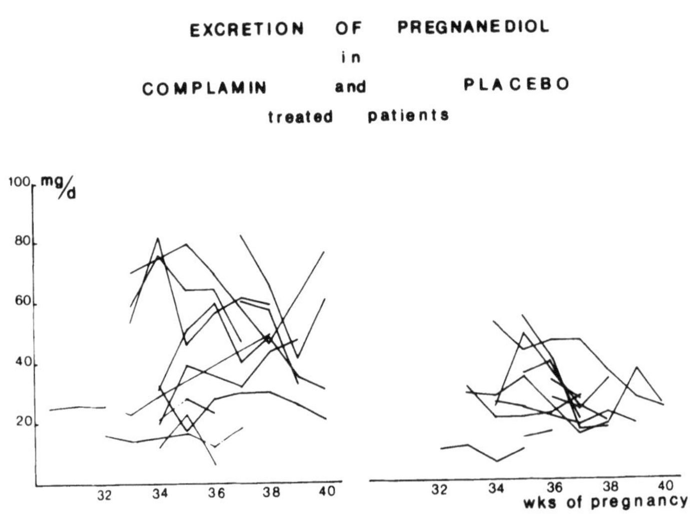

Fig. 1. This figure shows the consecutive weekly values for the excretion of pregnanediol for each patient in both the Complamin and the placebo group. The first point of each line represents the value obtained immediately before the start of the treatment in that patient. Excretion lines for patients from whom no pre-treatment measurement was obtained, are not shown in this figure

Table 1. The consecutive weekly values for the excretion of pregnanediol in the Complamin-treated and the placebo-receiving women. The pre-treatment values, when present, are underlined.

Weeks of pregnancy	30	31	32	33	34	35	36	37	38	39	40
Complamin group No.											
1								$\underline{60}$	57	33	
2								$\underline{82}$	65	41	60
3					$\underline{12}$	23	6				
4					$\underline{31}$	51	59	40	49	35	31
5				$\underline{58}$	$\underline{75}$	64	64	47			
6				$\underline{53}$	81	46	56	61	59		
7+				$\underline{70}$		79	69		46		76
8+					$\underline{32}$	17	28	30	30	26	21
9					$\underline{21}$	28	23				
10					$\underline{20}$	39		32	43	47	
11+	$\underline{25}$	26	26	23	29				49		
12			$\underline{16}$	14		17	12	18			
13				-	39	58	36	33	8	16	
Placebo group No.											
1						$\underline{14}$	16				
2				$\underline{31}$	21	21	22	27			
3			$\underline{10}$	11	6	10					
4							$\underline{27}$	23	33		
5					$\underline{24}$	48	36	23	19		
6					$\underline{52}$	43	46	46	35	27	24
7				-	67	51	51		56	58	
8					$\underline{26}$	24		18	22	18	
9				$\underline{29}$	28	34		15	19	36	24
10						$\underline{35}$	39	20			
11+						-	53	40	37		
12+							$\underline{33}$	27			
13						$\underline{54}$	40	17	17		
14						96		78	54	68	
15+					26	32	34		37		23
16			-			48	25	34			
17							$\underline{20}$		19		

The patients marked with^{+} , had normal values for serum creatinine throughout the trial.

Those women from whom no pre-treatment value was obtained, were omitted from this part of the study. For each week that the treatment lasted, the percentage values were collected for both groups (Table 2 and Fig. 2).

For each week of treatment it was tested whether the values in both groups gave an indication for higher pregnanediol excretion in Complamin-treated patients as compared to the excretion in non-Complamin-receiving patients. For this, the one sided tail-probability, P_L, was calculated by use of WILCOXONS's test. Also the frequency was noted of increased (> 100 %) or of decreased (< 100 %) excretions, for both groups for each week of treatment. On these 2 x 2 tables FISHER's test was applied, in order to investigate whether the increase of pregnanediol excretion is more frequent in Complamin-treated patients.

Table 2. The values of the excretion of pregnanediol, expressed as percentages of the pre-treatment values. For both the Complamin-treated and the placebo-receiving women, the values obtained per week of treatment for each woman, are grouped together and ranged from low to high.

Weeks of treatment	1		2		3		4		5		6	
Group	C	P	C	P	C	P	C	P	C	P	C	P
	53	68	50	32	73	32	75	52	66	52	66	46
	79	74	50	57	92	69	81	67	81	66	100	124
	88	82	55	60	94	71	94	79	111	69	196	
	95	83	87	68	99	88	115	85	112			
	104	85	88	88	106	96	116	87	113			
	129	92	104	95	106	100	158					
	133	97	110	117	110		215					
	153	110	110	122	129							
	165	111	113	150	160							
	192	114	190									
	195	200										
n	11	11	10	9	9	6	7	5	5	3	3	2

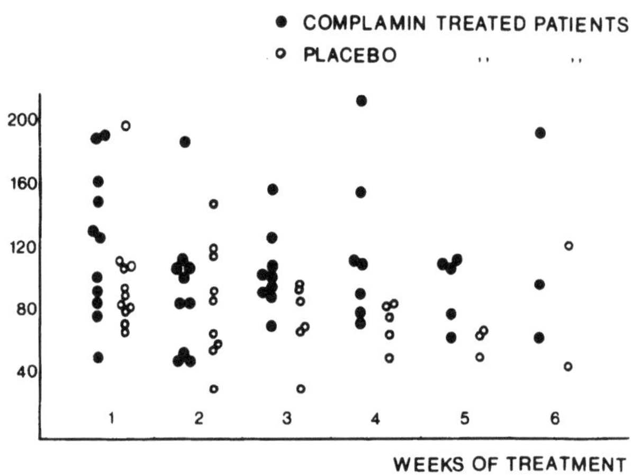

Fig. 2. Graphical display of the values given in Table 2

This statistical analysis revealed that in the third and following weeks of treatment the pregnanediol excretion is higher in Complamin-treated patients than in non-Complamin-receiving patients. In the 3rd and 4th week of treatment, increased values (as compared to the pre-treatment value) are seen more frequently in Complamin-treated patients (Table 3).

Table 3. The results of the statistical analysis of the percentage values for the excretion of pregnanediol, given in Table 2.

Excretion of Pregnanediol, Complamin vs Placebo		1	2	3	4	5
Weeks of treatment		1	2	3	4	5
WILCOXONS's test	P_L	0.11	>0.20	0.01	0.03	0.05
FISHER's test	P_L	0.20	0.40	0.04	0.07	0.18

The effect of Complamin on the excretion of oestrogens

The values for the excretion of oestrogens are given in Table 4 and Fig. 3. These values were transformed into percentages of the pre-treatment values as was done with those for the pregnanediol excretion (Table 5 and Fig. 4).

Statistical analysis of these figures provided no indication that treatment with Complamin leads to an increased excretion of oestrogens in women who are under treatment for suspected placental insufficiency (Table 6).

Table 4. The consecutive weekly values for the excretion of oestrogens of the Complamin-treated and the placebo-receiving women. The pre-treatment values, when present, are underlined.

Weeks of pregnancy	30	31	32	33	34	35	36	37	38	39	40
Complamin Group No.											
1								47	48	45	
2								31	29	37	41
3					107	121	117				
4					32	42	53	47	55	45	54
5				32	54	51	48	38			
6				78	91	72	73	80	37		
7+				37		49	46		54		66
8+					8	15	18	25	31	32	41
9					9	22	40				
10					21	31		47	50	47	
11+	23	34	23	28	27		38		50		
12			16	22	21	23	20	8			
13				30	26	43	46	51	36	37	
Placebo Group No.											
1						18	21				
2				23	27	26	25	36			
3			16	24	20	29					
4							30	33	43		
5					24	46	45	34	40		
6					31	36	36	47	54	66	64
7				-	53	51	61		60	77	
8					26	29	17	32	50	48	
9				28	28	36		36	41	37	43
10						12	62	55			
11+						44	31	30	30		
12+							22	19			
13						19	39	45	48	49	
14					-	52		47	40	64	
15+				-	31	34	31		31		38
16			17			22	25	27			
17							20	31	30		

The patients marked with +, had normal values for serum creatinine throughout the trial.

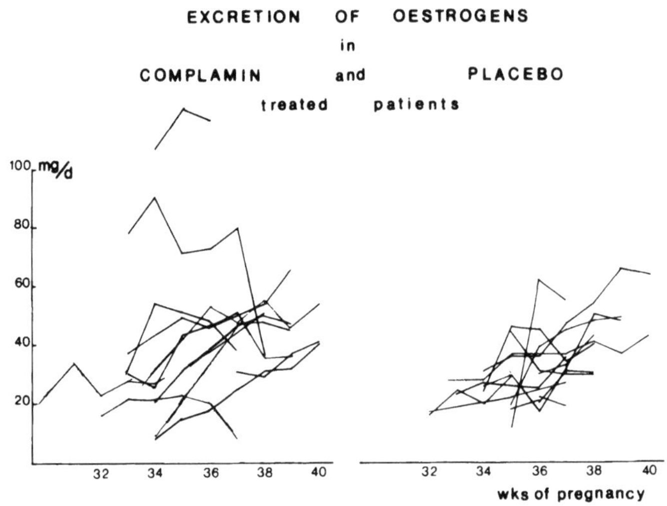

Fig. 3. This figure shows the consecutive weekly values for the excretion of oestrogens for each patient in both the Complamin and the placebo group.The first point of each line represents the value obtained immediately before the start of treatment in that patient. Excretion lines for patients from whom no pre-treatment value was obtained, are not shown in this figure

Table 5. The values of the excretion of oestrogens, expressed as percentages of the pre-treatment values. For both the Complamin-treated and the placebo-receiving women, the values obtained per week of treatment for each woman, are grouped together and ranged from low to high.

Weeks of treatment	1		2		3		4		5		6	
Group	C	P	C	P	C	P	C	P	C	P	C	P
	87	71	92	65	94	68	102	128	47	146	123	132
	94	86	96	68	122	109	117	147	50	159	165	206
	102	100	100	113	124	123	119	156	120	185	169	
	113	110	109	116	132	129	125	167	141	213	513	
	117	111	119	125	144	142	170	174	146			
	131	116	131	129	147	152	172	192	400			
	138	117	132	143	150	181	224	258				
	148	117	143	150	153	253	387					
	148	150	159	188	238							
	169	155	166	237	313							
	188	192	224	458								
	244	205	225									
		517	445									
n	12	13	13	11	10	8	8	7	6	4	4	2

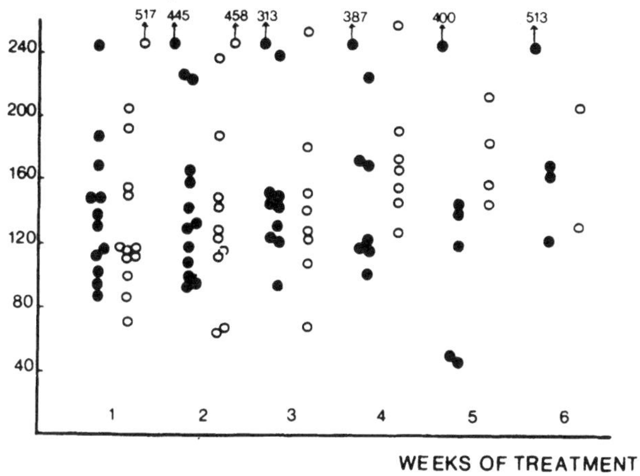

Fig. 4. Graphical display of the values given in Table 5

Table 6. The results of the statistical analysis of the percentage values of the excretion of oestrogens, given in Table 5.

Excretion of Oestrogens						
Complamin vs Placebo						
Weeks of treatment		1	2	3	4	5
WILCOXON's test	P_L	>0.20	>0.20	>0.20	>0.20	>0.20

The effect of Complamin on the birth weight

In order to enable a valid comparison between the birth-weights of the children born from the Complamin-treated patients and those from the placebo group, all children born with a gestational age of less than 38 weeks, were omitted from this part of the study. Likewise, we omitted the two twins who were born from women in the Complamin group. The weights of the mature newborns are given in Table 7 and Fig. 5.

Statistical analysis, again by use of WILCOXON's and FISHER's tests, showed that from these results no indication can be obtained that the use of Complamin in patients treated for suspected placental insufficiency leads to higher birth-weights (Table 8).

Further inspection of the data of the patients in both groups revealed a heterogeneity with regard to the renal function. In both groups (3 in the Complamin group and 2 in the placebo group) patients were present whose values for the serum creatinine were and remained normal (< 7.6 mg/l). Leaving out those patients, and again comparing the birth-weights between the groups, a value for P of 0.06 was obtained (Table 8).

Table 7. The weights of the neonates with a gestational age of 38 weeks or more (twins excluded), born from the Complamin-treated and the placebo-receiving women. The group and the number of each neonate's mother are given so that the corresponding values for the excretion of pregnanediol and oestrogens can be found in Table 1 and 4. The arrows indicate those mothers whose serum creatinine values remained normal throughout the study.

Complamin group		Placebo group	
No.	birth weight in g		No.
→11	2260	2400	4
9	2630	2450	13
→ 8	2740	2480	9
1	3060	2620	5
→ 7	3540	2690	17
10	3550	2830	8
5	3560	3090	11←
2	3620	3230	16
13	3650	3340	15←
4	3800	3440	6
		3530	7
		3730	14
		3920	10

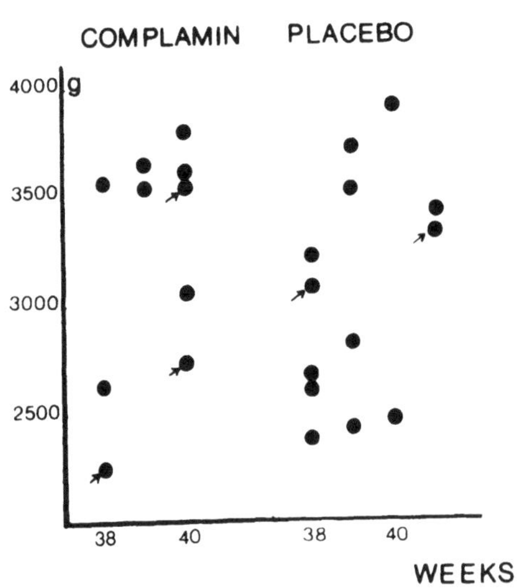

Fig. 5. Graphical display of the birth-weight given in Table 7

Table 8. The results of the statistical analysis of the birth-weights, given in Table 7.

Birthweights of mature newborns, Complamin v s Placebo		
	all	from mothers with abnormal serum creatinine
WILCOXONS's test P_L	>0.10	0.06
FISHER's test P_L	0.36	0.11

Discussion

In regard to the fact that no clear indication was obtained that the use of Complamin in the treatment of suspected placental insufficiency improves the effective function of the placenta, as judged by the weights of the neonates, the following factors must be taken into consideration:

1. Defective selection of the patients used in this double blind trial. The heterogeneity in respect to the maternal creatinine values and the presence of mature neonates of nearly 4000 g in the placebo group points in this direction. Moreover the groups may have been too small.
2. The birth-weight in general might not be an adequate expression of the effective placental function.
3. Complamin or Complamin in the dosage as used in this study is ineffective to improve placental function.

Arguments for the lack of effect of Complamin on the functioning of the feto-placental unit might be found from the values for the excretion of oestrogens which we observed in this trial. In addition to this it might be mentioned that SCHMID and KELLER (1972) did not find a change in the oestrogen excretion of toxaemic women, when treated intravenously with 1200 mg of Complamin for 3 days.

Nevertheless, we are faced with the fact that we observed evidence for an increased excretion of pregnanediol in Complamin-treated patients as compared to controls. In the trial of SCHMID and KELLER this effect of Complamin was not found. It can, however, not be ruled out that this is due to the short duration of medication in their study, whereas we observed the increase of pregnanediol excretion only after 2 weeks of treatment.

An increase of the excretion of pregnanediol does not necessarily reflect an increased secretion of progesterone by the placenta, but might be caused by an increased conversion of progesterone into pregnanediol. In women with placental insufficiency HENSSEN (1969) found this conversion lower than in women with normal pregnancies.

Finally it must be mentioned that there is no proof that the effect of Complamin on the pregnanediol excretion could not have been caused by nicotinate or nicotinate-containing complexes.

In conclusion we must state that the evidence for a salutary effect of Complamin in the treatment of placental dysfunction is insufficient.

One might endeavour to set up a new double-blind trial, carefully selecting homogeneous and comparable groups of patients with nephrogenic toxaemia along with placental insufficiency. The fetal outcome in such a trial could lead to the decision whether or not Complamin has to be added to the obstetrical therapeutic arsenal.

Summary

By means of a double-blind trial, it was investigated whether the use of xanthinol-nicotinate (Complamin) in the treatment of patients with suspected placental insufficiency was followed by an improvement of the placental function.

Excretion of pregnanediol, of total oestrogens and weight of the neonates were chosen as parameters of placental function. The values of the excretion were expressed as percentages of the pre-treatment values. For the comparison of the birth-weights, premature newborns and twins were excluded.

The observations provided neither arguments for increased excretion of oestrogens in Complamin-treated women with suspected placental insufficiency, nor for higher birthweights of children born from such patients, as compared to non-Complamin-treated patients. The excretion of pregnanediol seems to be higher in Complamin-treated patients, but this does not necessarily reflect an improvement of placental function.

References

BERGSTEIN, N. A. M., VAN KESSEL, H.: Xanthinol nicotinate and placental function. Lancet ii: 111 (1968).

BERGSTEIN, N. A. M.: Kann man durch Complamin-Retard die Placentafunktion beeinflussen? In: EPH Gestosis, page 321, Ed.: E.T. Rippmann and Ch. Rippmann, Berlin: Walter de Gruyter 1972.

BROSENS, I.: A study of the spiral arteries of the decidua basalis in normotensive and hypertensive pregnancies. J. Obstet. Gynaec. brit. Cwlth. 71, 222 (1964).

FREESE, U. E.: The utero-placental vascular relationship in the human. Amer. J. Obstet. Gynec., 101, 8 (1968).

HENSSEN, S. G. F.: "Progesteronsecretie tijdens de zwangerschap" Thesis, Nijmegen, 1969.

MARZETTI, L., BENAGIANO, G.: Valutazione clinica dell'impiego di un farmaco ad azione fibrinolitica nella terapia delle gestosi del terzo trimestre. La Clin. Obstet. Gin., 66, 429 (1964).

SCHMID, J., KELLER, P. J.: Isoxsuprinum, Dipyridamol und Nicotinsäurepräparate in der Behandlung mangelversorgter Feten. Arch. Gynäk. 212, 68 (1972).

VAN KESSEL, H., SEITZINGER, R., SCHREURS, J., VERSTEEG, M.: Oestrogens in late pregnancy assayed by an automated fluorometric procedure. Ned. T. Verlosk. 69, 81 (1969).

VAN KESSEL, H.: Automatisierte Oestrogen und semiautomatisierte Pregnandiolbestimmung zur Diagnostik der Plazentainsuffizienz. In: Fortschritte der Perinatalen Medizin. 2. Deutscher Kongreß für Perinatale Medizin 1969. Ed.: E. Saling and K. A. Hüter, Stuttgart: Georg Thieme Verlag 1971.

WALLENBURG, H. C. S.: Über den Zusammenhang zwischen Spätgestose und Placentarinfarkt. Arch. Gynäk. 208, 80 (1969).

WALLENBURG, H. C. S., STOLTE, L. A. M., JANSSENS, J.: Experimental infarcts in the placenta of the rhesus monkey. Europ. J. Obstet. Gynec. 1, 25 (1971).

WALLENBURG, H. C. S.: On the morphology and pathogenesis of placental infarcts. Thesis, Amsterdam, 1971.

The Therapy of EPH Gestosis with Xantinol-Nicotinat: Short-Term Reactions of Blood Coagulation, Fibrinolysis and Human Placental Lactogen

S. Kunz, E. Kidess, S. Heller, and H. Weber

Since several years new aspects concerning the treatment of EPH gestosis are becoming more and more important. Included in this framework is the therapy with vascular effective pharmaca. Several authors (among others BERGSTEIN, V. KESSEL) report on positive results with xantinol-nicotinat. In part the therapeutic effect is explained with the increase of the placenta perfusion based on the hemodynamic influence of the substance, in part with its effect on the blood coagulation and the fibrinolysis. Though the activation of the fibrinolysis is possible only over short periods the decrease of the maximum thrombus elasticity described in some reports and the increase of the antithrombin level could be of importance for a longer treatment. Being a placental parameter with a short half-value time HPL seems to be especially appropriate for the evaluation of both the short-term and the long-term alterations in the functional condition of the feto-placental unit.

26 pregnant women (15 gestosis patients and 11 probationers without gestosis symptoms) divided into 4 control groups got 3 x 300 mg Complamin per os every day. Several authors (e. g. CLOEREN) mention a temporary reduction of the uterus and placenta blood circulations after dispensing xantinol-nicotinat in the case of gestosis. This negative effect is explained with the relative hypovolemia present in some gestosises. Several probationers (4 patients ill with, 3 without EPH gestosis) therefore were additionally infused with 300 ml Dextran (Macrodex 6 %). Blood lettings were carried out with the fasting patients before and 30, 60, and 120 min after the dose of Complamin. In the present examinations the emphasis was put less on the question of the clinical success of the therapy than on the problem of the objectifyability and reproducibility of alterations of coagulation-physiological parameters and of the HPL level with the chosen test order.

Our results are the following:

Fig. 1 illustrates the behaviour of the HPL level. The initial values correspond to the through line 0, the individual points to the differences of the values after 30, 60, and 120 min. In our opinion only the control group treated with Complamin tends to positive differences.

The mean value of the examinations after 30 min is higher than the initial value by 0.25 micrograms, that after 60 min by 0.3, and that after 120 min still by 0.12 micrograms. However, because of the small number of cases these differences cannot be fixed statistically. 2 p for the two first groups correspond to only < 0.1. The values of the control group additionally treated with Macrodex did not change, i. e. in spite of the diluting effect there is no decrease.

In the group of the gestosis the mean value remains constant in all stages of the examination so that essential fluctuations can be excluded.

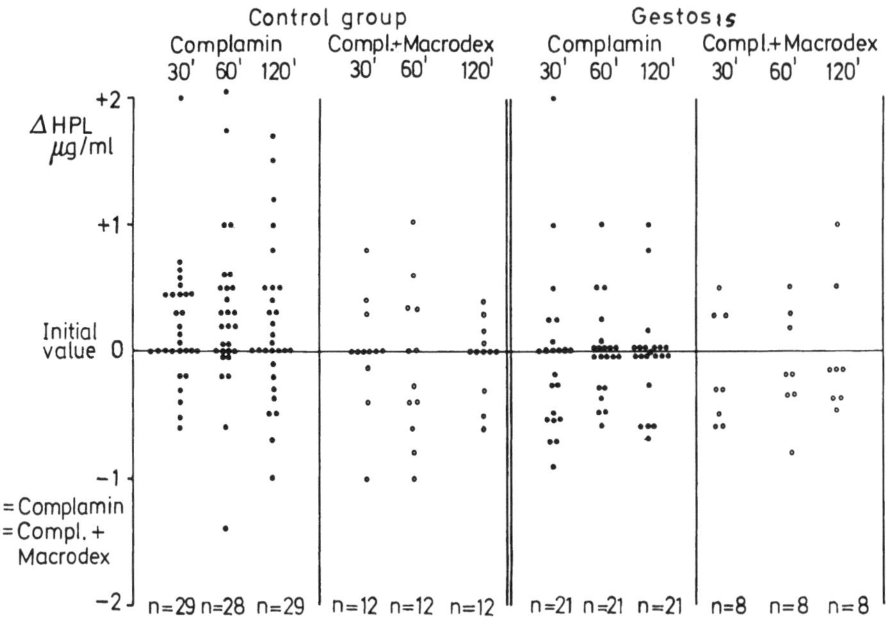

Fig. 1. Short-Term Alterations of the HPL Level after the Application of Complamin and Complamin + Macrodex

In all global tests of blood coagulation carried out, the reaction and coagulum formation times do not show significant alterations in the thrombelastogramm.

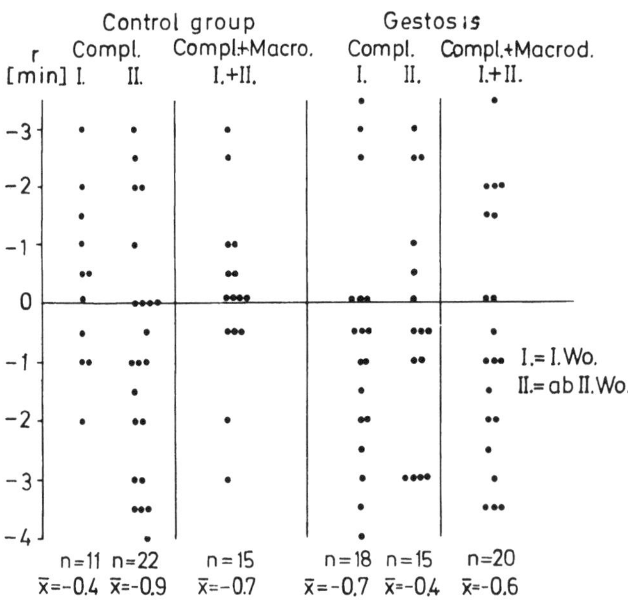

Fig. 2. Thrombelastogramm - Reaction Time Differences before and after the Application of Complamin (Macrodex)

The illustrated alterations of the maximum amplitude, i. e. of the coagulum consistence can be proven statistically. You can see that the Complamin groups here are subdivided: Under I we listed the differences before and after the dose of Complamin, under II those of the second week of therapy. In this way it can be demonstrated that the short-term effects are still traceable evan after a long period of treatment. The most evident decrease in the coagulum consistence is to be found with simultaneous infusion of Macrodex.

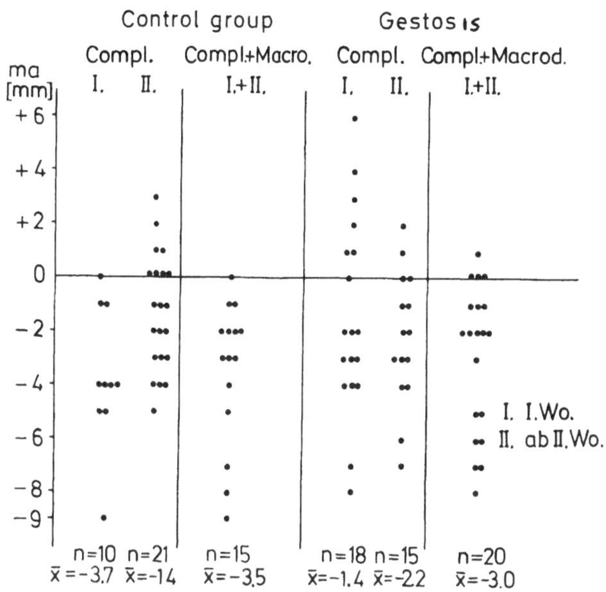

Fig. 3. Thrombelastogramm - Maximum Amplitude Differences before and after the Application of Complamin (Macrodex)

Traces of a complete lysis in the TEG could be found in none of the cases examinated. Also in only a few cases the amplitude narrowed to the half of the maximum within the recording time of 2 - 4 hours.

As expected the time of euglobulin lysis was prolonged (to 11 - 13 hours) without exception as regards the initial values, a consequence of the reduced fibrinolytical activity during pregnancy. The values of the patients in the control group and those of the gestosises do not differ essentially. The lysis time of 60 min after the Complamin dose reduces to 4 hours in the case of the first group and to 3 hours with additional Macrodex infusion. In the group of the EPH patients the corresponding values are 6 1/2 hours and 5 hours, respect. In no case a plasmin activity could be traced on the factor XIII and human fibrin plate free of plasminogen. Also the examinations on activator activity on the bovin fibrin plate were always negative with the exception of two control cases. We could not find out any difference in the behaviour of the proactivator before and after the application of Complamin.

We further examinated alterations of the thrombocyte numbers. Also here no significant differences were found. In the control group treated with Complamin + Macrodex and in the corresponding gestosis group the fibrinogen level just dropped by 10 and 15 %, respect. After the above mentioned lysis examinations this decrease is probably not a result of a fibrinogenolysis but of the increase of the circulating plasma volume caused by the oncotical effect of the dextran. In this connection the behaviour of the fibrin splitting products must be mentioned; they were checked by use of the staphylokokkal-clumping test. A proven titer increase as index to an activation of the fibrinolysis was not found. In the case of the gestosis patients treated with Complamin and Macrodex we determined in 8 cases an increase by 1 - 2 stages, in 5 cases unchanged and in 3 cases dropping titers with regard to the examination of 16 comparison groups.

To conclude, the results of the immunological determinations of the inhibitors are illustrated:

	Control group			Gestosis	
	Complamin	Compl.+Macrodex		Complamin	Compl.+Macrodex
α_1-Antitrypsin	O 495 mg % I 496 mg %	O 418 mg % I 406		O 503 mg % I 501	O 475 mg % I 429 2p<0.1>0.05
α_2-Makroglobulin	O 288 mg % I 279 mg %	O 279 I 251	2p<0.1>0.05	O 245 I 240	O 202 I 190 2p<0.1>0.05
Antithromb. III	O 28.1 mg % I 28.2 mg %			O 28.4 I 27.9	O 25.9 I 25.1

Fig. 4. Inhibitors - Values before (O) and 1 h after (I) the Application of Complamin (+Macrodex)

Neither the alpha-1-antitrypsin content nor the alpha-2-macroglobulin content changes for a short time under the influence of the therapy. Provided an only short-term activation of the fibrinolysis with the appearance of free plasmin, a decrease of the immediate antiplasmin alpha-2-macroglobulin should be stated as an index to a decreasing reaction. Also these examinations make clear that the combination of Complamin and Macrodex results in more striking alterations which, however, also in this case do not exceed the limit explicable by the hemodilution. Also the antithrombin-III-content shows no significant alterations in the different groups.

The following can be concluded:

1. The chosen dosage of xantinol-nicotinat did not produce any reproducible short-term alteration of the HPL level in the group of our gestosis patients. Further examinations are necessary in order to clarify the different behaviour of the control group.
2. Over a short, surely reproducible period a reduction of the coagulum consistence is produced in the thrombelastogramm. A relative shortening of the euglobulinlysis time can also be produced.
3. It was not possible to objectify traces of a free fibrinolytical activity by means of the tested parameters. As numerous examinations of non-pregnant women have shown that an activation of the fibrinolysis can be produced by the use of xantinol-nicotinat as well as by the use of low molecular dextrans, we are presently testing the effect of higher dosages.

Ultrasound Study of the Effect of Hydergin on Feto-Placental Insufficiency

D. Răzvan Ionascu

I have attempted to study the effect of Hydergin (Sandoz) on feto-placental insufficiency.

As Hydergin has a vasodilating effect, it seemed logical to use it in feto-placental insufficiency where there is a reduction in maternal blood flow to the placenta. This results in:
a) Reduction in placental perfusion and
b) Vasoconstriction in uterine arterial vessels.

With Hydergin I hoped to improve this second factor, attempting to encourage a normal fetal growth-rate.

I have treated feto-placental insufficiency due to pre-eclampsia and due to causes which were not determined.

The diagnosis of feto-placental insufficiency has been established by demonstrating a retarded growth-rate in the biparietal diameter of the fetus, using an ultrasonic method (B. P. D.). The effect of Hydergin on feto-placental insufficiency was checked by serial ultrasonic cephalometry, serial ultrasonic measurement of the thoracic diameter of the fetus (T. D.) and of the thickness of the placenta.

Patients and Methods

The apparatus used has been Combison A and B Kretztechnik. Measurement of the fetal biparietal diameter, the thoracic diameter and placental thickness has been made by the A Scane technique, from the 18 - 20th week of pregnancy and at two weekly intervals onwards. Photographs of the growth of the fetal head, fetal thorax and placenta have been made by the B Scane technique.

Results have been correlated with amnioscopy and with the stress, oxitoxin and atropine tests, described by me in 1968 and 1971. The results have also been correlated with records of the fetal heart rate, with the pH of fetal blood samples from the scalp, with the fetal weight for gestation at birth and with the one-minute Apgar Score.

I have investigated 150 patients and divided them into three groups:
1. those with retarded growth-rate of the B. P. D. and without any therapy,
2. those with retarded growth-rate of B. P. D on therapy,
3. those with normal growth-rate of B. P. D. on prophylactic therapy.

Results

1. In the first group there has been retarded growth of the fetal B. P. D. which has correlated either with stillbirths of 600 to 980 g occuring at 24 - 27 weeks (as in cases A_2, H_1, B_2), or with births of babies at 32 weeks weighing 1,800 g with a one-minute Apgar Score of 2

(as in the case B_1), or with births of babies at 40 weeks weighing 1,700 g, or more and with a one-minute Apgar Score of 4 (as in the case I_5). (See Fig. 1).

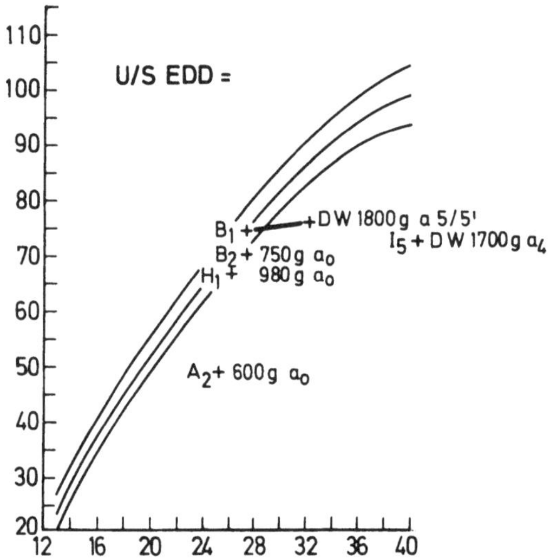

Fig. 1. Examples of retarded growth-rates of fetal biparietal diameter in patients in the control group. All were spontaneous deliveries, and the fetal birth-weight and one-minute Apgar Score are shown

In all the cases fetal tachycardia, green amniotic fluid at amnioscopy and fetal metabolic acidosis has been noted.

As an example of this group, case B_1, with a normal B. P. D. of 7.4 cm at 26 weeks is presented. Growth-rate became retarded, so that at 32 weeks it was 7.5 cm. An anterior placenta praevia was found. Delivery was spontaneous at 32 weeks and the fetal birth-weight was 1,800 g, with a one-minute Apgar Score of 2 and five-minute Apgar Score of 5. The pH of the fetal blood was 7.03 and the base excess - 13.4 m Eq/l. (See Fig. 2). Fig. 3 shows the B Scane of this case at 26 weeks.
2. Regarding the second group: there was initial retardation in the B. P. D. which gradually improved in cases I_3, D. K. R. The growth-rate of the T. D. and the thickness of placenta became normal after therapy.

The deliveries were spontaneous at 40 weeks and fetal birth-weights ranged from 2,800 to 3,200 g, with a one-minute Apgar Score of 7 to 10. I found clear amniotic fluid at amnioscopy, a normal fetal heart rate and a normal fetal blood pH. (See Fig. 4).

Case K is an example. The growth-rate of the B. P. D. was sub-normal. After therapy there was a gradual increase in the growth-rate of B. P. D. to normal of 9.8 cm at 40 weeks. The T. D. also increased. Spontaneous delivery occurred at 40 weeks. Fetal birth-weight was 3,100 g with a one-minute Apgar Score of 10. (Fig. 5). The B Scane of this case at 32, 36 and 38 weeks, as well as the fetal heart rate recorded by ultrasound technique at 38 weeks of gestation is shown in Figs. 6, 7, 8 and 9.

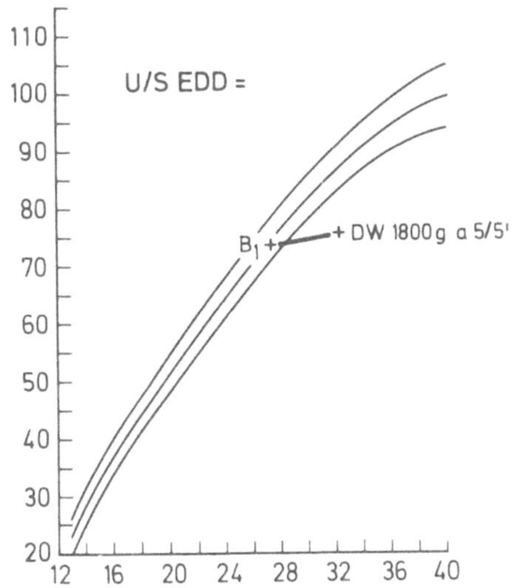

Fig. 2. The growth-rate of the fetal biparietal diameter of case B_1. Spontaneous delivery at 32 weeks. The fetal birth-weight: 1,800 g, one-minute Apgar Score: 2, and the five-minute Apgar Score: 5

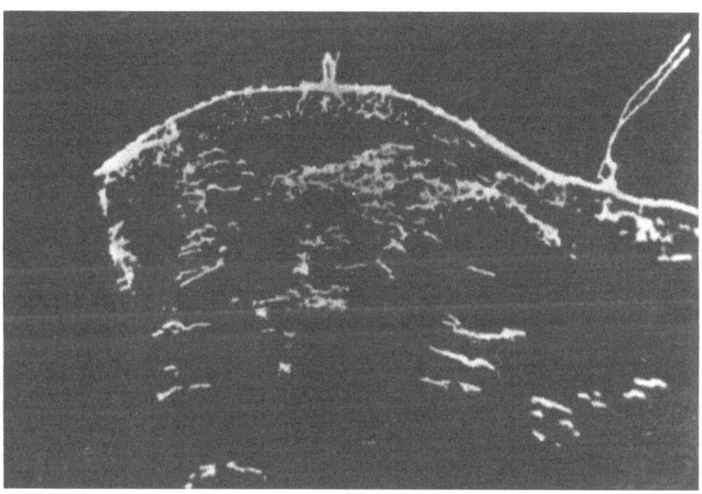

Fig. 3. B Scane L - 0 of case B_1, with a fetal biparietal diameter of 7.4 cm at 26 weeks and with an anterior placenta praevia

3. The third group treated prophylactically showed a normal growth-rate of B. P. D. rising to the upper limit of normal at 38 - 40 weeks of gestation, (seen in cases P. and T.).

The growth-rate of the T. D. and the thickness of placenta was normal. The deliveries were spontaneous at 40 weeks of gestation and fetal

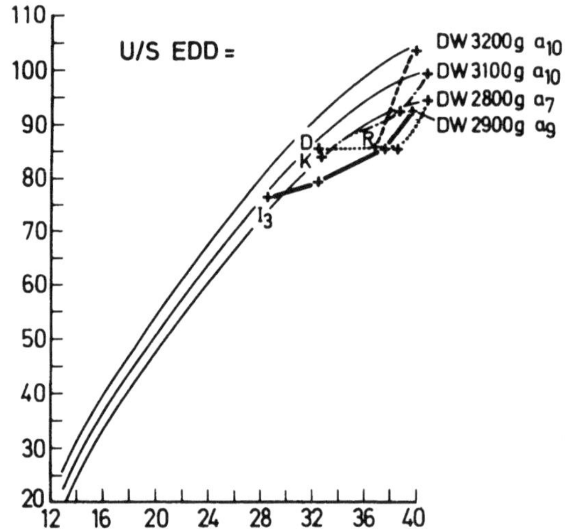

Fig. 4. Examples of growth-rates of the fetal biparietal diameters in patients from the second group. Spontaneous deliveries occurred at 40 weeks. The fetal birth-weights were 2,800 - 3,200 g and the one-minute Apgar Score was 7 - 10

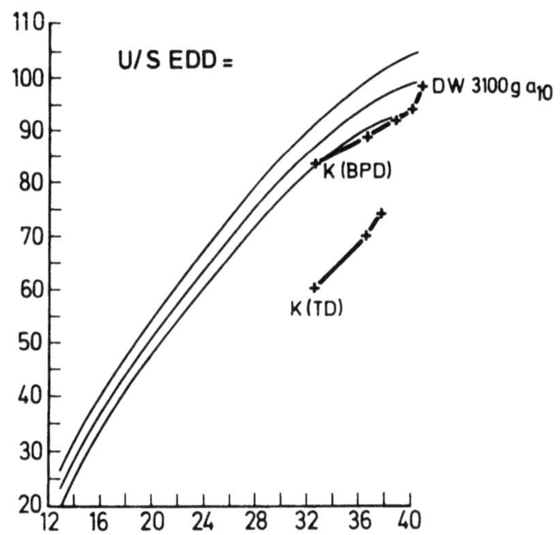

Fig. 5. A single example of the growth-rate of fetal biparietal diameter and of the fetal thoracic diameter in case K. Spontaneous delivery occurred at 40 weeks. The fetal birth-weight was 3,100 g and the one-minute Apgar Score was 10

birth-weights ranged from 3,300 to 3,600 g with a one-minute Apgar Score of 9 to 10. Amnioscopy, fetal heart rate recording and pH of fetal blood samples were normal (Fig. 10).

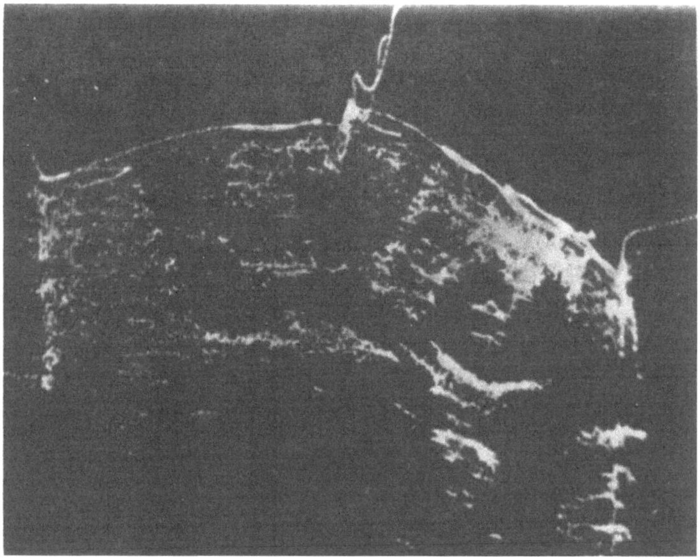

Fig. 6. B Scane L - O "Tilt 30 to the left" of case K, showing the fetal biparietal diameter of 8.3 cm and the fetal thoracic diameter of 6 cm at 32 weeks. Posterior placenta

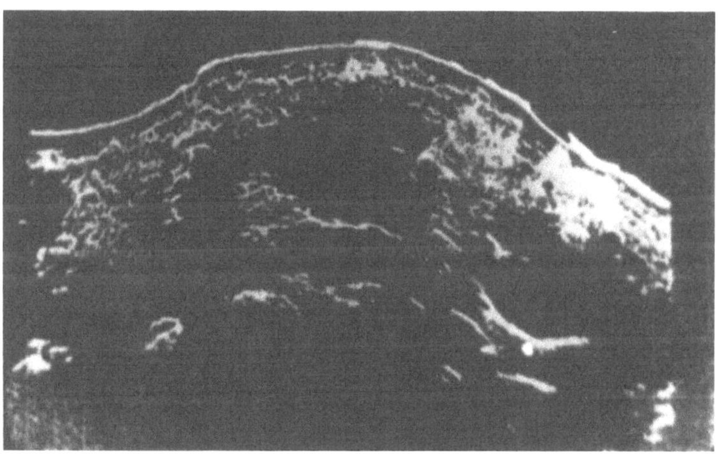

Fig. 7. B Scane L - O of case K at 36 weeks. The fetal biparietal diameter is 8.8 cm and the fetal thoracic diameter is 7 cm. Posterior placenta

Case T is presented as an example. Growth-rate of B. P. D., T. D. and placental thickness were exceptional. Spontaneous delivery occurred at 40 weeks, the fetal birth-weight was 3,600 g, with a one-minute Apgar Score of 10 and the placenta weighed 750 g (Fig. 11). Figs. 12 and 13 show the B Scane of this case at 36 and 39 weeks of gestation.

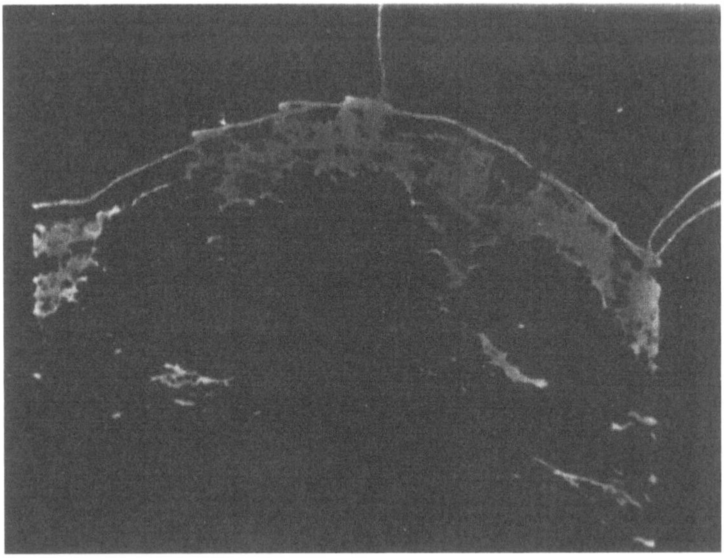

Fig. 8. B Scane L - O of case K at 38 weeks. The fetal biparietal diameter is 9.2 cm and the fetal thoracic diameter is 7.4 cm. Posterior placenta

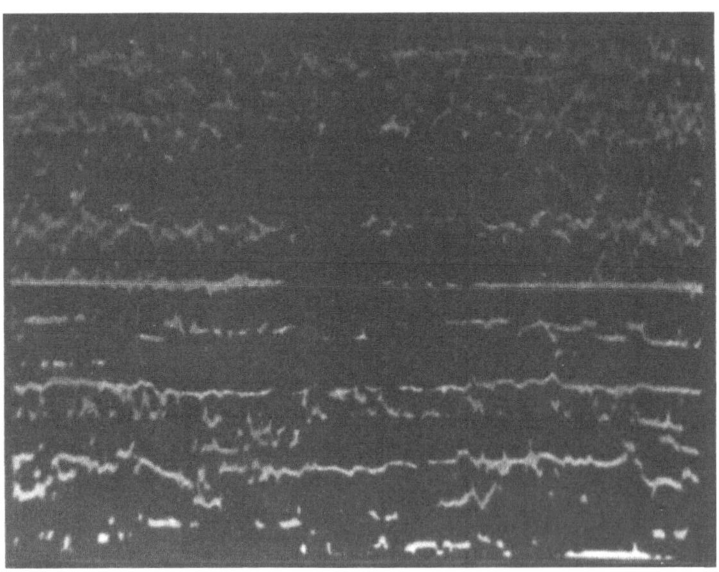

Fig. 9. A fetal heart rate recording of 150 beats per minute by an ultrasound technique in case K at 38 weeks

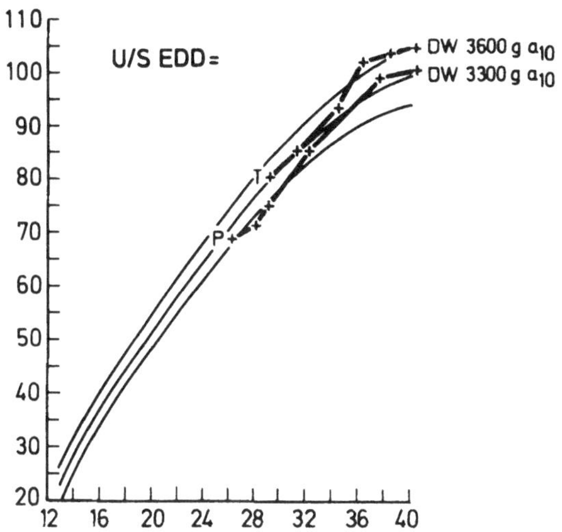

Fig. 10. Examples of growth-rates in fetal biparietal diameters in the third group. Spontaneous deliveries occurred at 40 weeks. The fetal birth-weights were 3,300 to 3,600 g. The one-minute Apgar Score was 10

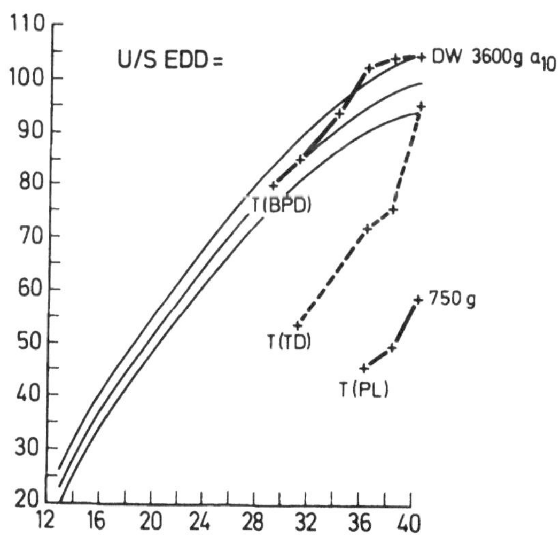

Fig. 11. This figure shows the growth-rate of the fetal biparietal diameter, the fetal thoracic diameter and the placental thickness in case T. Spontaneous delivery occurred at 40 weeks. The fetal birth-weight was 3,600 g and the one-minute Apgar Score: 10. The placenta weighed 750 g

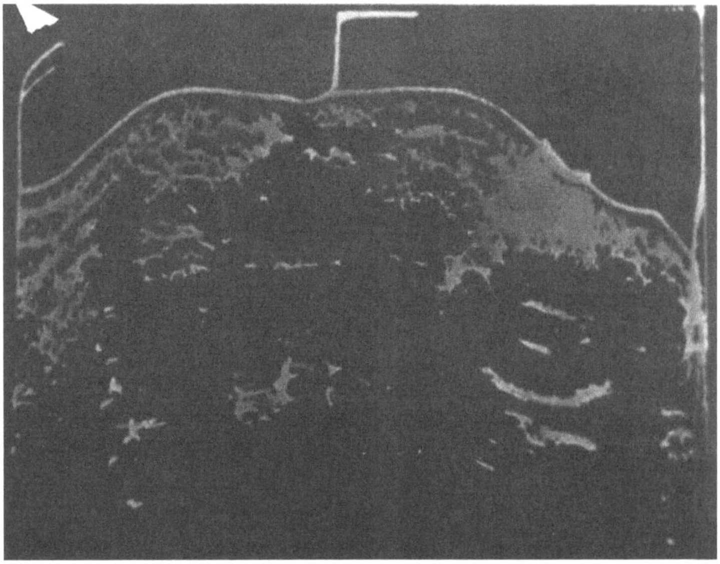

Fig. 12. B Scane L - 0 of case T showing a fetal biparietal diameter of 10.2 cm, the fetal thoracic diameter of 7.2 cm and the placental thickness of 4.5 cm at 36 weeks. Posterior placenta

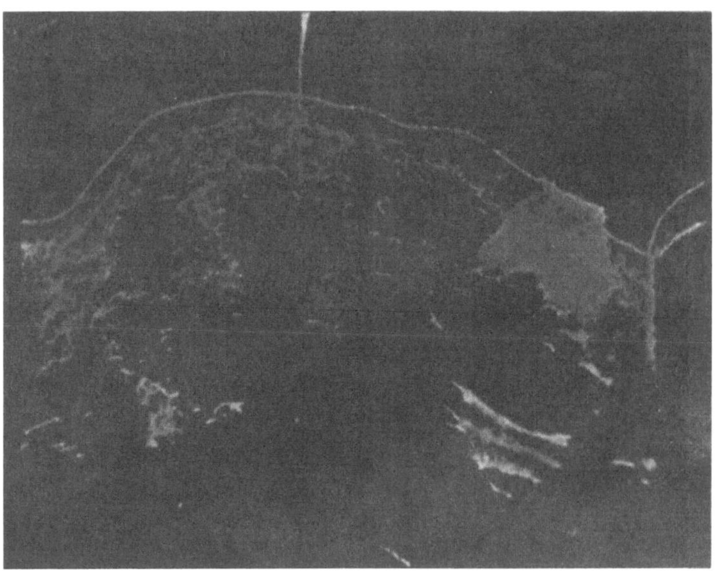

Fig. 13. B Scane L - 0 of case T showing a fetal biparietal diameter of 10.4 cm, a fetal thoracic diameter of 9.5 cm and the placental thickness of 5.8 cm at 39 weeks. Posterior placenta

Fig. 14 shows the growth-rate of the biparietal diameter of all three groups.

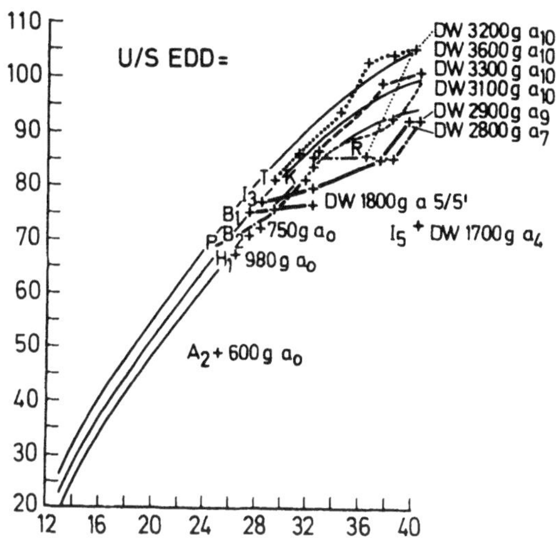

Fig. 14. Examples of growth-rates of fetal biparietal diameters from the three groups. All were spontaneous deliveries. The fetal birth-weights and the one-minute Apgar Scores are shown

I suggest that therapy with Hydergin produces a very important growth-rate in biparietal diameter, of thoracic diameter and of the placental thickness. This implies a normal fetal growth-rate. This result has been obtained by studying 150 cases, divided in three groups of 50 patients. Still-born or premature delivery cases occurred only in the first group without Hydergin treatment.

I recommend treatment with Hydergin to decrease or to eliminate the risk of placental failure and also for prophylactic therapy.

Hydergin has been given from 18 to 20 weeks until the end of the pregnancy. The dosage used has been either 3 mg orally daily or 15 - 20 drops (1 ml) 3 times per day, or a weekly intramuscular injection of one ampoule of 1 ml.

Summary

The aim of this work is to study the effect of Hydergin (Sandoz) on feto-placental insufficiency.

The diagnosis of feto-placental insufficiency has been established by retarded growth-rate of the fetal biparietal diameter measured ultrasonically.

The effect of Hydergin was checked by serial ultrasonic fetal cephalometry, serial ultrasonic measurement of the fetal thoracic diameter and by the thickness of the placenta. It has been found that therapy with Hydergin produces an increase in the growth-rate of the fetal biparietal diameter, the fetal thoracic diameter and the thickness of the placenta. This implies a normal fetal growth-rate and I suggest treatment with Hydergin to decrease or eliminate the risk of placental failure and for prophylactic use.

Therapy of Feto-Placental Insufficiency with Xantinol-Nicothinate, Glucose and Insulin

G. P. Mandruzzato, P. Spanio, F. Carli, G. Carlomagno, and F. Diversi

At the basis of a functional insufficiency of the feto-placental unit, there is usually an altered maternal-fetal exchange, or, more broadly speaking, a manifold reduction in the fetal supply lines. When chronic, fetal growth is impaired. Numerous attempts have been made to improve the precarious fetal situation.

Usually attempts have been made to intervene at different levels:
1. Improving the utero-placental circulation in order to facilitate the materno-fetal exchange.
2. Increasing the supply of glucose to the fetus, as it is the main source of energy during intra-uterine life.
3. Increasing the nutrition of the fetus by means of intra-amniotic amino-acid infusions.

In most reported series, urinary oestriol excretion has been chosen to assess the results of treatment.

We report here the results obtained from the treatment of pregnancy associated with reduced oestriol excretion and retarded growth of the fetus.

Materials and Methods

In order to obtain the maximum homogeneity, we chose our cases to be studied with care. We selected patients in whom the 24 hour oestriol excretion, measured according to BROWN and COYLE, was in the range of subnormally low and low according to BJORO; i. e. included within the first and second standard deviation or below the second standard deviation. In addition, those cases in which a conspicuous maternal pathology was evident, were excluded (Toxaemia, diabetics above WHITE's class A, uterine malformations, etc.).

The only cases taken into consideration were those in which the oestriol had been measured at least 4 times before treatment began, and in which treatment was continued until delivery.

Creatinine excretion was always measured with the oestriol, and samples in which the 24 hour creatinine was lower than 0.8 g were excluded.

In this way, we selected 7 cases of constantly abnormal oestriol, accompanied by retarded growth. All cases were in-patients from the beginning of treatment until delivery. The treatment consisted of Xantinol-Nicothenate 600 to 1200 mg orally daily, intravenous infusion of 500 ml of 20 % dextrose, and in 5 cases the use of intermediate- or rapid-acting insulin.

In the following tables, clinical features of the patients together with treatment and results are detailed.

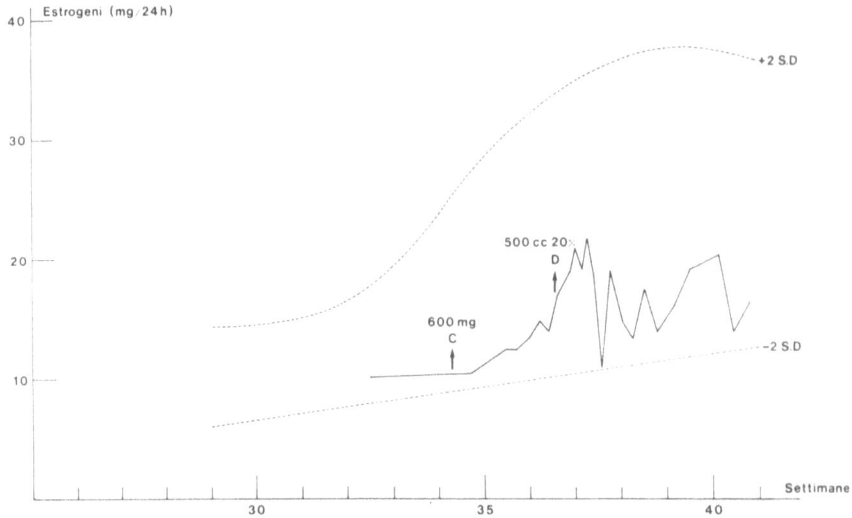

Fig. 1. S. A. a. 26 Gr. 2. P. 0
P/A 120/70 HB 12.1
K. 1. 77
A 40 settimane P.S. femmina 2780 Placenta 400 gr Apgar 8 - 10 pH 5' 7.23

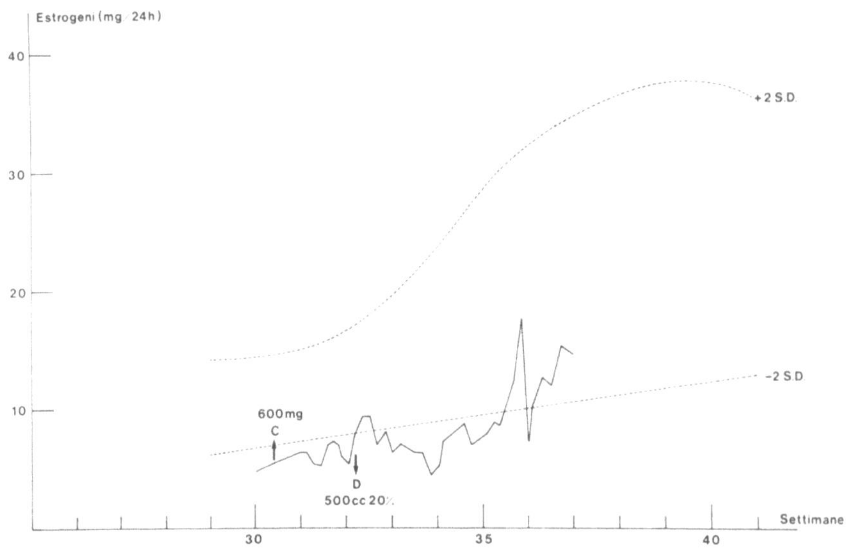

Fig. 2. D. P. L. a. 27 Gr. 2 P. 1 (Pregressa morte neonatale 1700 gr)
P. A. 105/65 HB. 12.1
K = 1.21
Uricult sterile
P. C. (podalica) femmina 2140 (malformata)
Placenta 360 gr Apgar 2 - 5

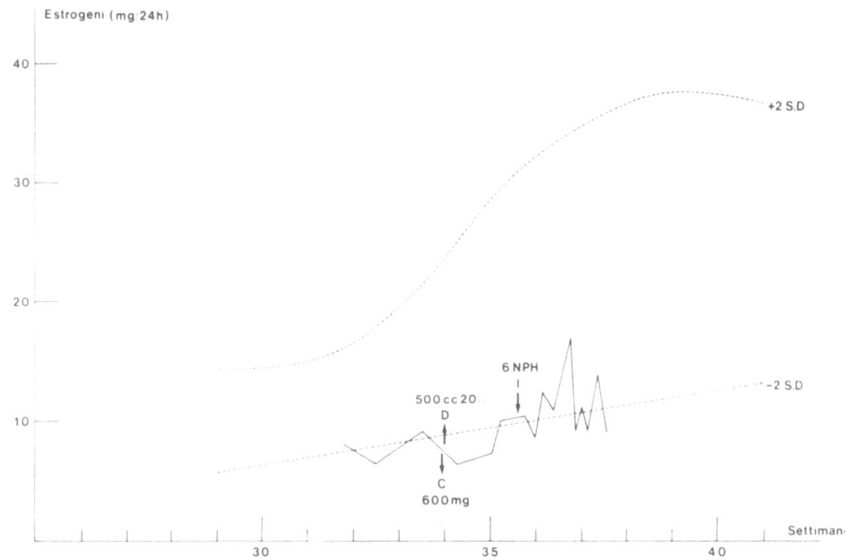

Fig. 3. M. M. a. 30 Gr. 1
P. A. 130/70 Hb 10
K = 1.38
P. C. femmina 2980 Placenta 430 Apgar 10 - 10 pH 7.22 a 5'

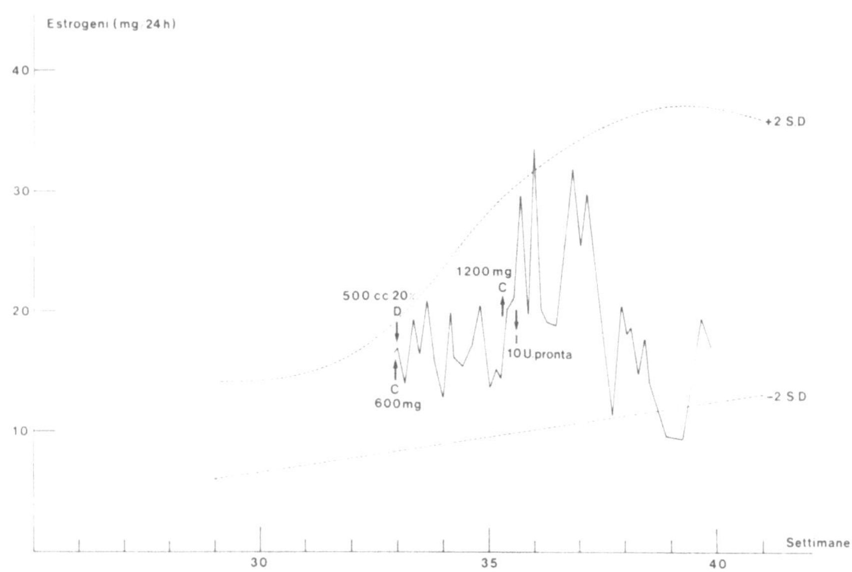

Fig. 4. P. L. a. 30 Gr. 2 P. 0
P. A. 120/70 HB. 12.8 FIGLU 0.55 K = 1.10
Amniocentesi 38 settimane: Estriolo 62.3 gamma L/S 1.97
Bil. 0.05
P. S. Femmina 2500 pH scalp 7.35 Placenta 510 gr Apgar 6 - 9 pH a 5' 7.11

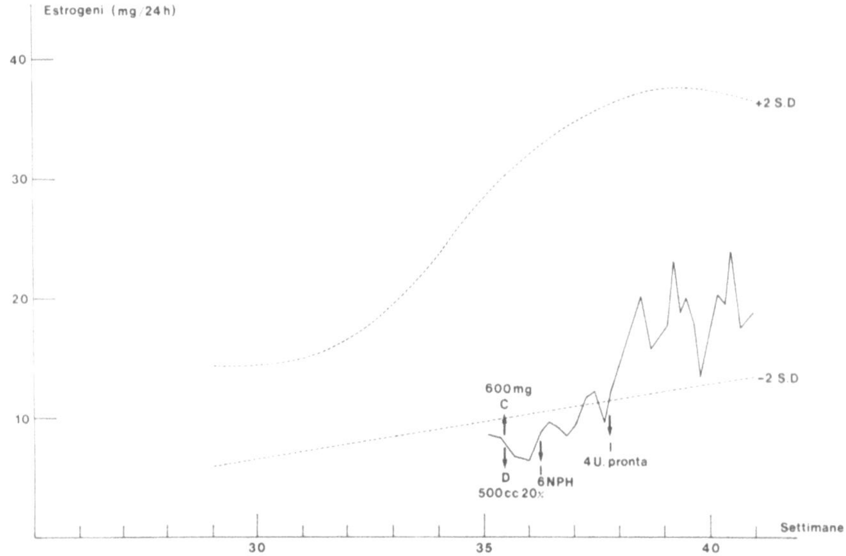

Fig. 5. M. L. a. 38 Gr. 5 P. 2
P. A. 120/70 Hb 10.6 FIGLU 0.6 Uricult 10^3 *K = 1.28*
P. S. maschio 2440 Placenta 350 gr Apgar 8 - 10 pH a 5' 7.18

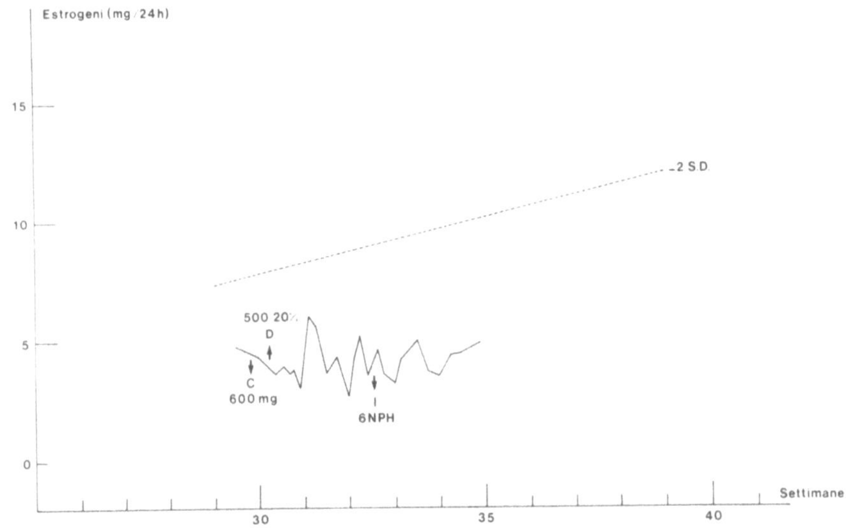

Fig. 6. A. T. a. 25 Gr. 2 P. 1 (morte intra-uterine per gestosi)
Cardiopatia N. Y. H. A. 2°
P. A. 140/70 Hb 10.9 Uricult sterile
K. 1.38
P. S. femmina 1650 pH scalp 7.04 a meno 5'
Apgar 6 - 8 pH 6.89 a 1' e 7.04 a 5'
Placenta a metà ipotrofica

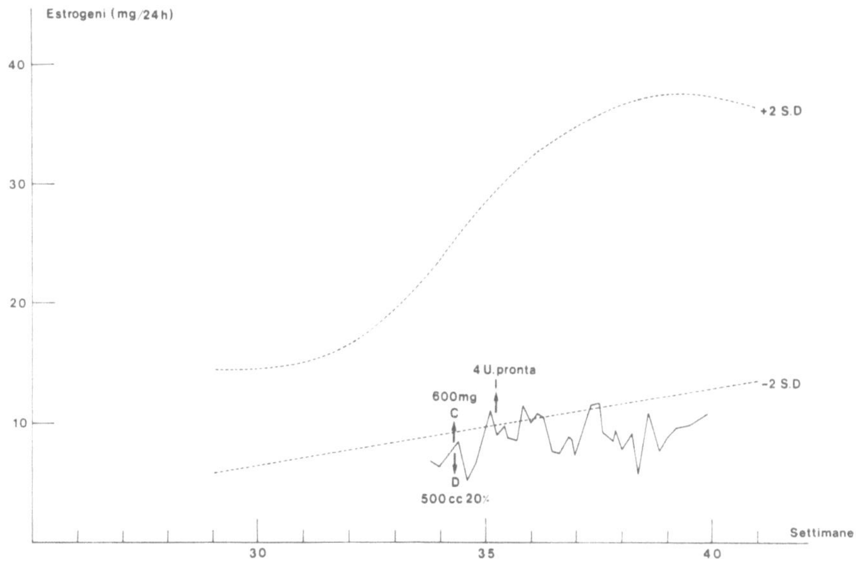

Fig. 7. C. M. a. 17 Gr. 1
P A 110/70 Hb 11.3 K. 1.54
Uricult sterile
A 38 settimane ammiosgrafia e amniocentesi
Parto indotto femmina 1270 Placenta 285 gr
Apgar 1 - 5 pH a 5' 7.06

Results

As is clearly shown in the tables, oestriol excretion was increased following treatment with Xantinol-Nicothenate and dextrose in case 1. In case 2, however, there was some increase - but not constant and only after prolonged treatment. In cases 3, 4 and 5 the oestriol excretion increased significantly only after treatment with insuline. In cases 6 and 7 there was no change. In case 2 a fetus was born with multiple malformations; in case 6 half of the placenta was distinctly hypotrophic (Figs. 8 and 9). In case 7 retarded growth was already marked at the time of the patient's admission and after 40 weeks of pregnancy a 1270 g baby was born.

It should be noted that the increase in the oestriol excretion is significant in that in all cases in which it increased, the ratio of oestriol to creatinine increased equally.

Discussion

Even if oestriol excretion as a measure of chronic fetal distress, and as an indirect measure of the outcome of treatment, has its limits, the correlation between oestriol, chronic fetal distress and retarded growth is quite good, especially in extreme cases (oestriol subnormally low or low). But low oestriol excretion may be improved merely by bed rest. Therefore, we considered only those cases where treatment began a few days after admission to hospital.

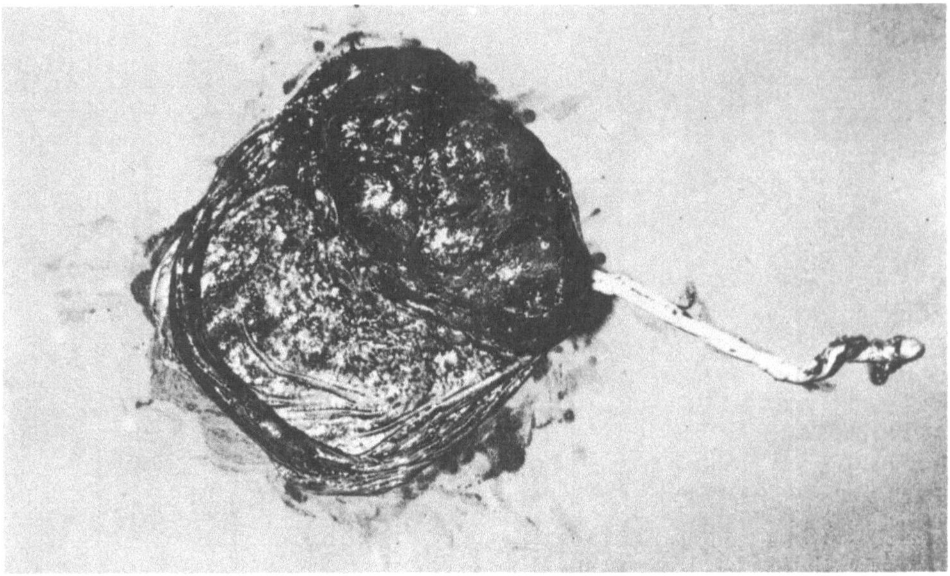

Fig. 8. Caso No. 6. Placenta, maternal surface

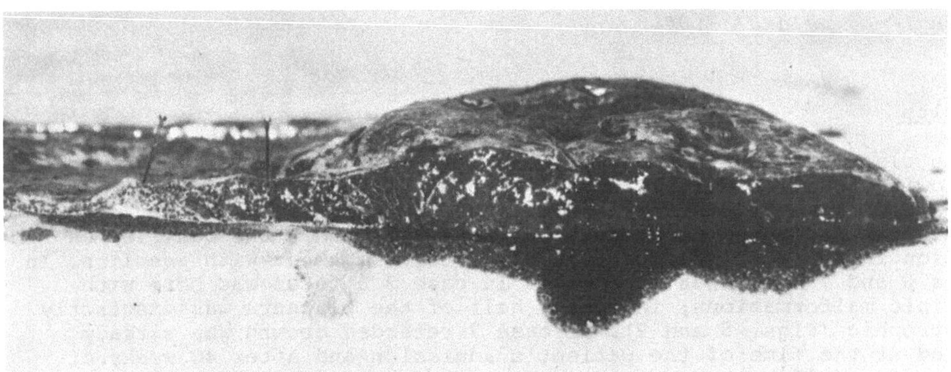

Fig. 9. Caso No. 6, Placenta, transverse section

As we did not notice any constant response to Xantinol-Nicothenate and dextrose we decided to add insulin because it encourages deposition of placental glycogen, and is likely to enhance the trans-placental transfer of glucose.

Results obtained, although from a small number of patients, would suggest that:
1. Low oestriol excretion can be increased by adding insulin to Xantinol-Nicothenate and dextrose treatment.
2. This observation may be of practical use in the treatment of chronic feto-placental insufficiency and of retarded growth.

References

1. BEISCHER, N. A.: O' Sullivan E. F., The effect of rest and intravenous infusion of hypertonic dextrose on subnormal estriol excretion in pregnancy. Am. J. Obstet. Gynec. 113, 6, 771 (1972).
2. BERGSTEIN, N. A. M.: Kessel Van H., Xanthinol nicotenate and placental function. Lancet 2, 111 (1968).
3. BJÖRO, K.: Oestriol Assay in obstetric Practice Acta Endocrinologica Suppl. 161 Copenhagen 1972.
4. BROTANEK, V., HODR, J.: The effect of isoxsuprine on utero-placental circulation in Horsky J. Stempera Z. K. Intra-uterine dangers to the foetus. Excerpta medica Foundation. Amsterdam 424 1967b.
5. BROWN, J. B., COYLE, M.: Urinary excretion of oestriol during pregnancy. A shortened procedure J. Obst. Gynec. Brit. Cwlth. 70, 219 (1963).
6. HOFFBAUER, H., BUSCH, W.: Die Erfolge einer Dauerheparinisierung bei intra-uteriner Mangelentwicklung Communication au IV Deutscher Kongreß für Perinatale Medizin, Berlin 1971.
7. RENAUD, R., BOOG, G., BRETTES, J. P., IRRMAN, M., DE MOT, E., SCHUMACHER, J. CL., GANDAR, R.: La souffrance Foetale. Aspects Thérapeutiques XXII Congrès National d'anesthésie et réanimation. Ed. Arnette Paris, 853, 2 (1972).
8. SISTEK, J., BOSSART, H.: Normalisation of fetal acid-base balance by glucose-insulin load to the mother. 3. European Congress of Oerinatal Medicine Lusanne, Ed. Hans Huber: Bern p. 319.

Maternal Excretion of Oestriol before and during Treatment of Placental Insufficiency with Xantinol-Nicotinate

E. Denzer and K. H. Mannherz

Recently BERGSTEIN and VAN KESSELS reported an increase of maternal urinary excretion of oestriol during treatment with xantinol-nicotinate in pre-eclamptic women. We therefore investigated the effect of this substance on the oestriol excretion of so far 14 patients with placental insufficiency also trying to look for clinical signs of improvement.

Material and methods

Patients showing low oestriol excretion and signs of placental insufficiency were treated for 3 to 14 days - on average 8 days - with xantinol-nicotinate. 4 x 500 mg of xantinol-nicotinate in the retard form was administered perorally to 12 patients per day. Two patients received glucose infusions supplemented with 1,500 mg and 3,000 mg xantinol-nicotinate respectively. The treatment occurred between the 25th and 41st week of pregnancy.

Nine patients suffered from EPH-gestose, two from hypertonia, no cause for placental insufficiency could be found for the remaining 3 patients.

Before starting our investigation we repeatedly estimated the value of oestriol excretion of these patients according to ITTRICH. On average 3 to 4 urines collected during 24 hours were evaluated per patient before treatment was started. During treatment about 5 estimates were made per patient, we thus collected 54 estimates before and 72 during treatment.

Results

In Fig. 1 the mean values of maternal urinary excretion of oestriol of 17 healthy pregnant women is plotted against duration of pregnancy. On the same graph the amount of oestriol excretion (mean values) of the 14 patients investigated is given by a pair of columns (open column before and filled column during treatment). The columns are positioned on the period of pregnancy during which treatment occurred.

The estimated mean values of oestriol excretion represent lower limits of normal excretion. During treatment an increase in oestriol excetion could only be measured in the cases I, II, III, V and VI. It amounted to 58 % in case I, to 36 % in case II, to 65 % in case III, to 25 % in case V and to 27 % in case VI. In all VI cases where an increase in oestriol excretion was obtained, treatment had been started before the 38th week of pregnancy. All other patients did not show an increase, but it should be noted that because of the low number of patients investigated in this prelimenary study a statistical computation cannot yet be undertaken. Therefore figs. 2 and 3 give the oestriol excretion profiles of two individual patients, namely case II and III, before and during administration of the substance. The last figure represents a patient (case XIV) showing an increase of 28 % in oestriol excretion. In this particular case treatment had already been started in the 25th

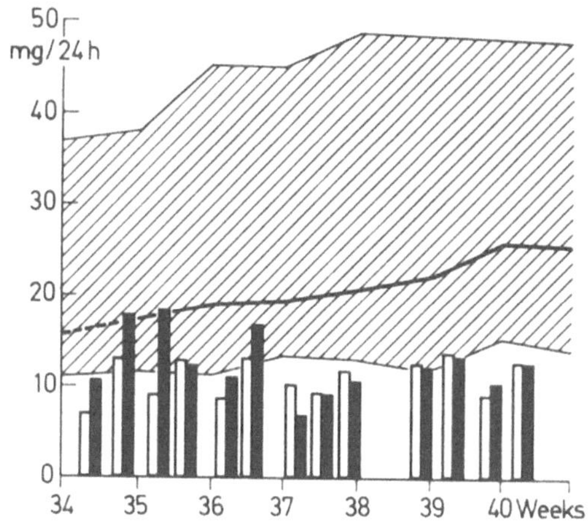

Fig. 1. Mean values of oestriol excretion before and during treatment with xantinol-nicotinate. See also text

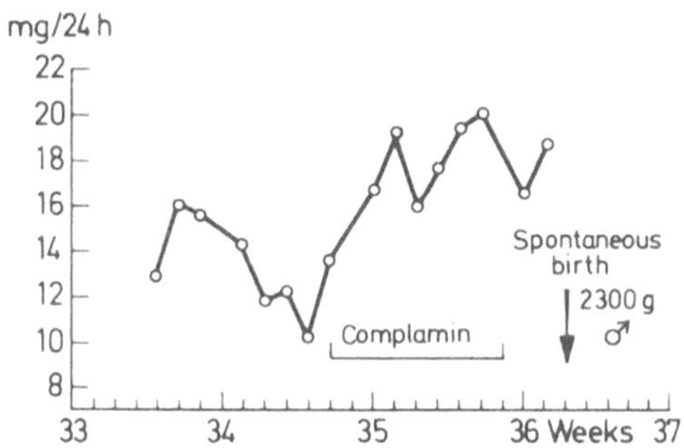

Fig. 2. Oestriol excretion profile of case II. Bar indicating duration of treatment

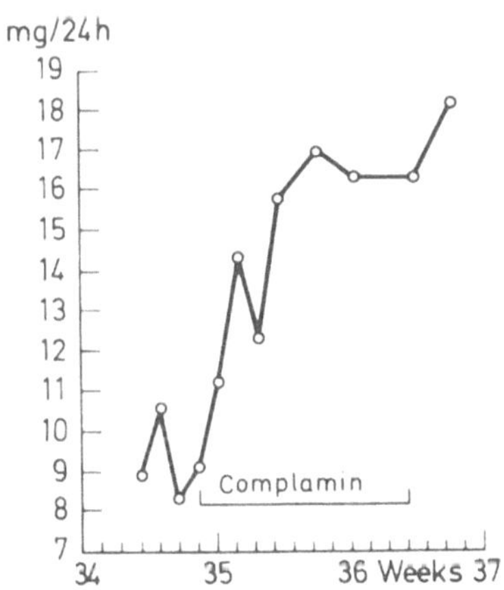

Fig. 3. Oestriol excretion profile of case III. Bar indicating duration of treatment

Pat. No. 14 V. M. 18 years 25. / 26. week of pregnancy		
	Oestriol mg / 24 h	H C S
Before treatment	1,4	2,4 mcg
After treatment	1,8	2,9 mcg

Fig. 4. Daily mean values of oestriol excretion before and during treatment of case XIV

week of pregnancy. Unfortunately we do not have fully reliable values of normal oestriol excretion occuring at this early stage of pregnancy. We have to state, however, that in some cases signs of placental insufficiency persisted as judged by pathological CTG-records, decrease in body circumference and/ or loss of weight in spite of an increase in maternal urinary oestriol excretion.

Summary

We investigated the effect of xantinol-nicotinate on urinary oestriol excretion of 14 pregnant women with signs of placental insufficiency. In six cases showing low values of oestriol excretion initially an increase ranging from 25 % to 65 % was observed during treatment, whereas in 8 cases no significant increase could be detected. We found that an increase in oestriol excretion could only be achieved when treatment with xantinol-nicotinate was started before the 38th week of pregnancy. In several cases, however, the increase in oestriol excretion was not paralleled by a relieve of clinical signs of placental insufficiency. Still, further investigations on the effects of this drug when administered at early stages of pregnancy are necessary, before morphological changes of the placental have yet taken place.

Xanthinol Nicotinate in the Treatment of EPH Gestosis

I. Marzetti, L. Zichella, P. Salmaggi, and E. Calzolari

A significant improvement in patients with EPH (edema - proteinuria - hypertonia) gestosis was shown by us (1964) following Xanthinol Nicotinate treatment. We have extended out studies to determine whether the fibrinolytic and haemokinetic action of the drug also improved the utero-placental flow hence increasing feto-placental function, as described by some authors (VAN KESSEL, BERGSTEIN).

In 9 patients with mono and polysymptomatic EPH gestosis Xanthinol-Nicotinate was administered by intravenous infusion of 900 mg a day in 500 ml of 5 % dextrose. The infusion rate was regulated according to maternal skin vasodilatation. Urinary oestriol excretion was used for assessment of fetal wellbeing and feto-placental function (Fig. 1).

Table 1 lists the obstetrical history and the clinical condition of patients at the beginning of the treatment and the administration period. In 7 cases of polysymptomatic EPH gestosis 5 premature fetuses were living and survived (2 spontaneous deliveries and 3 caesarean section). In 2 cases intra-uterine fetal death occurred (Fig. 1). In 2 cases of monosymptomatic EPH gestosis urinary oestriol excretion was normal; the 2 patients are still pregnant.

For the fetal prognosis serial assessments are necessary. In 3 cases (7, 8, 9) the increase in oestriol excretion at the beginning of treatment was followed by a sudden decrease. A caesarean section was conducted immediately . In 2 cases (2, 6) in which the oestriol excretion did not increase intra-uterine death occurred before the 31st and 24th week.

Benefical effects of xanthinol nicotinate are limited when there are extensive abnormalities of the placenta and its functions.

HOELZL and HAEFFELER recently found significant correlation between disturbed placental circulation and low levels of oestrogens in cases of EPH gestosis. PONTONNIER and LAGORGE, studying placental circulation in the intervillous space with 133 Xenon, found a decrease in blood flow in abnormal pregnancies. The same authors noted a satisfactory correlation between the decrease of placental blood flow and urinary oestriol excretion.

Table 1

No. patient	Obstetrical history	Before therapy Blood pressure	Proteinuria	Oedema	Weeks of therapy	Results
1 3257 1972	1 C. S.	130/ 85	1 %	+	from 32 to 35	V. D. 35th week living infant 2100 g
2 3365 1972	1 V. D.	140/ 90	1,5 %	++	from 28 to 30	Intra-uterine death 31st week 500 g
3 208 1973	1st pre- gnancy	150/100	1,5 %	+	from 32 to 35	V. D. 35th week living infant 1600 g
4 287 1973	2 V. D.	120/ 80	1 %	+	from 25 to 28	Still pregnant
5 704 1973	1 V. D. 1 C. S. 2 neonatal death	130/ 90	1 %	++	from 22 to 29	Still pregnant
6 756 1973	1st pre- gnancy	210/140	2 %	+	from 21 to 23	Intra-uterine death 24th week
7 795 1973	1st pre- gnancy	155/ 90	1 %	+	from 34 to 36	C. S. 36th week living infant 2400 g
8 815 1973	Intra-uterine death 34th week	150/100	2 %	++	from 34 to 35	C. S. 35th week living infant 1450 g
9 857 1973	2 abortions	180/100	7 %	++	from 37 to 39	C. S. 39th week living infant 1060 g

C. S.: Caesarean Section, V. D.: Vaginal Delivery

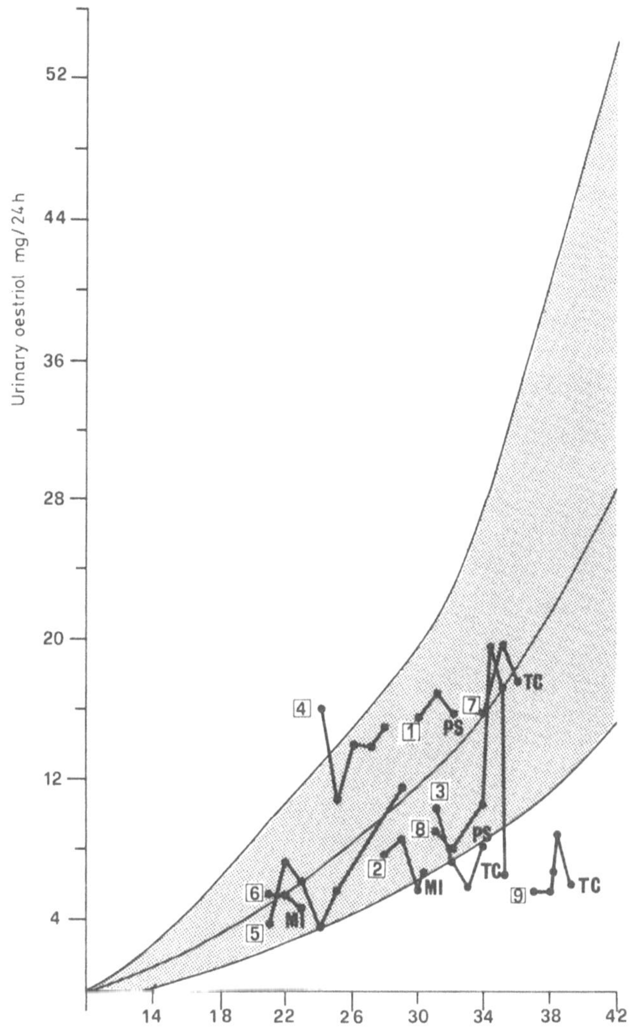

Fig. 1. Urinary oestriol excretion before and during xanthinol nicotinate treatment (PS = Vaginal Delivery, TC = Caesarean Section, MI = Intra-uterine Death)

References

1. BERGSTEIN, N. A. M.: Kann man durch Complamin-Retard die Placentafunktion beeinflussen? 2 EPH Gestosis Symposien.
2. BERGSTEIN, N. A. M., V. KESSEL, H. I. J. M.: Xanthinol Nicotinate and placental function, Lancet 13, 111 (1968).
3. HOELZL, M., HAEFFELER, R.: Rate of urinary oestrogen excretion correlated with placental morphology especially in respect to disturbance of maturation in cases of EPH gestosis. III Europ. Congr. Perinatal Med. Lausanne 1972.

4. MARZETTI, L.: Possibilità e vantaggi dei farmaci fibrinolitici nella terapia della nefropatia gravidica - Quaderni Clin. Ostet. ç Ginec. 19, 346 (1964).
5. MARZETTI, L., BENAGIANO, G.: Valutazione clinica dell' impiego di un farmaco ad azione fibrinolitica nella terapia delle gestosi del terzo trimestre. Clin. Ostet. ç Ginec. 66, 429 (1964).
6. PONTONNIER, G., GRANDJEAN, M.: Measurement of placental clearance of 133 Xenon - Methods and results. III Europ. Congr. Perinatal Med. Lausanne 1972.
7. PONTONNIER, G., LAGORCE, J.: Les Lésions rénales et l'hémodynamique placentaire dans les dysgravidies au gestoses. 3, EPH gestosis p. 217 Homel.

The Treatment of EPH-Gestosis with Xantinol-Nicotinat - Alterations of HPL and Coagulation-Physiological Alterations over Long Periods

H. Weber, S. Heller, S. Kunz, and E. Kidess

The alterations of HPL and coagulation-physiological parameters over short periods in the treatment of EPH-gestosis with xantinol-nicotinat have been handled.

In order to get a picture of the alterations of HPL and the blood coagulation over a long period we treated 26 pregnant women with this substance. There were 15 gestosis patients and 11 probationers without symptoms of gestosis. The women were observed over a period of two weeks. Further we treated a group of 5 gestosis patients with Complamin during 11 weeks and measured the HPL and coagulation values.

Because of the already mentioned presumption of a temporary hypovolumenia following the application of Complamin we maintained the former test order so that one group was infused with Macrodex 6 % in addition to the oral dose of Complamin. This happened to resume to the examinations conducted by GRANDJEAN-DELMAS who in the case of 16 pathological pregnancies with a significant reduction of the blood circulation in the placenta, found out that the circulation increased by 50 to 100 % after an infusion of 6 % dextran. In two cases the increase was only small and in 3 cases there was no alteration or reduction, respect. To evaluate the placental blood circulation we referred to the placenta scintigraphy with Xe^{133}.

In the case of our patients who were treated with Complamin over a period of more than two weeks we abandoned the infusion of Macrodex and measured the HPL and coagulation values every day before the dose of Complamin was given. In all cases 3 x 300 mg Complamin/die per os were applicated. Only the group of the 15 gestosis patients and the 11 probationers who were observed over a period of two weeks, were infused with 300 ml Macrodex 6 % each in addition to the first dose of Complamin. The HPL was determined according to the AMBERLITE Method after MEADE and KIDGAARD and by means of the Radio Immunassay of Mssrs. Hoechst.

The following alterations over a long period were stated:

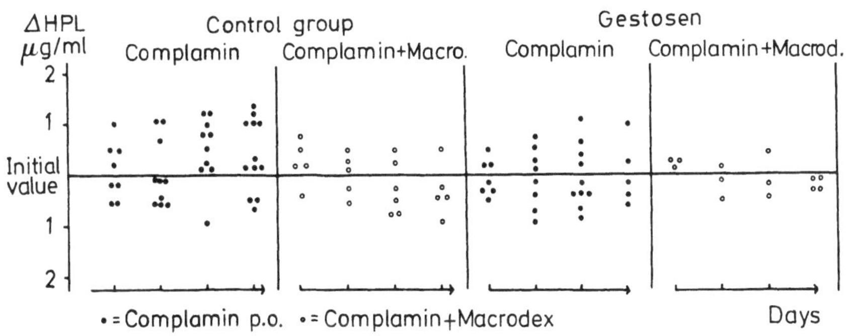

Fig. 1. HPL Alterations after the Application of Complamin and Complamin +Macrodex during the First Week of Therapy

During the first four days of the therapy the control group treated with Complamin shows a similar tendency in the first column as in the case of the short-term controls, the delta HPL increasing slightly in most of the cases. The control group in the second column treated with Complamin and Macrodex shows a certain tendency to the negative delta HPL which in our opinion is caused by the cumulation of the plasma expander, a fact stated also with the controls over short periods. The gestosis group, in contrary, shows an uniform dispersion of the delta HPL around the initial value in the course of 4 days.

The behaviour of the HPL level was remarkable during the therapy over long periods.

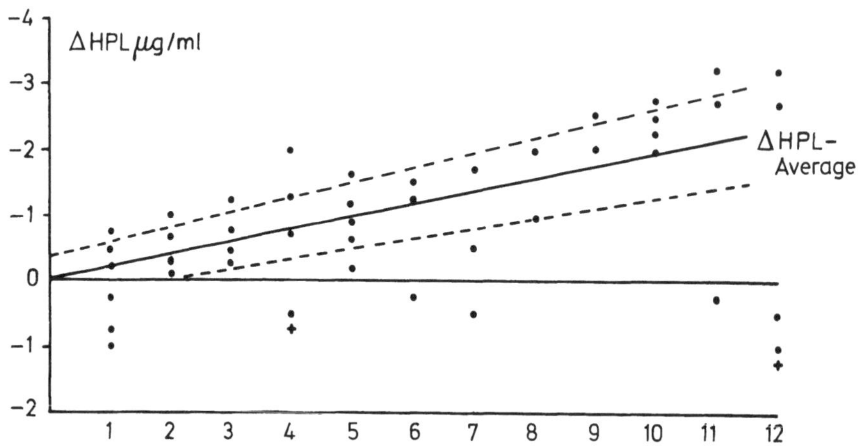

Fig. 2. HPL Alterations after Application of Complamin p. o. to Gestosis Patients over Long Periods during the Last Trimester of Pregnancy

The increase of the HPL - specific to our laboratories - can be seen from this figure. It illustrates the dispersion during the 30th and 40th week of pregnancy of our gestosis patients. Apart from a few exceptions - e. g. the fetuses of 2 patients necrosed - the therapy succeeded in an increase of the HPL values corresponding to the normal curve at least. Before the beginning of the therapy all 16 gestosis patients showed HPL values significantly lower than the standard values. In the course of the therapy over 11 weeks 3 patients reached normal values as regards the absolute HPL value as well as the delta HPL. Both pregnant women without increase of the HPL value had a death-birth.

Many scientists tested the behaviour of the blood coagulation of gestosis patients. Before all they stated a further increase of the hypercoagulability in comparison with the normal gravidities. The same applies to the reduction of the fibrinolytical activity. In our opinion this problem is of special importance with regard to the evaluation of the examinated alterations over long periods i. e. an effective therapy should result in a tendency towards a normalisation.

This finds its expression in a strong shortening of the reaction time in the thrombelastogramm and in an increase of the coagulum consistence. In the sense of a decreasing coagulopathy the result may be a measurable lost of fibrinogen caused by permanent fibrin deposits in the placenta. On the other hand also raised fibrinogen levels are described which are explained with an excessive production of new fibrinogen. In the case of our patients the alterations of the TEG values behave differently.

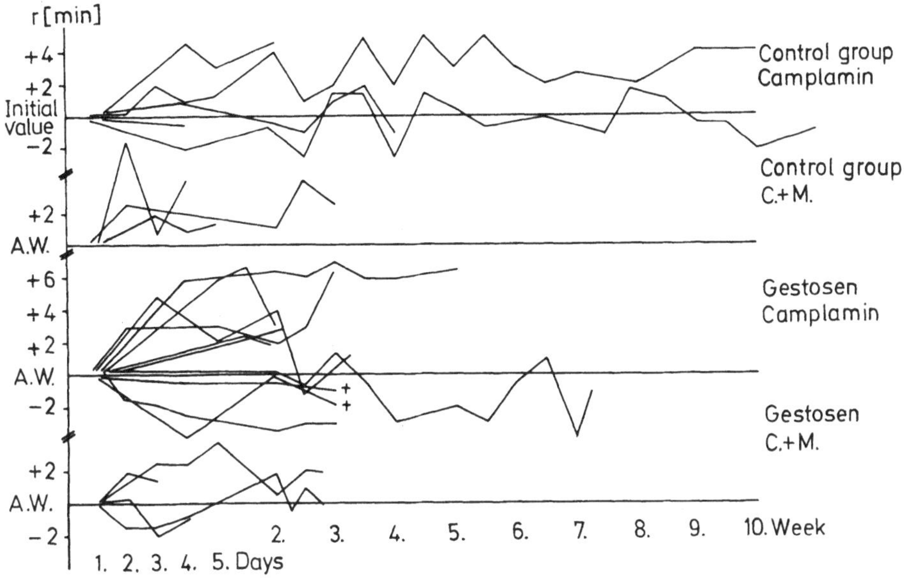

Fig. 3. TEG Reaction Time - Alterations over Long Periods (Difference to the Initial Value)

The difference between the reaction time and the initial value can be taken from this figure. Most of the patients, i. e. 6 from 9, showed a prolonged r-value after two weeks of therapy, only that of two patients was shortened. Also the coagulum consistence seems to reduce up to this moment what can be seen from Fig. 4.

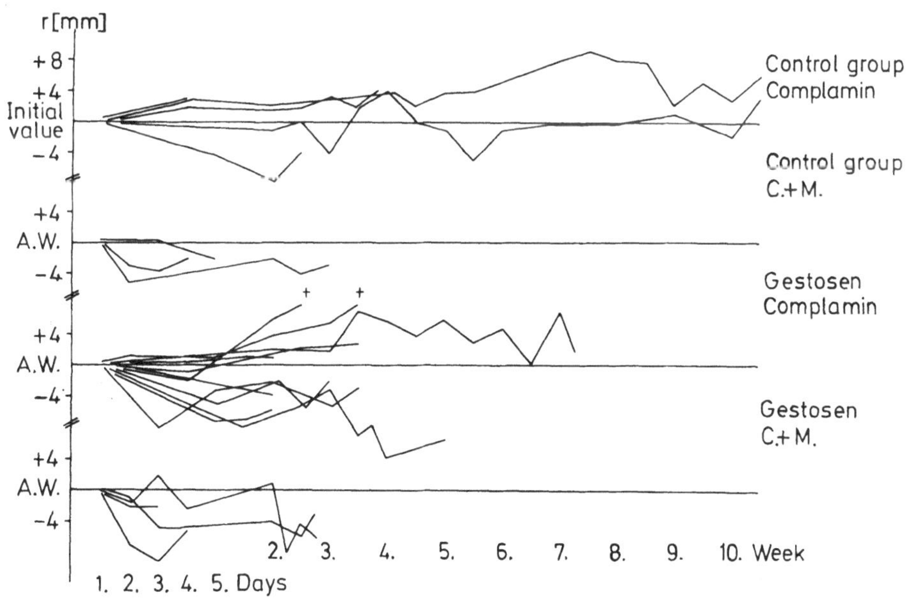

Fig. 4. TEG Maximum Amplitude
Alterations over Long Periods (Differences to the Initial Value)

The four cases who show an increase of the maximum amplitude comprise the above mentioned two patients whose fetuses died. However, it must be emphasized that this is only an interpretation as the difference of the group members does not allow a statistical statement.

A comparison of the cases with severe pathological HPL level had the remarkable result that all five patients had an extreme low fibrinogen level of 126 to 268 mg / %. Furthermore, the thrombocyte numbers are clearly lower. They amount to 135000 to 173000 instead of 192000, the average of the other patients.

During the therapy these values first increased but then dropped again distinctly when the fetuses of two patients died. The examinated parameters of the other patients as fibrinogen, plasmin inhibitors, and thrombocytes do not differ from those of a normal pregnancy. The blood platelet aggregation test after BREDDIN which resulted in 12 cases in the pathological stages 4 and 5, improved up to stage 3 in 5 cases and up to stage 2 in one case.

After a critical review of the results the following can be concluded:
1. In the case of two patients with severe placental insufficiency who did not show in improvement after a former therapy with diuretica, antihypertonica, and protein substitution, the fetuses died in spite of the Complamin dose. The HPL and coagulation values described a correspondingly negative curve.
2. In our opinion, a favorable effect of the therapy could be realized in the case of the other 14 patients.
3. In accordance with our tests conducted with respect to alterations over short periods we are now testing whether there exists a dose dependency in the therapy of gestosis with xantinol-nicotinat with respect to alterations over long periods.

The Behaviour of Serum Electrolytes, Serum Protein, and of the Substances to be Eliminated in the Case of Gestosis Treated with Xantinol-Nicotinat and Heparin

C. Bieling, E. Kidess, and S. Kunz

14 patients in the last trimester of pregnancy who were found to have EPH gestosis symptoms (edemata, hypertonus, proteinuria) on the occasion of the routine pregnancy examination were hospitalized until the symptoms disappeared or until delivery. Under untreated conditions, under therapy, and post partum the serum metabolites creatinine, urea, uric acid, bilirubin, protein, albumin, cholesterin, potassium, sodium, calcium, chlorine, and phosphorus were determined in intervals of one week. Rest in bed, diet containing much protein and small salt quantities, and 3 x 300 mg xantinol-nicotinat (Complamin) were prescribed after the first measurements. Furthermore, after one week seven patients were treated with heparin. For that purpose the preparation Cutherparin was injected subcutaneously into the abdominal wall three times a day, usually 2 x 0,5 ml corresponding to 20000 - 30000 USP units. The blood coagulation was observed by permanent controls of the TEG. A r-value of 20 min. was aspired.

The results of the examinations can be taken from the following figures, broken down to months of pregnancy and type of therapy. The 3rd trimester was included, from the 6th month of pregnancy up to the puerperium. After the breaking down to groups according to the type of therapy and post partum a statistical review was performed by a coupled mean value comparison by means of the t-test. A value of 2 p lower or equal to 0.10 was fixed as significance limit.

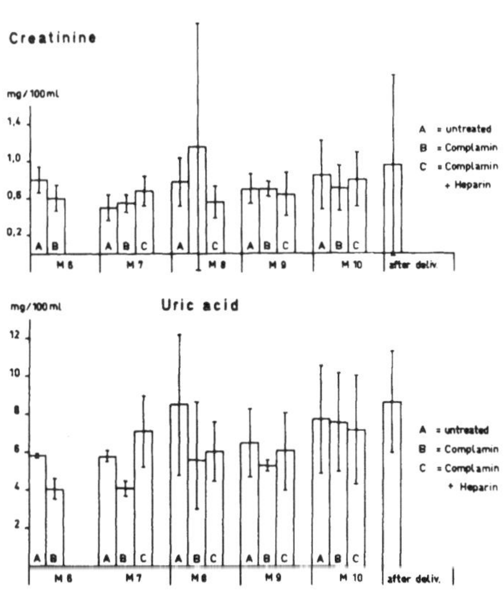

Fig. 1. Substances to be eliminated

The substances which must be eliminated were found to be of variable behaviour with extended dispersions. Most of the creatinine values are not situated in the pathological range. Pathological values only appear in the 8th and 9th months in which, however, the majority of the values is also situated within the normal range, the mean value being increased by only a few pathological values. This fact is proved by the standard deviations. Similar conditions were found with the urea, not illustrated. As to the uric acid before all untreated patients coming to an examination only in the 8th or 10th months show pathological values. The high uric acid values post partum should be caused by hemoconcentration and involution processes in the childbed. A group comparison of all groups with all groups did not establish significant differences between creatinine and urea. As regards the uric acid the values of the patients treated with Complamin were significantly higher than those of non-treated women, the values of the patients treated with Complamin + Heparin were significantly higher than those of the patients treated with Complamin only. There are no further tendencies to be stated as regards the course of pregnancy and the modus of treatment.

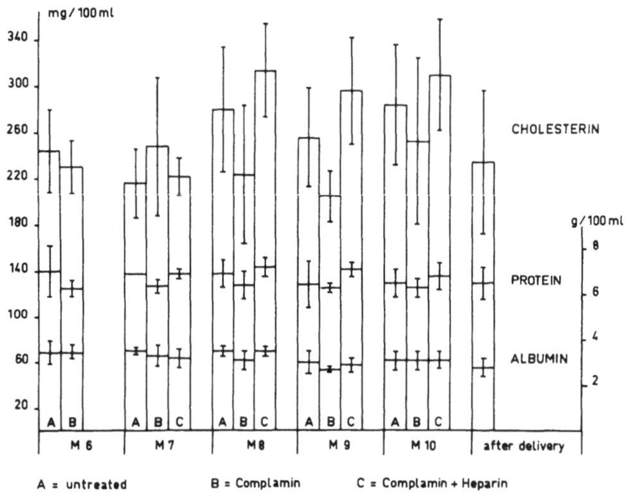

Fig. 2. Cholesterin

The values of cholesterin are very much dispersed in all groups. The dispersions and mean values partly penetrate very far into the pathological range of the hypercholesterinemia of normal non-pregnant women. Tendencies as regards the course of time cannot be taken from this figure. The statistical group comparison shows that the values of the non-treated women are significantly lower than those of the patients treated with Complamin + Heparin and of the lying-in women, and that the values of the patients treated with Complamin are lower than those of the patients treated with Complamin and Heparin.

The values of biliburin are all normal and insignificant, thus they are not illustrated.

Proteins

The mean values broken down to pregnancy months are all situated near the lower standard value of the 6.7 g/100 ml for normal non-pregnant women. The same applies to the albumin values which all do disperse near the lower standard value of 3.5 g/100 ml for normal non-pregnant women. The group comparison shows that the protein values of non-treated patients are located significantly lower than those of the patients treated with Complamin + Heparin. As regards the albumin the postpartal values are essentially lower than those of all pregnant women.

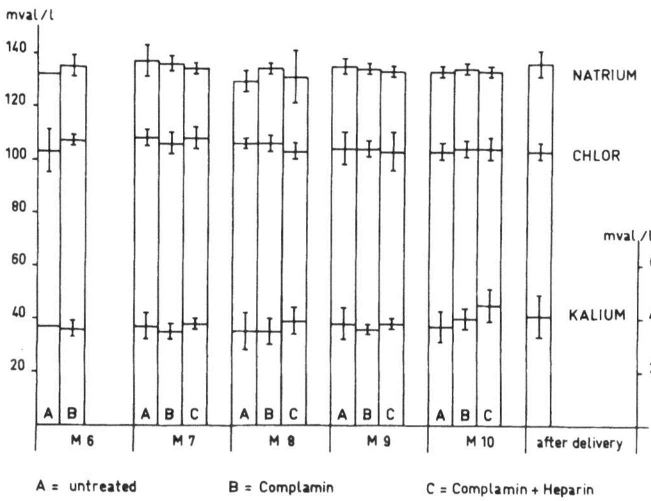

Fig. 3. Electrolytes

In spite of partly severe clinical appearances the behaviour of the electrolytes is uniform. The values of chlorine are normal as well as those of calcium and phosphorus. They are not illustrated and do not show any significant group difference. The values of sodium and potassium with a smaller dispersion range are all located in the lower third of the standard range for normal non-pregnant women. These findings tally with the alterations of the serum electrolytes during a normal pregnancy, mentioned in the relevant literature. The group comparison shows significantly lower values for potassium in the case of non-treated patients as compared with group C and post partum. The sodium values of the non-treated patients are essentially higher than those of the Complamin + Heparin-treated patients, which on their part are lower than those of the lying-in women.

Summary

In the case of 14 patients ill with EPH gestosis the serum concentrations of creatinine, urea, uric acid, bilirubin, protein, albumin, cholesterin, potassium, sodium, calcium, chlorine, and phosphorus were controlled under untreated conditions, with rest in bed, diet containing much protein and small salt quantities, and after one week with 3 x 300 mg xantinol-nicotinat (Complamin), and in seven cases with an additional heparinisation in weekly intervals and post partum. The concentrations were then compared after groups of months of pregnancy. In spite of partly severe clinical appearances the serum electrolytes and the bilirubin showed in all groups a constant behaviour in the lower standard range. Protein and albumin behaved constantly with little dispersions around the lower standard value of normal non-pregnant women. The values of the substances to be eliminated and of cholesterin showed extended dispersions with partly normal, partly highly pathological values.

Long Term Heparin Therapy for Placental Insufficiency

K. Wernicke, E. Halberstadt, R. Gerner, G. Bastert, and H. Eckert

Chronic placental insufficiency, as a course for fetal malnutrition and for increase in perinatal mortality, often follows from decrease in utero-placental bloodflow resulting in disturbances of the microcirculation in the intervillous space.

The attempt to increase the bloodflow in the intervillous space by treating the mother with vasodilating drugs has not been successful to date (1).

Another way to attempt to improve the placental microcirculation is to use anticoagulants as they are used in treating disturbances of the general microcirculation. Heparin reduces fibrinous plugs, resulting from the release of thrombin secondary to this disturbances of microcirculation (2).

Results are reported of treating a series of patients with varified placental insufficiency with continous heparin infusion of 20 000 units per day for 3 to 7 weeks; an amount insufficient to prolong clotting time. As control a non treated series of patients with placental insufficiency was used (Fig. 1).

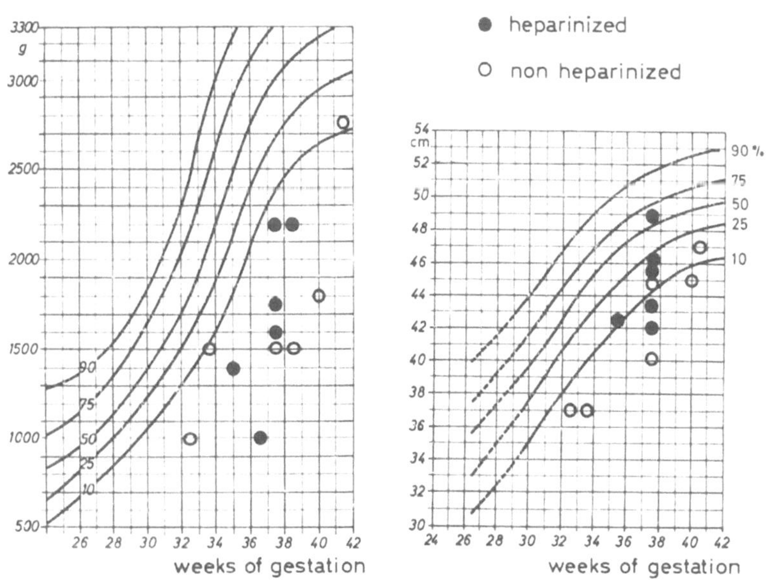

birth-weight in dependence of gestational age

(Lubchenko et al. 1966)

lenght (crown-heel) in dependence of gestational age

(Lubchenko et al. 1966)

Fig. 1

The discrepancy between size of the uterus and gestational age, as well as the deficit of biparital diameter as measured by ultrasound cephalometry, was unchanged by heparin therapy in all our cases. 24-hour estriol excretion in urin strongly increased shortly after the beginning of heparin therapy in the majority of our cases (Fig.2).

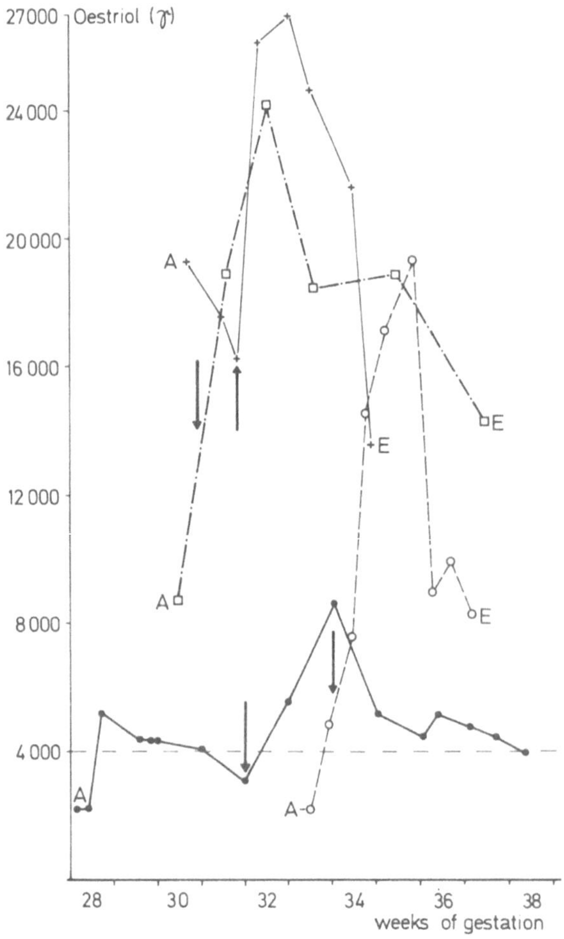

Fig. 2. Estriol levels (μg/24 hrs) in 4 cases of placental insufficiency treated with long term heparin infusions. A = day of hospitalization, E = delivery, ↑ = beginning of heparin therapy

No explanation can be given for this observation; bed rest was not the variable, since the control series, also at bed rest, did not show this early and marked increase in estriol excretion. A warning sign of respiratory insufficiency was a steep fall in estriol excretion independent of the absolut level.

The amount of placental lactogen, as a measure of placental function, in both series of cases were similar. Cases with placental lactogen below 4 μg/ml, indicating fetal danger, were seen in both series (Fig.3).

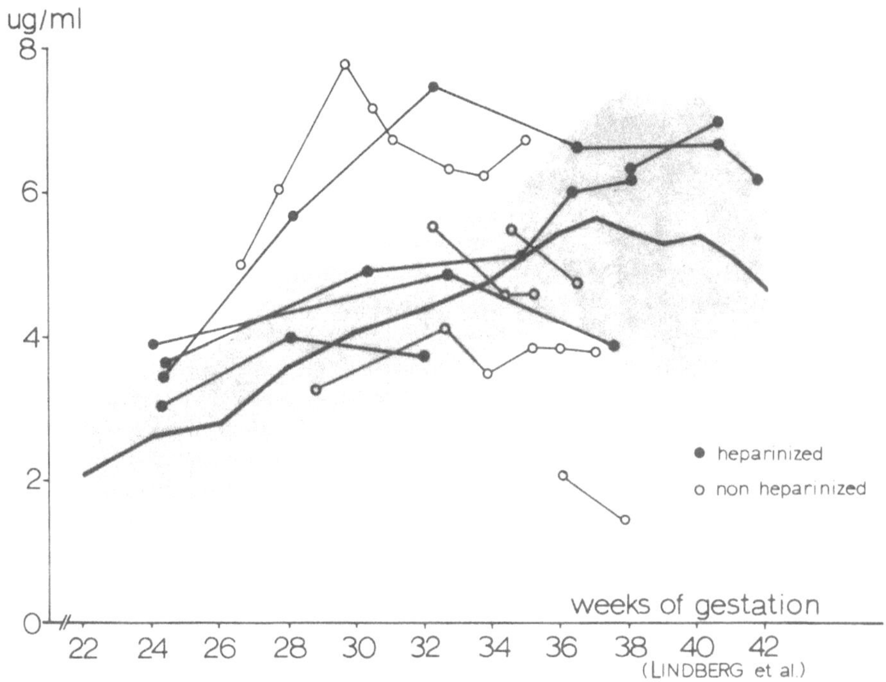

Fig. 3. Human Placental Lactogen (HPL)

In the same way the alkaline-leukocyte-phosphatase was not changed by heparin therapy. There were cases in both groups, in which a sudden fall in this enzyme indicated fetal danger.

The clotting factors (Table 1), which may affect fibrin deposition in the placenta, were investigated in both the heparinized and non heparinized patients. Only prothrombin was slightly reduced in some cases in the heparin treated series. Fibrinogen level increases slightly.

Table 1. Clotting factors

factor II
factor V
factor VII
factor X
fibrinogen
split products
cryofibrinogen
fibrin
platelets
alpha-1-antitrypsin
alpha-2-macroglobulin
euglobulin-lysis-time

Special interest was concerned with the enzyme levels of the insufficient placenta. The following enzyme activities were evaluated and their amount related to the amount of DNA in a defined quantity of tissue. Fig. 4 shows the differences between normal placentas and insufficient placentas of both groups. In the insufficient placentas higher levels than normal were seen in the activity of enzymes concerned with anaerobic glycolysis such as PK, ALD and LDH. On the other hand the enzymes of the citric-acid-cycle were reduced in both groups

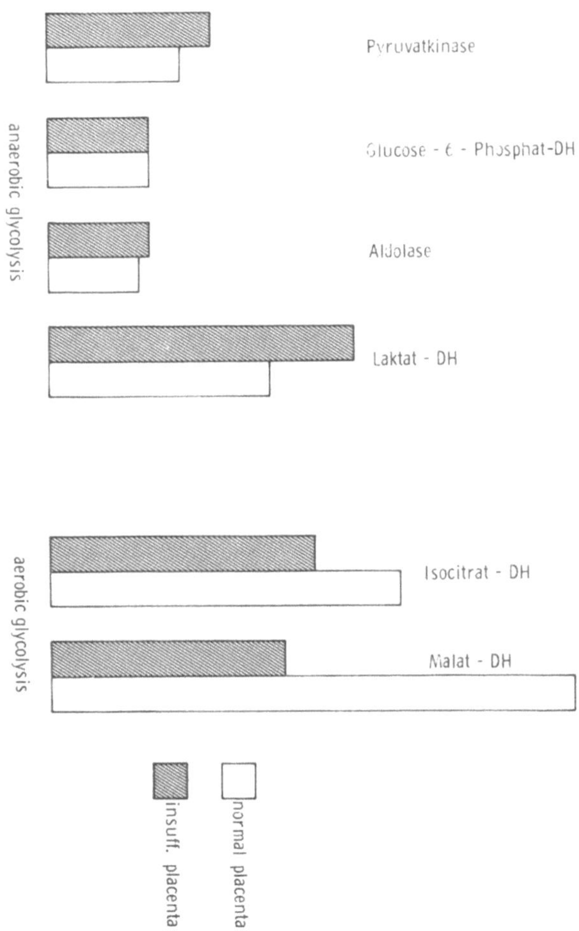

Fig. 4. Specific activities (µg DNA in 1 cm^3 tissue)

of insufficient placentas. In other words, long term heparin therapy is unable to reduce the increased anaerobic glycolysis in the insufficient placenta, nor to prevent the strong reduction of aerobic glycolysis and of all other anabolic reactions. The oxydative enzyme dysfunction, resulting in disturbance in energy balance and cell metabolism, was not improved nor prevented in cases of placental insufficiency by heparin therapy.

Similar results were found also in histological investigations, since no differences were seen between both groups. Lactatdehydrogenase, as a parameter of anaerobic glycolysis, was increased, while the oxygen labile enzyme, monoaminooxydase, was reduced (Fig. 5 a, 5 b).

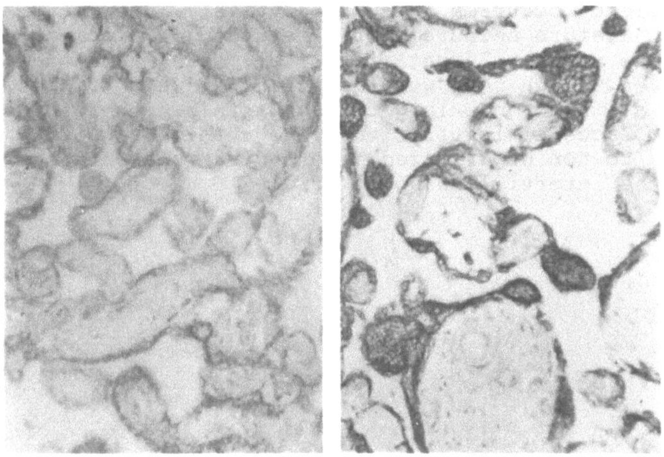

Fig. 5 a. Lactatedehydrogenase (left: normal placenta, right: insuff. placenta)

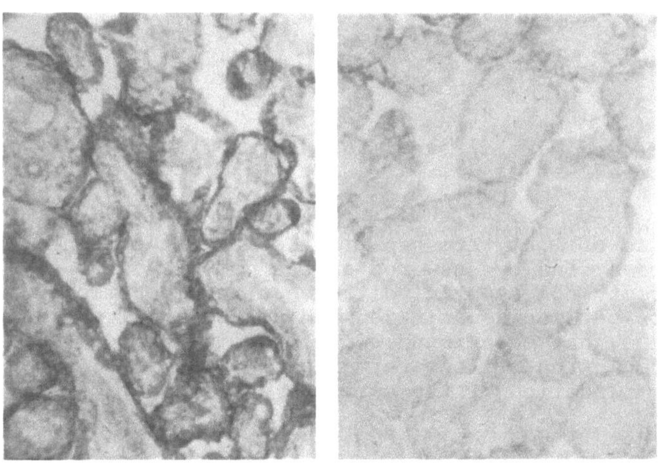

Fig. 5 b. Monoaminooxydase (left: normal placenta, right: insuff. placenta)

The biochemical and histochemical signs of decompensation of the placentas of both groups were to be expected, because in all cases pregnancy was terminated after the manifestion of respiratory insufficiency.

However clinically the results in the control group and the long term heparinized group were not always the same. In both series cardiotocography shows pathological slowing of the heart rate during oxytocin induced or spontaneous labor and diminution of fetal heart rate fluctuation. Nevertheless, in the heparinized group these cardiac signs of respiratory insufficiency occurred in a comparatively later stage of fetal development. Therefore because of the retarded development of the pathological state of the placenta relatively more mature newborns were delivered even though they were deficient in weight. Histologically one can find a hint of how long term heparinization retards the stage of metabolic placental insufficiency. Heparinized insufficient placenta compared to non heparinized insufficient placenta shows fewer fibrin-plugs in the intervillous space (Fig. 6).

Fig. 6. Fibrinous plugs in placental insufficiency (left: non heparinized, right: heparinized)

The question of the value of long term heparin therapy for placental insufficiency has not been finally answered on the grounds of these findings. Despite the fact, no essential difference in biochemical or histochemical parameters between heparinized and non heparinized cases of placental insufficiency has been found, we would like to commend the earliest possible beginning of long term heparin infusions, since the results suggest a retardation of the clinical development of placental insufficiency.

References

1. SCHMID, J., KELLER, P. J.: Saling, Dudenhausen: Perinatale Medizin, Band III, Stuttgart: Thieme 1971.
2. LASCH, H. G., KRECKE, H. J., RODRIQUEZ-ERDMANN, F., SESSNER, N., SCHÜTTERLE, G.: Verbrauchskoagulopathie, Folia haemat. (N. F.) 6, 325 (1961).

Therapy of Feto-Placental Insufficiency during Pregnancy the Effects of Drugs on Placental Function

J. Schmidt

Chronic placental insufficiency (10) leads to intra-uterine retardation of fetal growth, which results in intra-uterine death or in delivery of a newborn infant having a low birth weight for gestational age and with an increased morbidity (9, 10, 11). The primary cause is a placental dysfunction, and in most cases a decreased utero-placental blood-flow is present (6, 7, 10) which is isotopically demonstrable (7, 8, 19, 20). Fig. 1 shows three examples of measurement of placental blood-flow using Technetium 99.

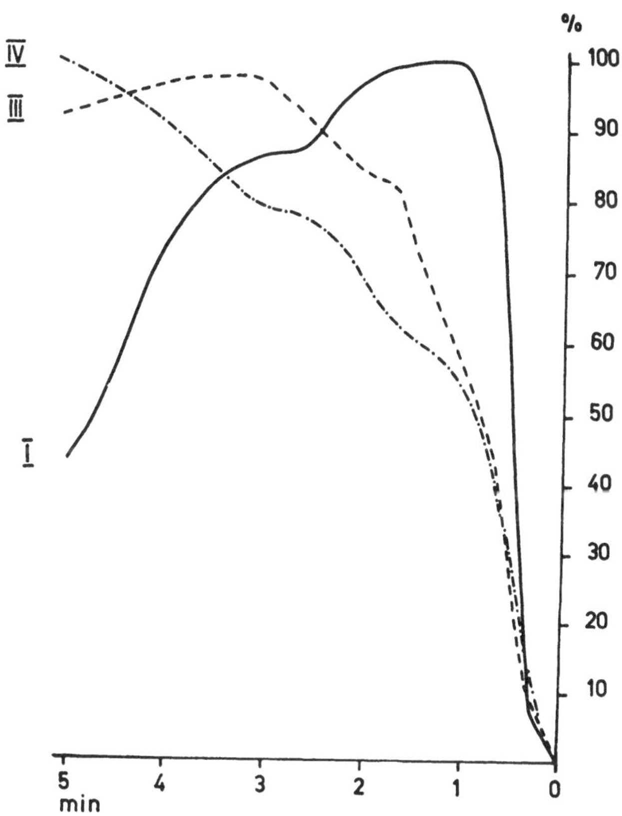

Fig. 1. 3 curves showing placental blood-flow measured by Technetium 99m

Curve I: Uncomplicated pregnancy
Curve III: Hypertensive pregnancy with intra-uterine growth retardation

Curve IV: Serious pre-eclampsia in the 32nd week of pregnancy with intra-uterine death three days after the measurement.

An attempt to improve the utero-placental blood-flow is indicated in those cases in which there is danger of intra-uterine death before the neonate is capable of an independent existence. We tested the following drugs with which an improvement in the placental carriage-capacity would be expected (Table 1): Adenosintriphosphoric acid (ATP) (13), Isoxsuprinum (5), Nicotinic-acid, Xanthinol-nicotinate (2), Nicotinyl-alcohol, Dipyridamol (15). The drugs were administered to the mother by intravenous drip. Effects were assessed by the following measurements: oestriol (Oe_3) and pregnandiol (P_2) in 24-hour urine; HCS = Human chorionicsomatomammotropin (HPL); HCG= Human Chorionicgonadotropin; progesterone (P) and heat-stable-alkaline phosphatase (HSAP) in the maternal serum.

Table 1. Drugs used

ATP	
Isoxsuprinum	(Duvadilan)
Nicotinic-acid	(Niconacid)
Xanthinol-nicotinate	(Complamin)
Nicotinyl-alcohol	(Ronicol)
Dipyridamol	(Persantin)
Heparin	
Heparin-dilydrin	

Fig. 2 shows the effect of ATP on these measurements. The ATP was given in a dose of 100 mg to 5 patients for three successive days. The individual patients are shown in different columns. The hormone concentrations are presented as a percentage of the average of the pre-therapeutic values.

We did not observe any significant increase after treatment (13 normal and 36 pathological pregnancies) (17, 18).

Recently reported studies (3, 14) indicate that fibrin deposition in the maternal vessels supplying the placenta impairs the utero-placental blood-flow and leads to a chronic feto-placental insufficiency. This could be the result of an increased consumption due to disseminated intravascular coagulation (4). Treatment by antithrombotic agents (heparin) should inhibit those clotting processes and improve the utero-placental blood-flow and thereby fetal growth (1, 12).

Patients and Methods

10 patients with clinical symptoms and / or pathological measurements suggesting feto-placental insufficiency were given heparin in a dose of 30,000 I.U. daily for a three week period by intravenous drip. 10 high-risk-pregnancies received the same dose of heparin and in addition 80 mg of an adrenergic beta-mimetic compound (Dilydrin) for three successive weeks.

The influence of heparin and heparin/Dilydrin on the placental function was assessed by the following parameters: oestriol and pregnandiol in 24-hour urine; HCS (HPL) and heat-stable alkaline phosphatase (HSAP) in the maternal serum. The growth of the fetal biparietal diameter was assessed and the fetal heart-rate continously monitored for 30 minutes once or twice every day. To avoid confusion of the results by bed rest and dietetic therapy, treatment was started 5 days after admission.

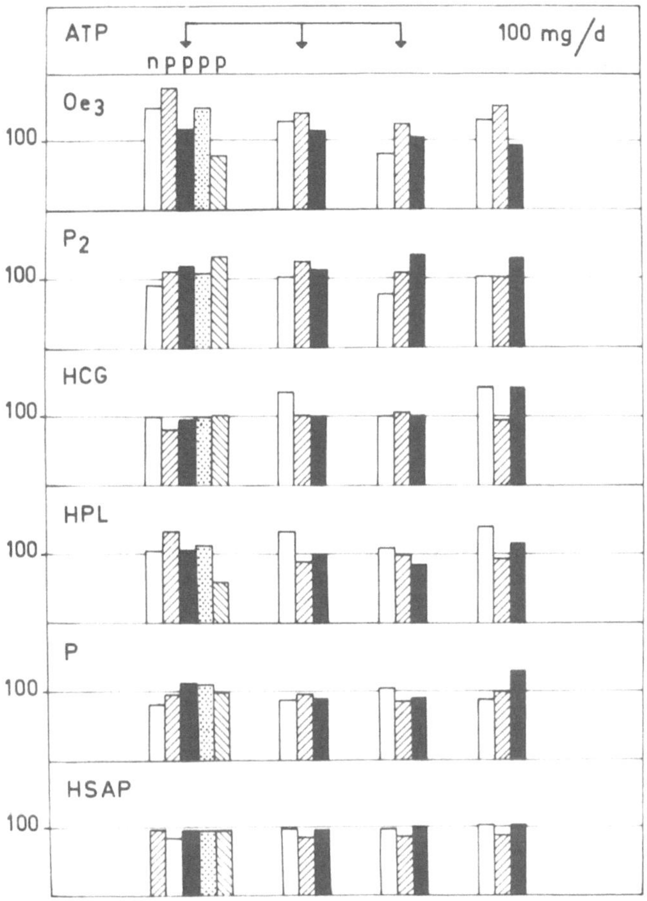

Fig. 2. The influence of 100 mg ATP on measured placental parameters. n = normal, p = pathological pregnancy

Results

The small number of cases together with small groups of different conditions prevented a statistical analysis of the results. Therefore the success of the treatment was calculated as follows: the average of the pre-therapeutic values was taken as 100 % and subsequent values are expressed as a percentage of the pre-therapeutic value.

Fig. 3 represents in one patient the expected and the effective values of oestriol. Despite treatment with heparin and Dilydrin for three weeks the values of oestriol are lower than expected.

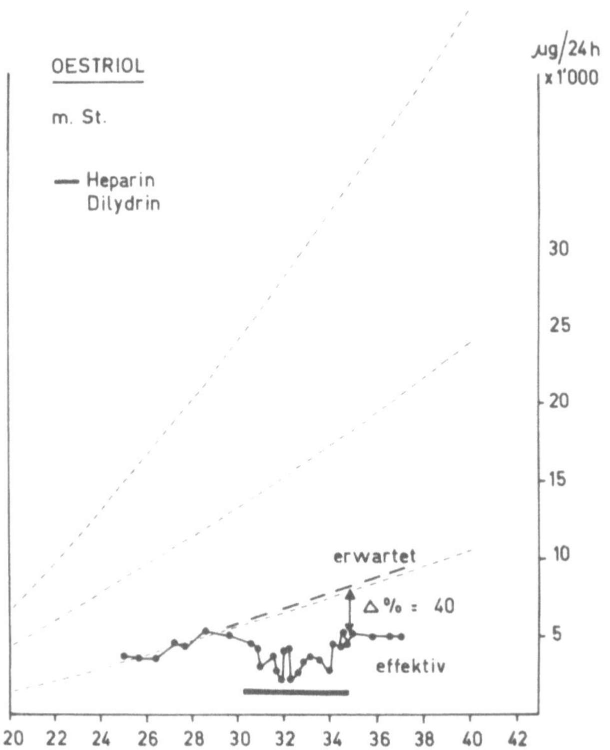

Fig. 3. Predicted and measured values of oestriol in a single patient

Fig. 4 shows HCS concentration in the same patient. Actual and predicted values agree. The results from 10 patients, who were given heparin 30,000 I.U. for three weeks are summarized in Tables 2, 3, 4 and 5. There is variation between predicted and measured values in all parameters. The excretion of oestriol (Table 2) demonstrated an insignificant increase in one case of toxaemia and in one case of intrauterine growth retardation.

The raised levels of oestriol in the case with Rh-Erythroblastosis is perhaps better explained by prenatal transfusions than by the heparin treatment (Table 2). Likewise the increased difference in the patients with diabetes mellitus can be explained by the strict insulin control.

Table 3 shows changes in the most sensitive measurement, HCS (HPL). Changes are inversely proportional to oestriol excretion. The largest increment was found after a second three weeks' treatment of an old primigravida and of a Rh-Erythroblastosis.

In Table 4 are shown the concentrations of heat-stable alkaline phosphatase. The results from patients with toxaemia were pathological. The other cases did not demonstrate any important differences except in case 7, in which the values decreased significantly after twelve weeks' treatment.

The fetal biparietal diameter growth also varies (Table 5). The growth was abnormal in one case of toxaemia and in one case of high-risk

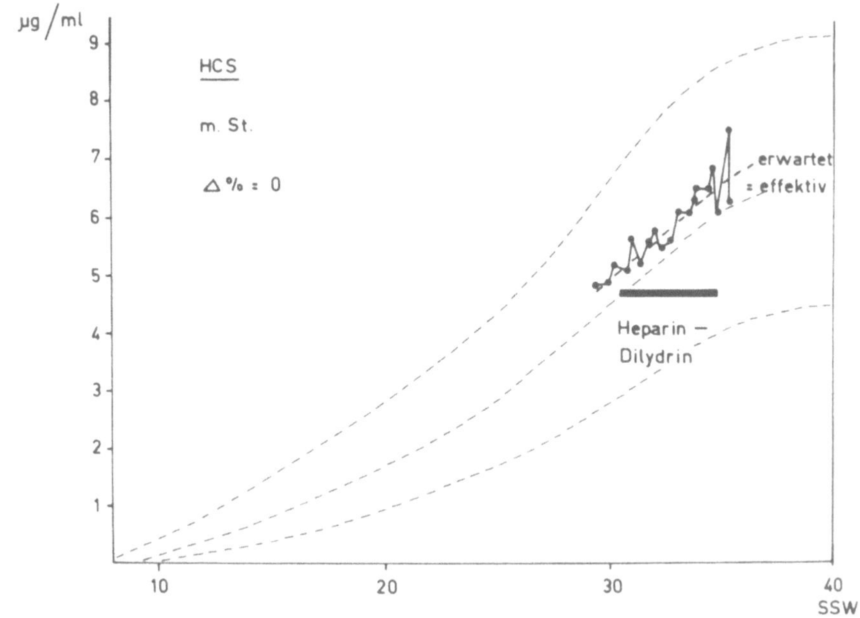

Fig. 4. Predicted (erwartet) and measured (effective) values of HCS (HPL) in the same patient as in Fig. 3

Table 2. Influence of Heparin on the estriol-values

No.	Diagnosis	Effective value %	Expected value %	Difference
1	EPH	155	155	0
2	EPH	82	125	- 43
3	EPH	125	122	+ 6
4	EPH	118	118	0
5	Fetal growth retardation	131	115	+ 16
6	Old primigravida	120	120	0
		108+	114	- 6
7	High risk pregnancy	147	147	0
		206++	268	- 62
8	Diabetes mellitus	120	113	+ 7
9	Diabetes mellitus	167	142	+ 25
10	Rh-erythroblastosis	180	118	+ 62

+Second treatment for three successive weeks
++Values after a treatment of twelve weeks

pregnancy in spite of heparin therapy. A significant increase was found only in one case of toxaemia. It was not possible to evaluate the monitored fetal heart-rate patterns.

The results in 5 patients, who were given heparin 30,000 I. U. and Dilydrin 80 mg daily are summarized in Tables 6, 7, 8, and 9. Oestriol excretion was below the expected level in all cases (Table 6). The HCS-values increased only in one case of toxaemia above the expected, whilst decreased significantly in the case of the Rh-erythroblastosis. The result was significantly below the normal value.

Table 3. Influence of Heparin on the HCS-values (HPL)

No.	Diagnosis	Effective value %	Expected value %	Difference
1	EPH	129	123	+ 6
2	EPH	143	126	+ 17
3	EPH	90	117	- 27
4	EPH	114	116	- 2
5	Fetal growth retardation	112	116	- 4
6	Old primigravida	124	119	+ 5
		152+	105	+ 47
7	High-risk pregnancy	100	139	- 39
		167++	258	- 91
8	Diabetes mellitus	89	102	- 13
9	Diabetes mellitus	64	113	- 49
10	Rh-erythroblastosis	143	121	+ 22

+Second treatment for three successive weeks
++Values after a treatment of twelve weeks

Table 4. Influence of Heparin on the HSAP-values

No.	Diagnosis	Effective value %	Expected value %	Difference
1	EPH	100	234	- 134
2	EPH	262	175	+ 87
3	EPH	115	170	- 55
4	EPH	123	174	- 51
5	Fetal growth retardation	110	134	- 24
6	Old primigravida	162	183	- 21
		167+	167	0
7	High-risk pregnancy	206	200	+ 6
		730++	950	- 220
8	Diabetes mellitus	136	119	+ 17
9	Diabetes mellitus	133	153	- 20
10	Rh-erythroblastosis	168	168	0

+Second treatment for three successive weeks
++Values after a treatment of twelve weeks

Table 5. Influence of Heparin on the growth of the fetal biparietal diameter

No.	Diagnosis	Effective value %	Expected value %	Difference
1	EPH	107	113	- 6
3	EPH	112	108	+ 4
4	EPH	103	103	0
5	Fetal growth retardation	105	104	+ 1
6	Old primigravida	106	109	- 3
7	High-risk pregnancy	153	158	- 5
8	Diabetes mellitus	105	104	+ 1
9	Diabetes mellitus	102	104	- 2
10	Rh-erythroblastosis	111	110	+ 1

The HSAP-values were pathological in three cases; (one uncomplicated pregnancy, one case with fetal retardation of growth, and in one case with Rh-Erythroblastosis) (Table 7).

Table 6. Influence of Heparin-dilydrin on the estriol-values

No.	Diagnosis	Effective value %	Expected value %	Difference
1	Normal pregnancy	104	119	- 15
2	EPH	82	117	- 35
3	Fetal growth retardation	152	172	- 20
4	Fetal growth retardation	154	114	- 40
5	Rh-erythroblastosis	100	133	- 13

Table 7. Influence of Heparin-dilydrin on the HCS-values (HPL)

No.	Diagnosis	Effective value %	Expected value %	Difference
1	Normal pregnancy	125	117	+ 11
2	EPH	166	115	+ 51
3	Fetal growth retardation	142	126	+ 16
4	Fetal growth retardation	122	122	0
5	Rh-erythroblastosis	136	166	- 30

A significant reduction in the growth of the fetal biparietal diameter (below normal) was found in case 3 (Table 9). Pregnandiol excretion was very variable and an evaluation was not possible (Table 8 and 9).

Table 8. Influence of Heparin-dilydrin on the HSAP-values

No.	Diagnosis	Effective value %	Expected value %	Difference
1	Normal pregnancy	120	170	- 50
2	EPH	113	120	- 7
3	Fetal growth retardation	110	146	- 36
4	Fetal growth retardation	153	166	- 13
5	Rh-erythroblastosis	100	170	- 70

Table 9. Influence of Heparin-dilydrin on the growth of the fetal biparietal diameter

No.	Diagnosis	Effective value %	Expected value %	Difference
1	Normal pregnancy	105	106	- 1
2	EPH	107	106	+ 1
3	Fetal growth retardation	113	107	+ 6
4	Fetal growth retardation	107	110	- 3

Discussion

The results must be interpreted with caution because of the big variations in the figures obtained. An improvement in the placental function cannot be demonstrated in one case by these results. It is of value to try and estimate the degree of fetal placental insufficiency when therapy has been commenced late. Heparin might inhibit further thrombosis, so that placental function would remain in the pre-therapeutic condition. Extensive fibrin deposition in the vessels of the placenta cannot be altered and morphological abnormalities could not be changed by heparin.

From our figures it is not possible to show that the treatment was of any value although a large clinical trial might demonstrate some benefit. If fibrin deposition in the utero-placental vessels is a primary cause of the impairment of placental blood-flow, the use of antithrombotic agents might inhibit the clotting process. It therefore seemed reasonable to treat patients with heparin or heparin / dilydrin who previously had a still-birth or had a pregnancy suggestive of utero-placental insufficiency.

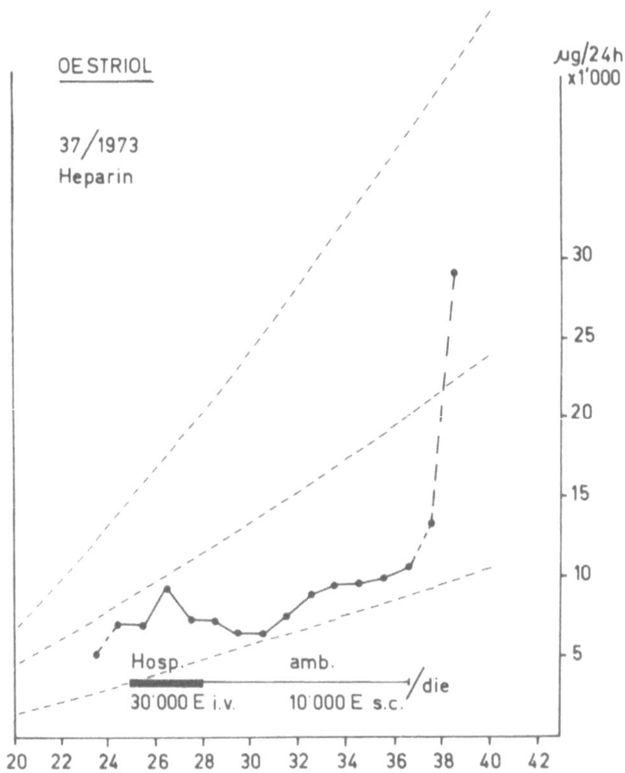

Fig. 5. Values of oestriol during treatment with Heparin. 30,000 units daily for three weeks by intravenous drip (i.v.). 10,000 units daily for nine weeks by sub-cutaneous injection (s.c.)

These show the changes in oestriol, pregnanediol, HCS and HSAP in a 28-year old patient, pregnant for the second time, who received 30,000 I. U. of heparin by intravenous drip for three weeks and after that 10,000 I. U. Depot-Heparin subcutaneously for 9 weeks. The first pregnancy resulted in a still-birth, weighed 1620 g and measured 41 cm long. The second pregnancy produced a full-term baby, weighing 3150 g and measuring 51 cm long. The Apgar score was 8/10. The successful result of the second pregnancy may be quite independent of the heparin treatment.

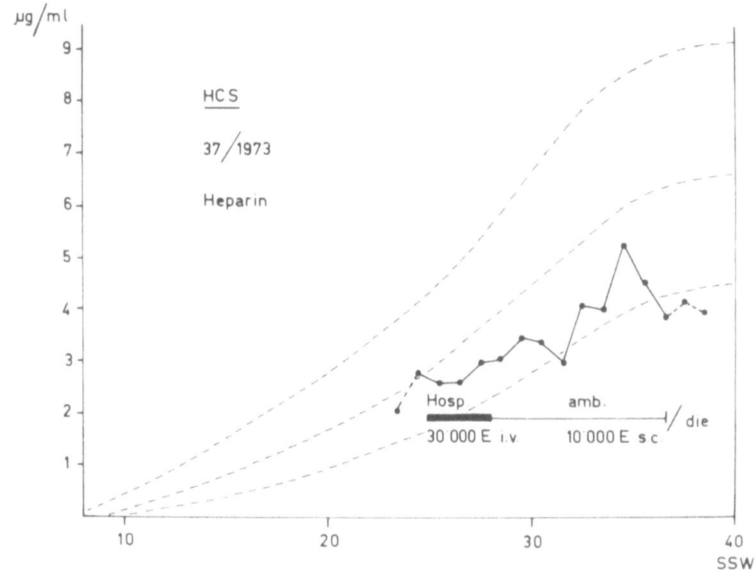

Fig. 6. Values of HCS (HPL) during a treatment with Heparin

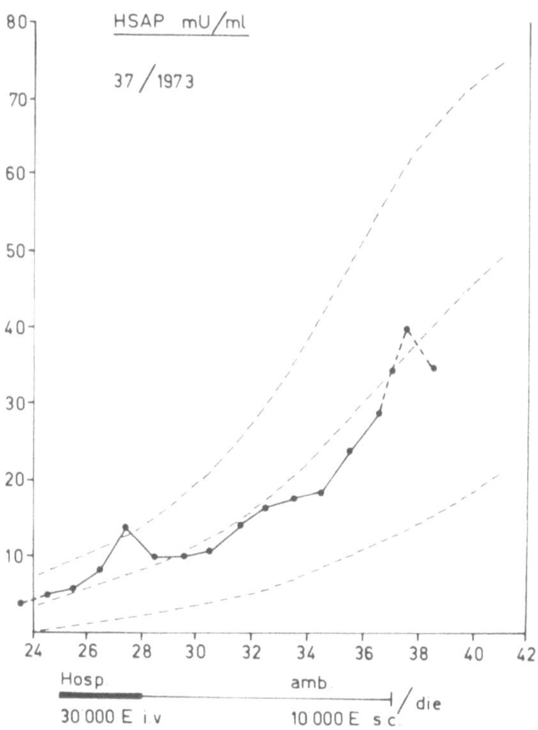

Fig. 7. Values of HSAP during treatment with Heparin

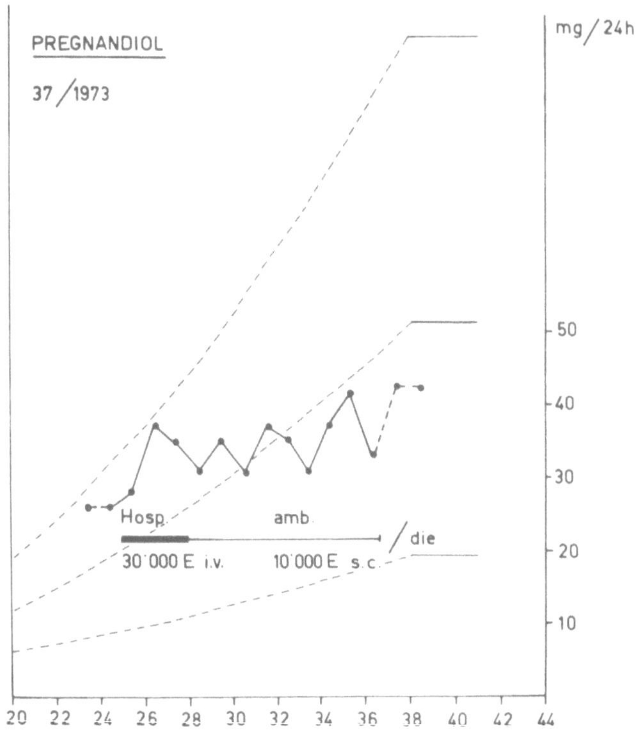

Fig. 8. Values of pregnanediol during a treatment with Heparin

Summary

Heparin, 30,000 I. U. daily, was given to 10 high-risk pregnant patients for three successive weeks by intravenous drip. Five other patients reveiced, in addition, 80 mg of an adrenergic beta-mimetic compound (Dilydrin) daily.

The influence of these drugs on placental function was assessed by following parameters: 24-hour excretion of oestriol and pregnandiol in the urine; HCS (HPL) and heat-stable alkaline phosphatase (HSAP) in the maternal serum; growth of the fetal biparietal diameter; and cardiotocographic tracings.

The treatment appeared to be without effect.

References

1. BAERTSCHI, U., SCHMID, J., KELLER, P. J.: Der Einfluß kurz- und langfristiger Heparingaben auf die Plazentafunktion. In: Perinatale Medizin, Bd. IV Stuttgart: Thieme.
2. BERGSTEIN, N. A. M., VON KESSER, H.: Xanthinol nicotinate and placental function. Lancet II, 111 (1968).

3. BONNAR, J., MC NICOL, G. P., DOUGLAS, A. S.: Coagulation and Fibrinolytic Systems in Pre-eclampsia and Eclampsia. Brit. Med. J. 2, 12 (1971).
4. BREHM, R., JANISCH, H.: Heparintherapie der EPH-Gestose. Dtsch. med. Wschr. 97, 417 (1972).
5. BROTANEK, V., HODR, J.: The effect of isoxsuprine on utero-placental circulation. In: Intra-uterine dangers to the foetus. Excerpta medica Foundation 1966.
6. DIXON, H. G., ROBERTSON, W. B.: A study of the vessels of the placental bed in normotensive and hypertensive women. J. Obstet. Gynaec. Brit. Emp. 65, 803 (1958).
7. DIXON, H. G., BROWNE, J. C., DAVEY, D. A.: Choriodecidual and myometrial blood-flow. Lancet II, 369 (1963).
8. GITSCH, E., JANISCH, H.: Durchströmungsmessung der Plazenta mit Radioisotopen. Z. Geburtsh. Gynäk. 174, 169 (1971).
9. GRUENWALD, P.: Abnormalities of placental vascularity in relation to intra-uterine deprivation and retardation of fetal growth. Significance of a vascular chorionic villi. N. Y. State J. Med. 61, 1508 (1961).
10. GRUENWALD, P.: Chronic fetal distress and placental insufficiency Biol. Neonate 5, 215 (1963).
11. GRUENWALD, P.: Abnormal growth in twins and infants of mothers with diabetes, hypertension, or isoimmunisation. Amer. J. Obstet. Gynec. 94, 1120 (1966).
12. HOFFBAUER, H., BUSCH, W.: Die Erfolge einer Dauerheparinisierung bei intra-uteriner Mangelentwicklung. Perinatale Medizin Bd. III, Stuttgart: Thieme 1971.
13. HORSKA, S., HODR, J., BROTANEK, V.: The mechanism of action of exogenous ATP for the treatment of fetal hypoxia during delivery. J. Obstet. Gynaec. Brit. Cwlth. 77, 994 (1970).
14. LUDWIG, H.: Pathologische Fibrinierung bei der Spätgestose. In: Die Spätgestose, Ed.: Rippman, E. T., Schwabe, Basel-Stuttgart. 1970.
15. MICHEL, C. F.: Die konservative Therapie der intra-uterinen Asphyxie. Perinatale Medizin. Bd. III, Stuttgart: Thieme 1971.
16. ROBERTSON, W. B., DIXON, H. G.: Utero-placental pathology. In: Fetus and placenta. Ed.: Klopper, A., Diczfalusy, E. Blackwell, Oxford, 1969.
17. SCHMID, J., KELLER, P. J.: Der Einfluß von ATP auf dic hormonale Parameter der Placenta. Arch. Gynäk. 212, 75 (1972).
18. SCHMID, J., KELLER, P. J.: Isoxsuprinum, Dipyridamol und Nicotinsäurepräparate in der Behandlung mangelversorgter Feten. Arch. Gynäk. 212, 68 (1972).
19. SCHMID, J., SCHWYTER, H.: Durchblutungsmessung der Plazenta mit Technetium-99 m. Gynäk. Rdsch. 13, 140 (1973).
20. WIGGLESWORTH, J. S.: Fetal growth retardation. Brit. med. Bull. 22, 13 (1966).

Intra-Uterine Growth of Newborn Infants of Parma

G. Bevilacqua and M. Moretti

In recent years the study of newborn infants has shown a great number of associations between neonatal disorders and abnormalities either of the gestation period or of intra-uterine growth.

In order to evaluate intra-uterine growth in the various ages of gestation it is necessary to plot a normal curve to use it as a standard reference. In many neonatal wards the growth curve of (4) is used; it was plotted in Denver, Colorado, and it was recommended by the American Academy of Pediatrics in 1967. Other curves are less frequently used, (YERUSHALMY, 1967; USHER and MC LEAN, 1969; BABSON, 1970).

The use of a standard curve should take into account geographical, socio-economic and racial conditions. The use of the American curve is justifiable in Italy, only because of our lack of a national standard. It was, therefore, necessary to carefully prepare an intra-uterine growth curve based on the data obtained in the city of Parma, and its environs. All the patients used are from the Institute for Child-welfare and Neonatal Medicine, Parma, and the newborn infants from the Clinic of Obstetrics and Gynaecology, from November 1970 to February 1973. A short but recent period has been chosen in order to avoid any eventual variation that might spoil the sample.

7.008 unselected neonates were used for the sample. The Institute for Child-welfare treats all abnormal newborn infants for the city and suburbs, being the only neonatal unit in the enitre zone. The Obstetric Clinic treats unselected pregnancies, which constitute a fairly representative sample of both city and area. Sufficient data was obtained to plot a weight curve from the 28th to 43rd weeks.

The gestation age was calculated from the first day of the last regular menstrual cycle of the mother and is calculated in weeks. The weight was obtained from the clinic card. About 1.500 cases were discarded: those cases in which it was not possible to have exact dates concerning the duration of pregnancy and all cases in which the weights within the first 12 hours of life were not available. Furthermore, all newborn infants with malformations that could affect the weight (hydrocephalic, anencephalic, etc.) twins, children of different nationalities were rejected. We included the newborn infants of mothers who were pre-diabetic or diabetic.

The curves have been plotted according to the method used by LUBCHENCO; plotting for every week of gestation single cases and successively considering the 10 % of the lowest weight of each week of gestation as the 10th percentile; likewise as has been done for the other percentage values.

Table 1 represents the gestation age from the 28th to 43rd weeks, the average weight, values and the weight for the 10th, 25th, 50th, 75th, 90th percentiles of 3.421 newborn female infants. Table 2 represents the average values for the 3.667 male infants.

Table 1. Intra-uterine growth standard: females

Gestational age (wk)	No. of cases	Mean weight	Percentiles 10th	25th	50th	75th	90th
28	6	812	600	720	800	850	940
29	7	1185	700	1000	1150	1400	1400
30	12	1604	1040	1400	1500	1650	1810
31	13	1626	930	1150	1550	1700	2295
32	27	1890	1470	1700	1800	2000	2330
33	34	1985	1500	1800	2000	2200	2360
34	45	2361	1700	2000	2100	2600	3200
35	65	2403	1700	2100	2400	2690	2925
36	111	2592	2000	2300	2575	2850	3190
37	154	2889	2100	2525	2800	3100	3450
38	323	3022	2265	2700	3000	3300	3650
39	653	3248	2750	3000	3250	3500	3750
40	1019	3400	2900	3100	3400	3650	3950
41	744	3425	2900	3150	3400	3650	4000
42	162	3477	2900	3100	3450	3750	4000
43	31	3456	2720	3075	3400	3575	4130

Table 2. Intra-uterine growth standard: males

Gestational age (wk)	No. of cases	Mean weight	Percentiles 10th	25th	50th	75th	90th
28	8	1037	800	850	1000	1100	1180
29	13	1484	1000	1125	1350	1800	2070
30	22	1709	1320	1400	1500	1600	2810
31	26	1769	1400	1500	1800	1900	2110
32	26	2092	1460	1850	2000	2300	2550
33	42	2103	1700	1800	2000	2250	2780
34	51	2227	1610	2000	2200	2500	2690
35	71	2551	2110	2300	2500	2800	3000
36	124	2700	2120	2400	2650	3000	3300
37	201	2922	2200	2600	2925	3400	3700
38	375	3141	2400	2850	3200	3450	3750
39	735	3380	2850	3100	3350	3650	3900
40	1060	3545	3000	3250	3550	3850	4100
41	707	3581	3000	3300	3400	3700	3850
42	176	3569	2950	3250	3600	3900	4200
43	21	3561	2610	3250	3600	3900	4300

In Fig. 1 the graphic representation of percentiles for both sexes is shown together; the curves were interpolated by means of a calculator with a polynomial of 4° degrees. From the analysis of the reported data a few deductions can be drawn; no substantial weight differences exist between the male and female infants even if the values of the latter tend to be slightly less than the male values in the corresponding gestational age.

Such differences rarely exceed 100 grams. This data allows consideration of males and females together in order to obtain a more representative sample.

Comparing the percentile curves for both sexes, of Parma and Colorado, the principal observation is that LUBCHENCO's figures were drawn from a neonatal clinic, and in some way they could represent a selected

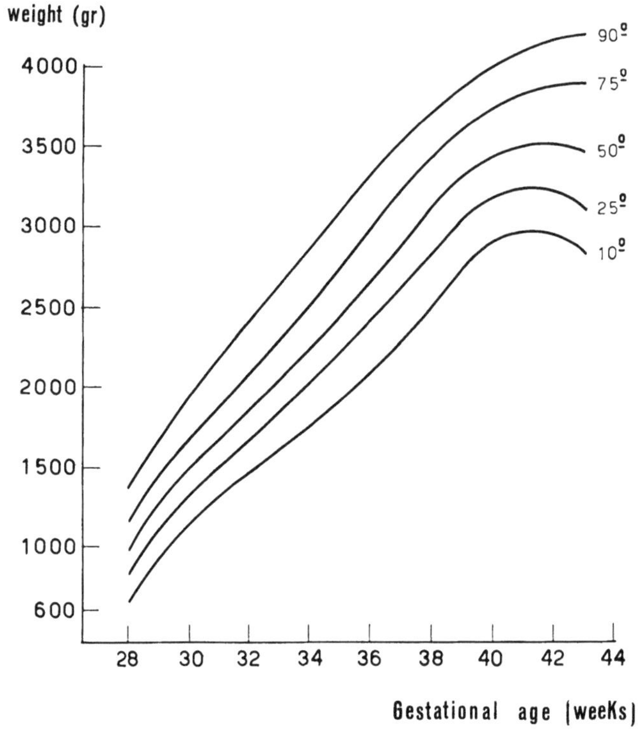

Fig. 1. Smoothed curves values for the percentiles of birth weight against gestational age of the neonates in Parma. Males and females are plotted together

sample, because fetal abnormalities might have influenced the weights. Eighty percent of our figures were taken from the nursery for normal newborn. Comparing the Parma and Denver curves we were struck by the lack of deflections between the 32nd and 35th week of gestation in the LUBCHENCO curve. Perhaps these deflections reflected serious fetal pathology.

The average weight of our infants with a gestation age of 40 weeks results in a weight higher by 244 g compared with the neonates of the same gestation age in Denver (3.474 g against 3.232 g).

The average weight in Parma is also higher than those noted by GRUENWALD in Baltimore (3.318 g) and slightly higher than those in Birmingham which were 3.434 g (MC KEOWN-GIBSON, 1951). Differences of the same order are found at 42 weeks of gestation. Our data did not support the idea of the existance of weight differences between different geographical conditions. LUBCHENCO suggested that the high altitude (over 10.000 ft) from which 30 % of the cases came may have had an effect in keeping the average values low. It is also possible that socio-economic and racial factors may also have influenced these differences.

The difference in weights from population to population confirms the usefulness of different standard curves according to the different local conditions. As the province of Parma is mainly agricultural with an almost negligible immigration and has average socio-economic conditions for Northern Italy, one can reasonably hold that the sample obtained would be applicable to other Italian zones where the curve could be used for clinical practice.

References

1. American Academy of Pediatrics. Committee on fetus and newborn. Nomenclature for duration of gestation, birth weight and intra-uterine growth. Pediatrics 39, 935 (1967).
2. BABSON, S. G.: Growth of low-birth-weight infants. J. Pediat. 77, 11 (1970).
3. GRUENWALD, P.: Chronic fetal distress and placental insufficiency. Biol. Neonat. 5, 215 (1963).
4. LUBCHENCO, L. O., HAUSMAN, C., DRESSLER, M., BOYD, E.: Intra-uterine growth as estimated from liveborn birth-weight data at 24 to 42 weeks of gestation. Pediatrics 32, 793 (1963).
5. MC KEOWN, T., GIBSON, J. R.: Observations on all births (23, 970) in Birmingham, 1947. IV., "Premature birth". Brit. Med. J. 2, 513 (1951).
6. USHER, R., MC LEAN, F.: Intra-uterine growth of live-born caucasian infants at sea level: standards obtained from measurements in 7 dimensions of infants born between 25 and 44 weeks of gestation. J. Pediat. 74, 901 (1969).
7. YERUSHALMY, J.: The classification of newborn infants by birth weight and gestational age. J. Pediat. 71, 164 (1967).

Maternal Hypertonic Dextrose Infusion in a Patient with Idiopathic Recurrent Placental Insufficiency and Low Urinary Oestrogens

S. N. Campbell, J. D. Andrew, and D. Donaldson

Maternal urinary oestrogen assay is an accepted method of assessing placental function and foetal well-being. Low values may reflect intra uterine growth retardation (IGR), (1). In apparently normal pregnancy, idiopathic IGR or previous unexplained foetal loss, which may recur, may be related to low fasting blood sugar levels and a flat glucose tolerance curve (2, 3).

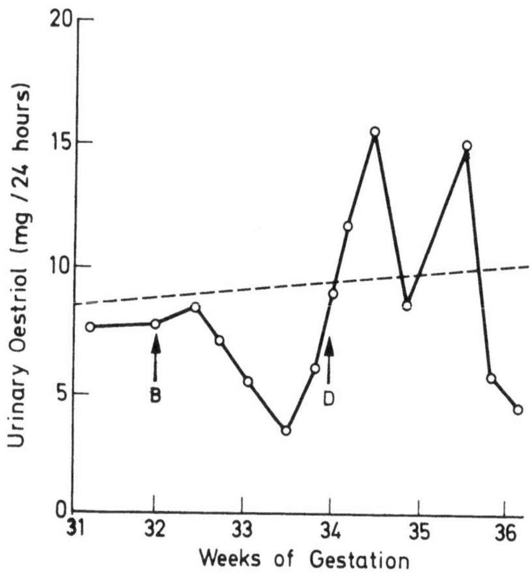

Fig. 1

In IGR, there is an absence of umbilical veno-arterial difference in glucose levels (4). In normal labour, maternal glucose load increases the normal umbilical veno-arterial difference in glucose levels (9). Foetal insulin, which may stimulate foetal growth (5), responds to maternal glucose load (6, 7).

Intrapartum and perinatal mortality of IGR with prematurity is high (8). Intra-uterine feeding, to gain maturity and improve foetal condition, merits attention.

Case Summary

A 32 year old secundigravida, with previous foetal loss associated with IGR, was admitted at 32 weeks gestation with a fundus of 30 weeks and a low oestrogen value of 7.5 mg/24 hours; otherwise the pregnancy was normal. An oral glucose tolerance test (50 g) revealed blood glucose values of 65 mg/100 ml (fasting) 80, 87, 100, 57 mg/100 ml at half hourly intervals; glycosuria occurred when fasting, and at one and two hours.

After two weeks bed rest, urine oestrogen values had fallen serially to 3.6 mg/24 hours and fundal height was static. Foetal palpation induced bradycardia. At 34.0 weeks, 4 litres of 25 % dextrose were infused by maternal intravenous administration, continuously for 48 hours, in addition to normal diet (2).

During infusion, maternal blood glucose levels ranged between 85 and 110 mg/100 ml, an average increase of 45 % above ante natal fasting levels and glycosuria was not detected. Urine oestrogen values increased immediately to 9.8 and 11.3 mg/24 hours. The patient volunteered that breast secretions and a 'sense of pregnancy' had returned, having subsided four weeks beforehand, as occurred prior to previous intra-uterine death. Foetal movements immediately became 'more purposeful'. Urine oestrogen levels further improved to 15.8 mg/24 hours and were sustained for eight days before serial subsidence to 3.6 mg/24 hours at 36.1 weeks. The symptoms of pregnancy and foetal movements followed the pattern of oestrogen excretion. By this time foetal growth seemed clinically to have increased. A post infusion glucose tolerance test at 35.3 weeks had produced levels of 60 (fasting), 76, 132, 130, and 84 mg/100 ml, without glycosuria.

At 36.3 weeks, a healthy but dysmature infant, weighing 2557 g, was delivered at elective Caesarean section, the circumvallate placenta weighing 545 g.

Neonatal hypoglycaemia did not occur. Birth weight had doubled at eight weeks, when maternal glucose tolerance test was 82 (fasting), 113, 122, 80 and 82 mg/100 ml, again without glycosuria.

Restoration of pregnancy symptoms with increased urinary oestrogen implies improved foeto-placental metabolism. Maintenance of improved levels for two weeks only, unlike other recorded cases (2) suggests that administration of 1000 G glucose overcame placental insufficiency temporarily. It has been estimated that 80 G glucose crosses the placenta daily for foetal energy requirements during normal pregnancy (9).

The hypothesis that low fasting blood sugars and flat glucose tolerance curves are related to idiopathic IGR implies that maternal adaptation to pituitary, adrenal, pancreatic and placental hormones may lead to disordered glucose homeostasis. This could result in glucose levels inadequate for normal foeto-placental metabolism, including early glycogen synthesis and storage.

Non recurrence of IGR in subsequent pregnancies suggests the importance of the individual placental factors in disordering glucose homeostasis, whereas recurrence suggests the possibility of a primary disorder in maternal glucose homeostasis.

Such disordered glucose homeostasis may be affected by inadequate first trimester absorption of glucose and amino acids (11) or undetected intermittent glycosuria in late pregnancy (12).

Absolute hypoglycaemia (<45 mg/100 ml) may not occur. Foetoplacental disturbance perhaps occurs at slightly higher glucose levels. Glucose levels <60 mg/100 ml are common in pregnancy and the pregnancy fasting level is normally about 10 mg/100 ml lower than in the non pregnant state (11).

Wide individual variation in glucose tolerance curves during normal pregnancy (13) may cause difficulty in reproduction of the flat curve. This perhaps reflects the truly fluctuating biological situation. The flat curve is more common in early pregnancy and may reflect an over vigorous maternal insulin response to pregnancy (11). Hypertonic dextrose infusion may symptomatically restore adequate glucose levels.

In conclusion, idiopathic IGR may be related to a disorder of maternal glucose hoemostasis; hypertonic dextrose infusion may contribute to foetal survival and consequent improved growth may enable safer delivery.

References

1. BEISCHER, N. A., BROWN, J. B.: Obstetrics and Gynaecology Survey 27, 303.
2. BEISCHER, N. A., O' SULLIVAN, E. F.: American Journal of Obstetrics and Gynaecology 113, 823 (1972).
3. CAMPBELL, N., PYKE, D. A., TAYLOR, R. W.: Journal of Obstetrics and Gynaecology of the British Commonwealth 78, 498 (1971).
4. MELICHAN, NOVAK, KAHN: Intra-uterine dangers to the foetus. Excerpta Medical Foundation. (Editors J. HORSKY and S. K. STEMBERA) (1967).
5. LITTLE, W. A., NASSER, D., SPELLACY, W. N.: American Journal of Obstetrics and Gynaecology 109, 732 (1971).
6. CRENSHAW, C., Jr.: Clinical Obstetrics and Gynaecology 13, 579 (1970).
7. COLTART, T. H., BEARD, R. W., TURNER, R. C., OAKLEY, N. W.: British Medical Journal 4, 17 (1969).
8. LUGO, G., CASSADY, G.: Amercian Journal of Obstetrics and Gynaecology 109, 615 (1971).
9. SHEATH, J., GRIMWADE, J., WALDRON, K., BICKLEY, M., TAFT, P., WOOD, C.: American Journal of Obstetrics and Gynaecology 113, 358 (1972).
10. MARKS, V.: British Medical Journal 1, 430 (1972).
11. HYTTEN, F. E., LEITCH, I.: The Physiology of Human Pregnancy (1971).
12. LIND, T., HYTTEN, F. E.: Journal of Obstetrics and Gynaecology of the British Commonwealth 76, 961 (1972).
13. LIND, T., CHEYNE, G. A., BILLEWICZ, W. Z., FAIRWEATHER, D. V. I.: Journal of Obstetrics and Gynaecology of the British Commonwealth 75, 540.

Improvements in Uterine-Placental Blood-Flow by Long-Term Treatment of EPH-Gestosis with Anti-Hypertensive Drugs

F. Nagl, O. Dubler, and E. Hochuli

We have shown in EPH-gestosis that the renal blood-flow can be improved by Reserpine and 1.4-Dihydrophthalazin (5) if the blood pressure is reduced slowly (see Figs. 1 and 2).

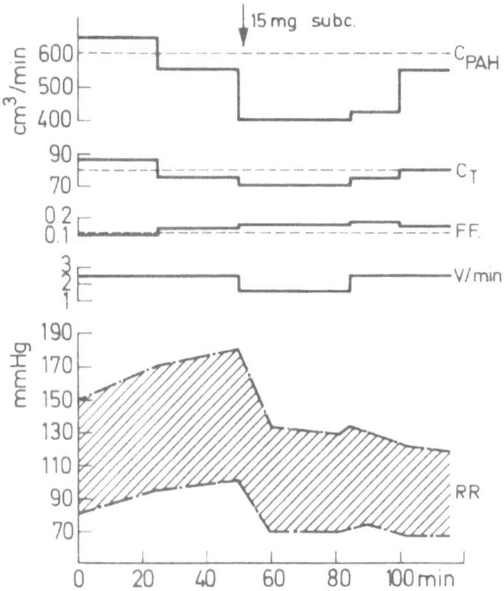

Fig. 1

BROWN and MORRIS (2) also showed an improvement in reduced uterine-placental blood-flow in gestosis (1, 3, 9) with antihypertensive therapy. From these results we suggest that blood-flow to the kidneys, placenta and uterus can probably be improved during pregnancy by a long-term-medication with hypotensive drugs. This is being shown in the following study (see Fig. 3).

In a woman who had chronic pyelonephritis and suffered an intra-uterine death of the foetus during the first pregnancy, renal function was not further reduced by long-term hypotensive treatment during the following pregnancy (6).

In case of chronic hypertension, especially of high diastolic pressure, the uterine-placental circulation is probably already lowered at a very early stage. This leads to irreversible damage of the uterine-placental vessels, as LUDWIG showed with the aid of an electron microscope (8). Hoping to prevent these alterations of the vessels and thus

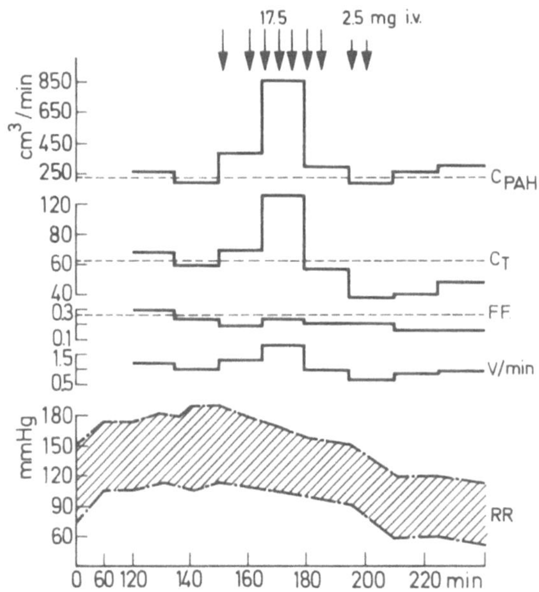

Fig. 2

maintain a sufficient blood-flow from the beginning, we started hypotensive treatment before the 24th week of pregnancy. We chose a diastolic pressure of 90 and a systolic blood-pressure of 150 mm/Hg as therapeutic indications. These blood-pressure figures are derived from BROWNS's diagrams (4), which show that perinatal mortality increases if the diastolic pressure is above 85 - 90 and the systolic pressure is above 150 - 170 mm/Hg (see Figs. 4 and 5).

Results

From January, 1963 to April, 1973 we treated 64 pregnant patients with pre-existing hypertension and controlled their blood pressure continously (see Table 1).

Table 1

Number of cases		64
Hospitalisation during pregnancy		9
Hypotensiv therapy sub partu		7
Delivery spontaneous	42	
operativ vaginal	10	
abdominal	12	
Average of birth weight		3053
Dysmaturity		1
Average of weight of placenta		570
Perinatal death		2

In 7 cases additional hypotensive medication had to be given during delivery. 42 women delivered spontaneously, 22 were delivered by operative procedures (10 vaginal and 12 abdominal). The frequency of

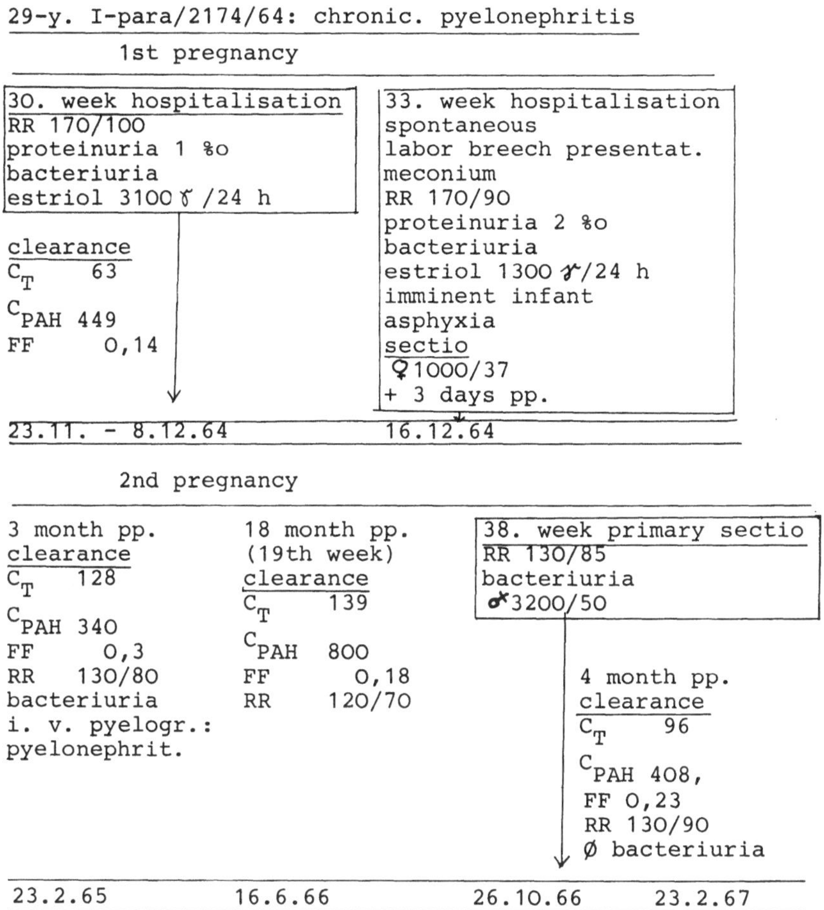
29-y. I-para/2174/64: chronic. pyelonephritis
1st pregnancy
30. week hospitalisation
RR 170/100
proteinuria 1 ‰
bacteriuria
estriol 3100 γ /24 h
clearance
C_T 63
C_PAH 449
FF 0,14
33. week hospitalisation
spontaneous
labor breech presentat.
meconium
RR 170/90
proteinuria 2 ‰
bacteriuria
estriol 1300 γ/24 h
imminent infant
asphyxia
sectio
♀1000/37
+ 3 days pp.
23.11. - 8.12.64
16.12.64
2nd pregnancy
3 month pp.
clearance
C_T 128
C_PAH 340
FF 0,3
RR 130/80
bacteriuria
i. v. pyelogr.:
pyelonephrit.
18 month pp.
(19th week)
clearance
C_T 139
C_PAH 800
FF 0,18
RR 120/70
38. week primary sectio
RR 130/85
bacteriuria
♂3200/50
4 month pp.
clearance
C_T 96
C_PAH 408,
FF 0,23
RR 130/90
Ø bacteriuria
23.2.65
16.6.66
26.10.66
23.2.67

Fig. 3

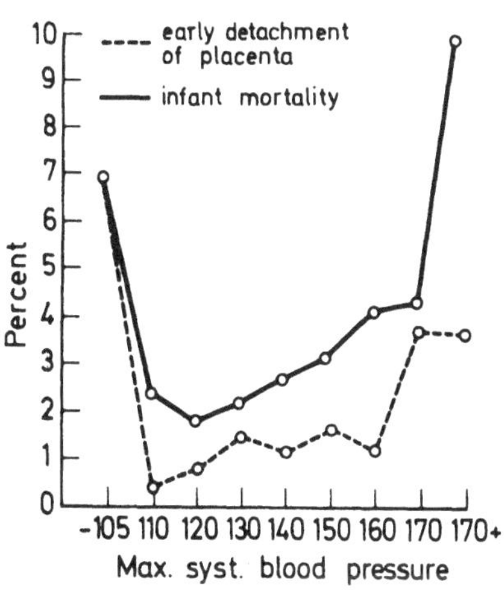
early detachment of placenta
infant mortality
Percent
0
1
2
3
4
5
6
7
8
9
10
-105 110 120 130 140 150 160 170 170+
Max. syst. blood pressure

Fig. 4

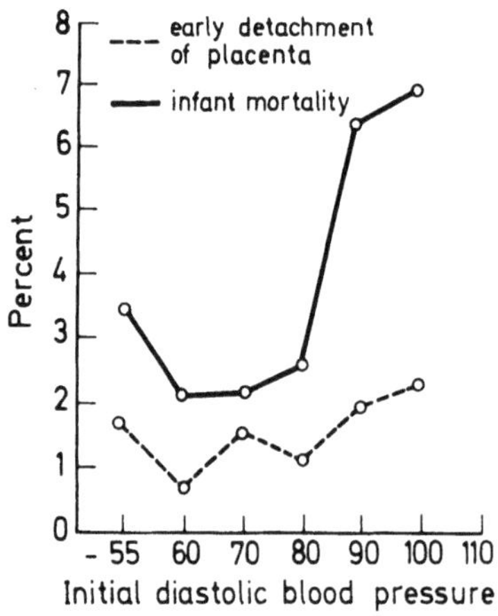

Fig. 5

intervention is high in this group. In only a third of these operatively-delivered cases, is there a causal connection between operative delivery and gestosis. The birth-weight (of those who were born alive including 4 premature births and one twin-birth) was 3053 g (between the 25th and 50th percentile of birth-weight at term). Only in one case did the neonate have signs suggesting "small for dates". The average weight of the placenta was normal at 570 g. There were two fetal deaths. In one case the mother, pregnant for the first time, was 25 years old, had pyelonephritis and was sub-fertile for one and a half years. Hypotensive control was difficult and the fetus died in the 33rd week of pregnancy. It weighed 860 g and was 35 cm long. The placenta weighed 135 g and had many infarcts). In the second case of fetal death, the hypertension was adequately controlled with reserpin (0.25 - 0.50 mg/day) but the fetus died in the 30th week of pregnancy. In this case, this may have been an acute exacerbation of a basic disease (possibly a phaechromocytoma) which was not diagnosed. These studies show that not all cases are successful. Fig. 6 shows one successful treated case with a severe primary hypertension.

The diagram shows our treatment using a combined preparation. Fig. 7 shows the child's growth in this case, assessed by ultrasonic measurements of the skull and the 24-hour urinary oestriol-excretion.

Conclusion

Our results in patients with bad medical histories are satisfactory. In our hands the perinatal mortality does not worsen with long-term treatment with hypotensive drugs, contrary to LANDESMANN's views (7). We did not notice any side effects of the hypotensives on the neonates. The mothers infrequently mentioned side effects due to the medication. The frequency of hospital admissions could be kept low during pregnancy with only 9 out of 64 cases admitted.

In our opinion long-term hypotensive treatment during pregnancy is, among other measures, of value to both mothers and children.

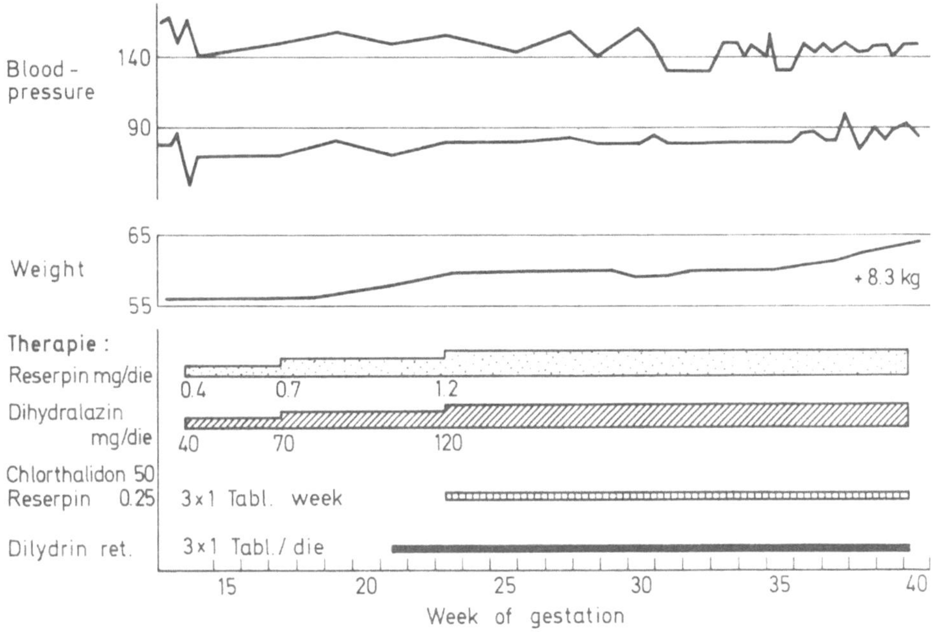

Blood - pressure
140
90
Weight
65
55
+ 8.3 kg
Therapie :
Reserpin mg/die
0.4
0.7
1.2
Dihydralazin mg/die
40
70
120
Chlorthalidon 50
Reserpin 0.25
3 x 1 Tabl. week
Dilydrin ret.
3 x 1 Tabl. / die
15
20
25
30
35
40
Week of gestation

Fig. 6

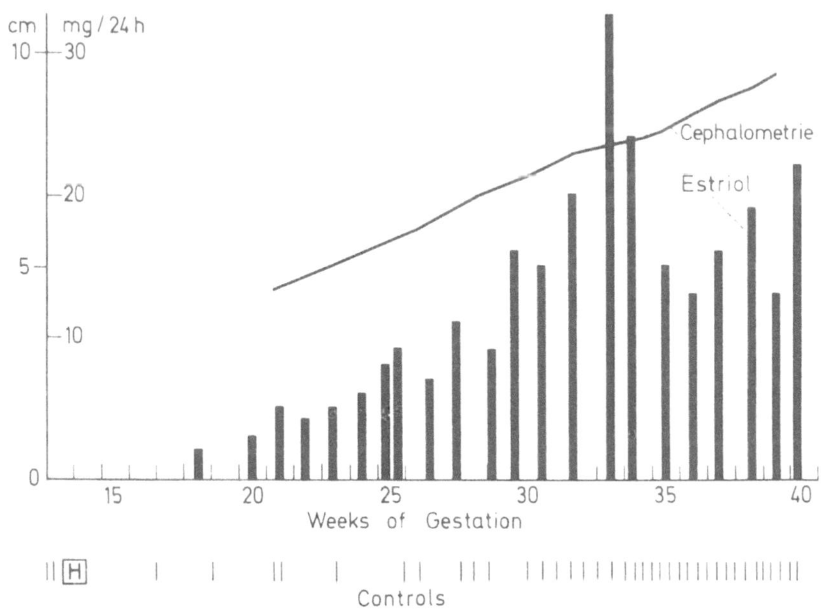

cm
mg / 24 h
10
30
20
5
10
0
Cephalometrie
Estriol
15
20
25
30
35
40
Weeks of Gestation
H
Controls

Fig. 7

References

1. ASSALI, N. S.: Measurement of uterine blood flow and uterine metabolism. Amer. J. Obstet. Gynec. 66, 3 (1953).
2. BROWNE, F. J.: Reaction to pressor substances in normal and toxaemic women. J. Obstet. Gynaec. Brit. Emp. 50, 254 (1943).
3. BROWNE, J. C. M., VEALL, N.: Maternal placental blood flow in normotensive and hypertensive women. J. Obstet. Gynaec. Brit. Emp. 60, 141 (1953).
4. BROWNE, J. C. M.: Survey of eclampsia; clinical aspects. Path. Microbiol. 24, 542 (1961).
5. HOCHULI, E.: Der Einfluß verschiedener hypotensiver Substanzen auf die Nieren-Clearence bei Schwangerschaftstoxikosen. Diss. Univ. Basel. Schwabe u. Co. Verlag 1955.
6. HOCHULI, E., WEICHE, V.: Zur Dauermedikation mit hypotensiven Substanzen in graviditate. Geburtsh. u. Frauenheilk. 1, 32 (1972).
7. LANDESMANN, R., MC LAREN, W. D., OLLSTEIN, R. N., MENDELSOHN, B.: Reserpin in toxaemia of pregnancy. Obstet. Gynaec. 9, 377 (1957).
8. LUDWIG, H.: Surface structure of the human term placenta and of the uterine wall post partum in the screen scan electron microscope. Amer. J. Obstet. Gynec. 111, 328 (1971).
9. MORRIS, N., HART, A.: Effective uterine blood-flow during exercise in normal and pre-eclamptic pregnancies. Lancet II, 481 (1956).

Vasoactive or Phosphorilated Glycide Therapy in Placental Insufficiency

P. Grella and E. Zardini

We have studied the effects of two treatment regimes in placental insufficiency. The first regime improves placental blood flow and the second stimulates placental metabolism of 1.6 diphosphate fructose.

We have assessed effects of treatment by radio-immunoassay of human chorionic gonadotrophin (HCG) and human placental lactogen (HPL) using Serono and Scavo kits. Normal values for HCG and HPL have been taken from the literature and from our own figures obtained from sera of normal pregnant females. We have treated those patients in whom the titre of HPL and HCG was below the second standard deviation (2 SD). As controls, we treated patients with normal titres of HPL and HCG.

Treatment

Two groups were selected. The first group received a mixture of Isoxuprine 50 mg, Xantinol Nicotinate 900 mg and Dipiridamal 100 mg (I.X.D.) made up in 500 ml 5 % glucose and given intravenously, daily, for seven days. The second group received 10 g of 1.6 diphosphate fructose (D. F.) intravenously, daily, for seven days.

Results

We have treated too few patients for a statistical evaluation to be possible. Using the I. X. D. regime in six cases the titre of HPL has increased by 27 % and the HCG titre by a mean of 30 %, in four patients. No change occurred in the other two patients. In the D. F. group, HPL increased by a mean of 24 %, and HCG by 12 %.

Conclusions

We tentatively suggest that treatment with 1.6 diphosphate fructose is superior to hypertonic dextrose with insulin and also to beta-mimetic drugs for placental insufficiency. In D. F. the sugar is already phosphorilated and hence can be better taken up by the placenta. There is evidence of abnormal carbohydrate metabolism in placental insufficiency - low fasting blood sugars and flat glucose tolerance curves. It is possible that D. F. would enter directly into placental anaerobic glycolisis to supply energy rich phosphate bonds. We also avoid the possible hazards of insulin therapy.

Effects of Synthetic Luteinizing Hormone-Releasing Hormone (LH-RH) on Serum Gonadotrophin, Prolactin and Chorionic Somatomammotrophin (HCS) during the Last Trimester of Pregnancy

P. Pujol-Amat, O. Gamissans, L. Cabero, P. P. Pérez-López,
E. Benito, J. Calaf, and C. Robyn

Intravenous injection of the synthetic decapeptide corresponding to LH-RH isolated from porcine hypothalami induces the release of both luteinizing hormone (LH) and follicle stimulating hormone (FSH) in men and non-pregnant women (SCHALLY et al. 1973). So far, no data on the effect of synthetic LH-RH during pregnancy have been reported. We have investigated whether synthetic LH-RH affects serum concentration of gonadotrophins, prolactin and HCS in pregnant women.

Ten women with normal pregnancies were investigated between the 30th and 40th weeks of gestation. One case of severe iso-immunisation, one case of pre-eclamptic toxaemia and one case of diabetes corresponding to class B of WHITE's classification (1949) were also tested during same period of pregnancy.

Synthetic LH-RH was kindly supplied by Farbwerke Hoechst (Frankfurt am Main, Germany). 100 µg was dissolved in 2 ml saline and injected intravenously within 1 minute. In all cases the injection of LH-RH took place at 12 a. m. Blood was collected before the injection at 30, 15 and at zero time. Samples were then taken at 5, 10, 20, 45, 60, 75, 90, 105 and 120 minutes later. Serum was separated by centrifugation after overnight storage at 4° C and stored at -20° C before being assayed. Prolactin, HCG, FSH and HCS were measured by radioimmunoassays using the double antibody technique (L'HERMITE et al. 1972; ROBYN et al. 1971; ODELL and HESCOX 1971; FRIESEN et al. 1970).

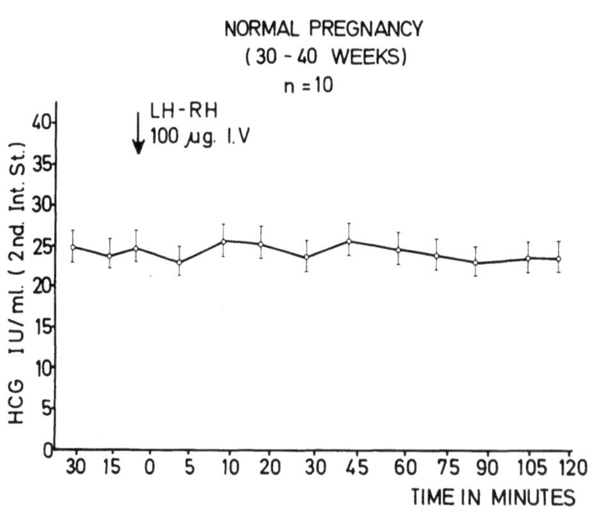

Fig. 1. Effect of LH-RH administration in serum concentration of HCG during the last trimester of normal pregnancy (Mean ± S.E.M.)

Prolactin results were expressed in mU; 1.0 mU is the amount of prolactin contained in 1.0 μl of a pool of sera rich in prolactin. For HCG and FSH the results were expressed in mIU with reference to the Second International Standard of HCG and to the Second International Reference Preparation of Human Menopausal Gonadotrophins, respectively. For HCS the results were expressed in μg of a laboratory standard (HCS, Biochemical Nutritional. USA). For each hormone, all the samples of the same woman were tested at the same assay. The assay results were calculated on a CDC 6400 computer according to RODBARD et al. (1968). No changes in serum levels of HCG or HCS occurred. The FSH values were very low, frequently under 1.0 mlU/ml. In only 5 out of 10 women with a normal pregnancy was there a minor increase in serum FSH between 5 and 45 minutes after injection. No significant variation in serum prolactin concentration was induced by the exogenous LH-RH. Also in the three pathological cases, no significant variations in serum HCG, FSH, prolactin or HCS have been found after LH-RH injection.

It can be concluded that during the last trimester of pregnancy a dose of 100 μg of LH-RH does not affect serum concentration of gonadotrophins. Thus, it seems that LH-RH does not influence the secretion of HCG by the trophoblast. Suppresion of FSH release could be due to a refractoriness of the releasing hormone of the pituitary gonadotrophic cells during pregnancy. An alternative explanation would be a much shorter half-life of LH-RH in the circulation related to a much higher aminopeptidase activity found in blood during gestation.

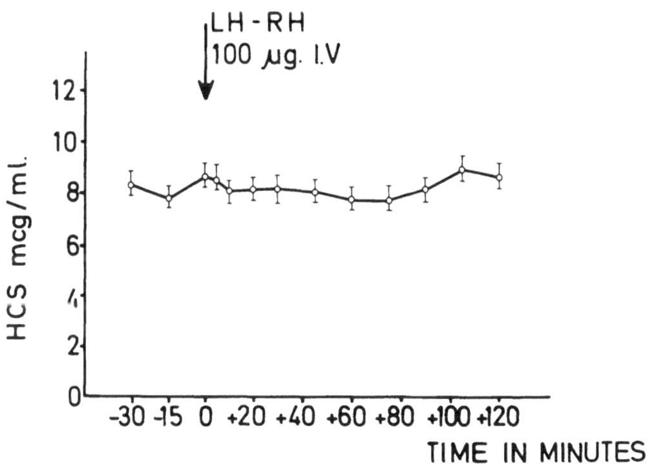

Fig. 2. Effect of LH-RH administration on serum concentration of HCS during the last trimester of normal pregnancy (Mean ± S.E.M.; n = 10)

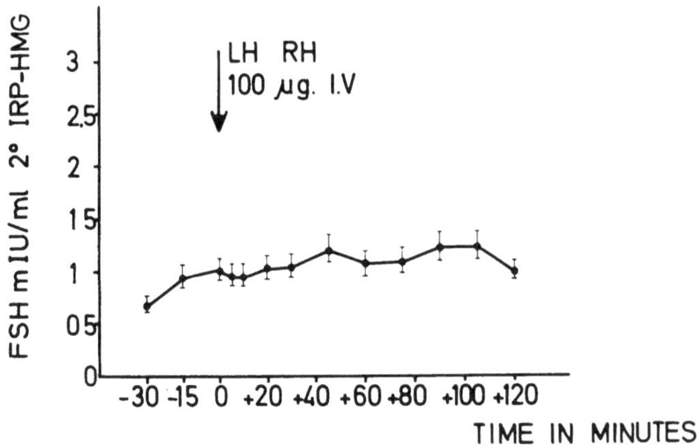

Fig. 3. Effect of LH-RH administration on serum concentration of FSH during the last trimester of normal pregnancy (Mean ± S.E.M.; n = 10)

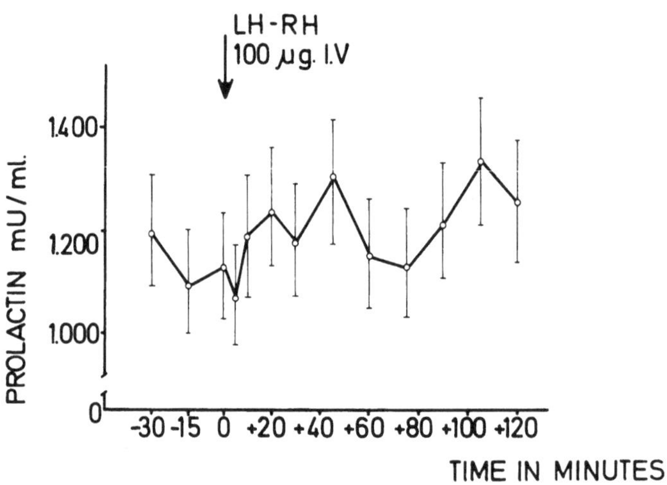

Fig. 4. Effect of LH-RH administration on serum concentration of prolactin, during the last trimester of normal pregnancy (Mean ± S. E. M.; n = 10)

References

L'HERMITE, M., DELVOYE, P., NOKIN, L., VEKEMANS, M., ROBYN, C.: Human Prolactin secretion, as studied by radioimmunoassay: some aspects of its regulation. A. O. A. Publishing. Prolactin and carcinogenesis (4th Tenovus workshop). Cardiff U. K. 1972.

ODELL, W. D., HESCOX, M. A.: Structure and activity relationships of Protein and Polypeptide hormones I.C.S. 241. M. MARGOULIES and F. C. GREENWOOD. Ed. Excerpta Medica Foundation. Amsterdam. P. 139.

ROBYN, C., L'HERMITE, M., PETRUTZ, P., DICZFALUZY, E.: Acta endocrinologica (Kbh) 67, 417 (1971).

RODBARD, D., RAYFORD, P. L., COOPER, J. A., ROSS, G. T.: Statistical quality control of Radioimmunoassay. Jelin Endocrinol. Metab. 28, 1412 (1968).
SCHALLY, A. V., ARIMURA, A., KASTIN, A. J.: Hypothalamic regulatory Hormones. Science Vol. 179, 241 (1973).
WHITE, P.: Pregnancy complicating diabetes. Am. J. Med. 7, 609 (1949).

Trial of Treatment of Chronic Fetal Distress by Naftidrofuryl

J. M. Thoulon

Using Naftidrofuryl (Praxilene) as a treatment of premature labour, an increase in urinary oestriol has been noted. I have used this vasodilating and utero-relaxing drug as a treatment of chronic fetal distress.

Three groups of patients were treated because of high risk pregnancies (diabetes, premature labour, 'small for date' babies) or abnormal levels of urinary oestriol.

Groups I (19 cases) and II (20 cases) were treated with an intravenous infusion of 8 ampoules of Naftidrofuryl in 500 ml of 5 % dextrose over 3 to 4 hours. Urinary oestriol concentration was measured before the treatment, and over the day following the treatment. The effect of treatment was assessed by measuring the urinary oestriol level. In group II, a double-blind method was used. In groupIII the infusion was maintained for 5 days. Urinary oestriol was measured over two days and the day before the beginning of treatment and over the third and fourth day of the infusion, and finally the day following the end of treatment.

Results of group I. In 10 cases out of 19, urinary oestriol increased more than 30 per cent, in 5 cases the increase lay between 0 to 30 per cent and in 4 cases there was no alteration.

Results of group II. Control series (9 cases): in 3 cases the urinary oestriol increase was more than 30 per cent, in 3 cases it was between 0 and 30 % and in 3 cases there was no alteration. In the Naftidrofuryl-treated patients (11 cases), 1 patient showed an increase of 30 %, 5 patients showed an increase of between 0 - 30 %, and in 4 cases there was no change.

Results of group III (19 patients; 24 infusions). In 14 cases the increase was more than 30 %; it was between 0 and 30 % in 3 cases and no increase occurred in seven patients. Of these seven patients five had 'small for date' babies. The Naftidrofuryl effect is transitory. In 11 cases out of 13, urinary oestriol decreased in 2 to 4 days following the last infusion. In 12 cases I noted an increase in urinary oestriol. In 11 cases a falling excretion could be made to rise.

To summarise, Praxilene increases urinary oestriol excretion although the mechanism is unknown and this may be without any fetal benefit. Multiple infusions produce a greater oestriol excretion. The results is transitory but with Praxilene a falling concentration may rise.

The biochemical results were good in the presence of toxaemia or a premature labour, but no change occurred in cases of 'small for date' babies. More work may show whether an increased urinary oestriol is of any benefit to the fetus.

Chronic Fetal Distress. Research on Placental Blood Flow and Therapy

G. Pontonnier, H. Grandjean, M. F. Sarramon, J. Degoy,
R. Guiraud, and R. Favretto

Introduction

The importance of placental haemodynamic disturbances in causing chronic foetal distress is today widely acknowledged among obstetricians. The result is that numerous drugs, supposedly active on the placental circulation, are suggested as therapy for chronic fetal distress.

But in our present state of knowledge it seems very difficult to demonstrate objectively the effect of such a drug or of any other factor (tobacco, physical exercise, for example) upon the growth and vitality of the human foetus in utero.

It would therefore be very interesting to use a method which allows the absolute or relative measurement of the placental circulation in order to verify the haemodynamic effect of the treatments which are regularly suggested.

It is with this hope, speaking more of the method rather than the results, that I am taking the liberty of publishing the research of my team working on the placental circulation.

Methods of Studying the Placental Haemodynamics

The exact measurement of the blood flow of an organ can be made only if the organ has a single feed artery and if one can measure the quantity of blood which passes through it within a given period of time. This anatomical arrangement is rarely encountered in human medicine where the measurement of visceral flow remains accordingly far from perfect. With the placenta the problem is still more complex as this organ is made up of two juxtaposed circulatory systems, the one foetal and inaccessible to clinical examination, the other maternal, i. e. the intervillous space which is fed by a multitude of arterioles. These arterioles stem indirectly from the different arteries which supply the uterus; the percentage of blood in these arteries which ends up in the placenta is unknown.

This anatomical peculiarity explains why it has never been possible to measure the placental flow during human pregnancy. Three sorts of attempt have been made:

METCALFE and ASSALI calculated the quantity of blood supplying the whole of the uterus, foetus and adnexa using a gas tracer, nitrous oxide (N 2O). One of the many negative aspects of this method is that of not distinguishing the placental flow from the flow of the other ovular centres; after all, it is mainly the placental flow which it is interesting to know, for it is closely connected with the state of the foetus in utero.

MC CLURE and WEALL, in order to overcome this shortcoming, measured the placental clearance of sodium 24. But this isotope is a poor tracer for haemodynamic studies as it is not biologically inert.

More recently VASICKA and then HINSELMAN and LIPPERT measured the variations in the volume of the intervillous space. The variations after injecting vasomotor drugs could make up a test of the placental haemodynamics. The studies are still only preliminary and deserve being followed up.

Personal Works

Scope

We ourselves carried out this research to produce an index of the placental circulation by measuring the clearance of Xenon 133. The method is based upon the principle of KETTY and SCHMIDT, according to which the elimination of a tracer which is biologically inert when injected into a tissue is a function of the flow of that tissue.

As the tracer we chose Xenon 133 which is:
-biologically inert,
-rapidly diffused,
-eliminated after its first pulmonary passage,
which avoids the inconvenience of recirculation of the tracer and explains the mild dose of radioactivity encountered during measurement.

Method

As a first stage the placenta is located ultrasonically or by low powered profile X-ray which shows well the opacity of the placenta in relation to surrounding soft parts if it is in a frontal position.

If the placenta is in a frontal position a dose of 250 microcuries of Xenon 133 in liquid form is injected transabdominally into the intervillous space.

A scintillation detector placed facing the point of injection registers the decrease in radioactivity at this level. It is connected to a recorder.

A curve is obtained of the basically bi-exponential kind with an initial phase of rapid ascent and a second phase of slow fall. These two phases appear clearly as semilogarithmic coordinates. The placental clearance is calculated from the first phase when it is enough to measure the slope to arrive at the local flow which is expressed in ml/100 g/min or in T 1/2.

Measurement

- 75 measurements were made during normal pregnancy.
- 127 measurements were made during pathological pregnancy.
- 15 measurements were repeated at 15 minute intervals on the same woman.

Results

In normal pregnancy the mean value for local placental flow is 135 ml $\pm$ 47/100 g/min from the 28th to the 41st week.

As can be seen from Table 1, the mean value for the placental clearance of Xenon 133 is lower and statistically significantly so in all the pathological groups studied, except in cases of moderate permanent hypertension. But as is shown by the magnitude of standard deviation, there are major variations from one measurement to another.

Table 1. Mean values during pathologic pregnancies

Diagnostic	Number of measurements	Mean values (ml/100/min)
- Mild hypertensive disease	17	110 ± 42
- Severe hypertensive disease	14	60 ± 20
- Pre-eclampsia - eclampsia	20	88 ± 23
- Superimposed pre-eclampsia	12	55 ± 20
- Pyelonephritis	17	67 ± 12
- Diabetis	19	72 ± 20
- Post-term pregnancy	4	48 ± 12
- Fetal Hypotrophy	24	63 ± 18

This is confirmed by the 15 measurements repeated at quarter hourly intervals on the same woman (Table 2).

Table 2. Repeated measurements without any drug

Name	1st measurement ml/100 g/min	2nd measurement ml/100 g/min	Name	1st measurement ml/100 g/min	2nd measurement ml/100 g/min
R. A.	150	160	V. I.	138	138
G. A.	49	46	POR	110	70
E. M.	99	86	DUP	115	140
L. L.	140	100	BRU	87	139
R. I.	57	57	DEL	50	37
V. A.	160	127	FAL	92	115
J. E.	40	69	FAL	63	57
D. U.	34	31			

These variations are clearly regrettable as they prevent giving a value to any individual result.

We have tried to understand the reason for these variations by means of a series of investigations.

Discussion

The first question to be put is that of where does the Xenon 133 go when it is injected into the intervillous space.

According to our working hypothesis, it is eliminated through the utero-placental veins; the speed of this disposal depends on the flow at the point of injection. But can the Xenon not diffuse into the neighbouring areas, and is this diffusion not a cause of error in our calculation?

Theoretically the Xenon can diffuse towards:
- the non-injected zones of the intervillous space,
- the foetus,

- the amniotic cavity,
- the myometrium.

We tried the systematic injection of Xenon 133 into the amniotic liquid and the drop in radioactivity is very slow; it can have only a negligible influence upon the slope of the curve recorded for the placenta.

Injecting Xenon 133 into the myometrium gives a curve with a slope similar to the one for the slow phase of our placental curves. We think that this slow phase represents to a great extent the flow of the myometrium.

It is not possible to measure the quantitiy of Xenon which passes to the foetus in a pregnant woman. We have studied this passage with pregnant sheep by removing the foetus while leaving it attached to the mother through the placental circulation; Xenon 133 is injected into the uterine artery and its passage is investigated on the foetus side. This passage does take place and occurs during the first minute, representing some 10 % of the injected dose. Given the physiological and anatomical conditions of the experiment it is clearly impossible to extrapolate these results obtained with a sheep to the pregnant woman. However, the results lead us to think that the diffusion of Xenon towards the foetus is rapid but small.

To complete these data we studied what happens to Xenon 133 injected into the intervillous space, using a gamma camera. We made the following observations:

The injected area has a diameter of some 6 cm.

If one studies the evolution of the radioactivity over a period of time in the intervillous, one sees that at the end of the injection the radioactivity is at a peak and that the injected area is of a certain breadth.

60 seconds later the radioactivity has clearly dropped, but the patch has not widened. One can thus conclude that the number of strokes counted at the point of injection falls not as a result of Xenon 133 diffusing within the intervillous space but as a result of this isotope leaving this very space.

Finally, with the doses used in these cases, of the order of 500 - 1.000 microcuries, a diffusion to the foetus of more than 10 % of the injected dose would have produced a radioactive foetal image. We never observed this.

In order to obtain the percentage variations due to the method, we then devised a system permitting the experimental reconstruction of the placental circulation by the in vitro perfusion of a placental cotyledon from the side of the foetus and of the mother. Thirteen placentae were thus perfused with a constant flow; the clearance of the Xenon 133 injected into the intervillous space was measured twice for each placenta; the variations from one measurement to another are between 15 - 20 %; the passage of Xenon towards the foetus does not exceed 10 % of the injected dose.

In terms of this research and our clinical experience, the decrease in placental clearance is considered abnormal only if it is more than 50 % and if it is found during several measurements. We are not reaching any therapeutic decision on the results of the placental clearance any more so than we are on the plasmatic or urinary dosage of oestriol, or on the study of the foetus' heartbeat. Only the combined results of these different tests reveal, in our opinion, a certain value. In any case we do not think that the measurement of the placental clearance can become a routine examination to be carried out when trying to assess the vitality of the foetus in utero. In fact this measurement is ultimately possible in only a small percentage of cases, since it can only be carried out if the placenta is in a frontal position and provided that the pregnant person is Rh + allowing the possibility of foeto-maternal transfusion and that it is not a case of either placenta praevia or of threatened premature birth.

However, this method can be used for studying the influence of certain factors on the placental circulation such as drugs or tobacco. We have thus begun a series of experiments the preliminary results of which we are passing to you.

In an initial series of experiments we studied the effect of Rheomacrodex on the placental clearance of Xenon 133. In fact certain researchers, and in particular CHARTIER and BARRIER, have recommended the use of this substance in the treatment of foetal distress.

With 16 pregnant cases we took an initial measurement of the placental clearance; a perfusion of 500 ml of Rheomacrodex was then administered; a second measurement of the clearance was taken at the end of the perfusion. One can see from Table 3 that if one accepts an increase of 50 % in the local flow as being significant then this is found in 12 of the 16 cases.

Table 3. Rheomacrodex effect on placental 133 Xenon clearance

Name	Diagnostic	local P. B. F. ml/100 g/min Before	After	Results
LL	Normal pregnancy	99	115	no action
TO	Pre-eclampsia	40	92	x2
LO	Superimposed pre-eclampsia	35	130	X3,5
BL	Superimposed pre-eclampsia	60	126	x2
MA	Hypertensive disease	77	126	+ 80 %
SA	Hypertensive disease	40	70	+ 75 %
ES	Pyelonephritis	60	90	+ 50 %
gi	Pyelonephritis	77	115	+ 60 %

Name	Diagnostic	local P. B. F. ml/100 g/min Before	After	Results
gA	Diabetis	40	200	x5
De	Diabetis	45	40	no action
Du	Posterm pregnancy	43	35	no action
Du	Hypotrophy	40	77	+ 90 %
VA	Hypotrophy	40	50	no action
Del	Pre-eclampsia	65	135	x2
Bol	Diabetis	70	170	x2,5
Mar	Chronic nephritis	60	100	x2

In a second series of experiments beginning at the moment, we have studied in the same way the effect of Praxilene and tobacco.

Praxilene was administered in a dose of 320 mg diluted in 500 ml of serum with 10 % glucose. Perfusion took place over 4 hours. In the three cases where this treatment was carried out one sees an increase in the local placental flow (Table 4). But this increase is not significant in relation to variations resulting from the method.

The placental clearance of Xenon 133 was measured among pregnant persons who are smokers and who volunteered. Two measurements were taken, one before and one after smoking a cigarette. The results obtained are conflicting (Table 5).

Table 4. Praxilene effect on placental 133 Xenon clearance

Name	Diagnostic	Local placental blood flow ml 100 g/min Before	After	Results
CHU	Hypotrophy	50	75	+ 25 %
MAR	Chronic nephritis	50	60	+ 10 %
LOR	Hypotrophy	60	85	+ 40 %

Table 5. Tobacco effect on placental 133 Xenon clearance

Name	Local placental blood flow ml/100 g/min Before	After	Results
VER	90	70	- 15 %
BOU	100	110	+ 10 %
SOU	85	60	- 20 %
CLO	150	110	- 30 %
EIS	230	230	0 %

It is quite clear that it is not possible to draw conclusions from these experiments which covered too small a number of cases. Research in this field is continuing at the present time.

Conclusions

When we carried out the first measurements of the placental clearance of Xenon 133 we were hoping to be able to produce a method to pinpoint and observe chronic foetal distress, which could be used in daily practice. This hope has in part not been fulfilled.

However, this research has not been in vain for it highlights the possibilities and limitations of our present means of investigation. It also shows one of the directions of research likely to resolve the problem posed by the human placental haemodynamics. In our opinion it is on the solution of this problem that there depends a better understanding of the physio-pathology of chronic foetal distress, an understanding which is an essential requirement for producing an efficacious treatment for this syndrome.

Work of the A and B Obstetric Clinics (Professors A. PONTONNIER and M. MONROZIES) and of the Isotope Laboratory (Prof. BRU) with the help of the D. G. R. S. T. contract No. 70 02 288 and of the INSERM contract No. 71 1 4905.

The Effect of Abdominal Decompression on the Newborn

W. Gruber, K. Baumgarten, and H. Fröhlich

Abdominal Decompression, first published by HEYNS in 1959, causes reduction of the intraabdominal pressure by decrease of the athmospheric pressure on the abdomen. On the other hand, pressure on the legs is increased. These changes in hemodynamics are followed by increased blood flow in the pelvic organs and in the placenta. An anticipated improvement of oxygenation of fetal blood could not be proved in the investigations of MATHEWS and LOEFFLER (1968).

HEYNS found relief of labour-pain and an acceleration of mental and physical development of the children following abdominal decompression during pregnancy. We tried to find out, whether abdominal decompression has any influence on the birth weight or Apgar score of the newborn.

Our material consists of 91 women, 60 primiparous and 31 multiparous patients, who used abdominal decompression in the second half of pregnancy for 10 to 38 times, on an average of 21 times for 30 minutes each time. All of them were delivered vaginally in the years from 1970 to 1972 at the second Department of Obstetrics and Gynecology at the University Clinic of Vienna. As reference group we used 100 women of the same social standing, who received the same prenatal care, but no abdominal decompression and were delivered in the same period of time at the same clinic under the same conditions. In both abdominal decompression-group and reference-group we compared

1. birth weights of the newborn
2. Apgar scores of the newborn and
3. duration of delivery

There was no difference in birth weight, either in primiparous or in multiparous patients with or without abdominal decompression.

There was also no difference in Apgar scores.

Delivery period in primiparous patients after abdominal decompression was 0.71 hours, i. e. 43 minutes shorter than in patients without abdominal decompression. This difference proved to be statistically insignificant, due to the small number of cases.

In multiparae the duration of delivery after abdominal decompression during pregnancy was 1.42 hours, i. e. 1 hour and 25 minutes less than without decompression. This difference is significant on the 5 % borderline.

In our study we could not prove any influence of abdominal decompression on the birth weight or the Apgar score of the newborn, in accordance with BLECHER's findings. On the other hand, an acceleration of delivery after abdominal decompression was demonstrable, though not significant, in primiparous patients and of statistical significance in multiparous patients. This acceleration seems to be caused by the psychoprophylactic effect of abdominal decompression during pregnancy.

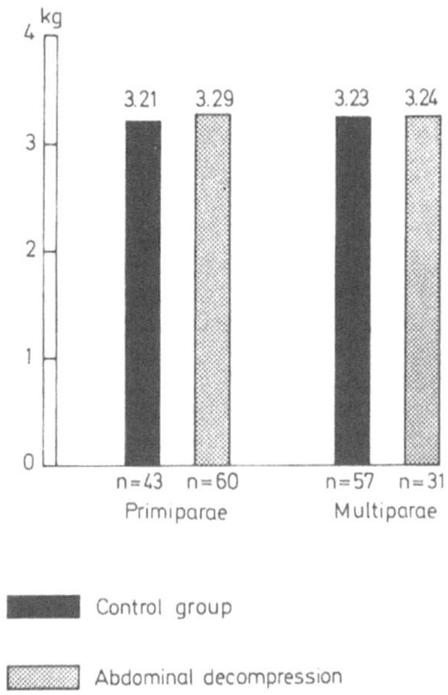

Fig. 1. Birth weight

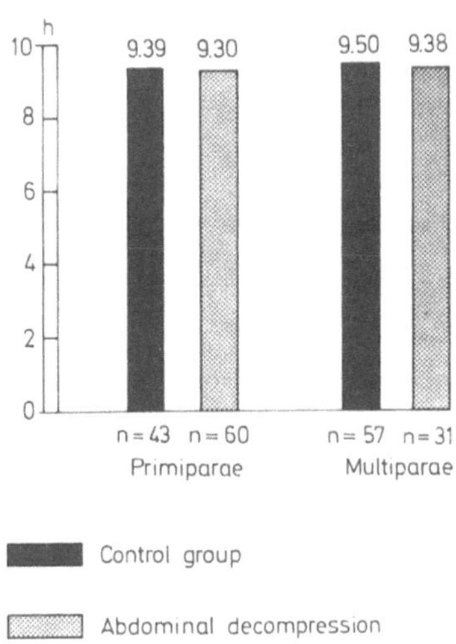

Fig. 2. Apgar Score

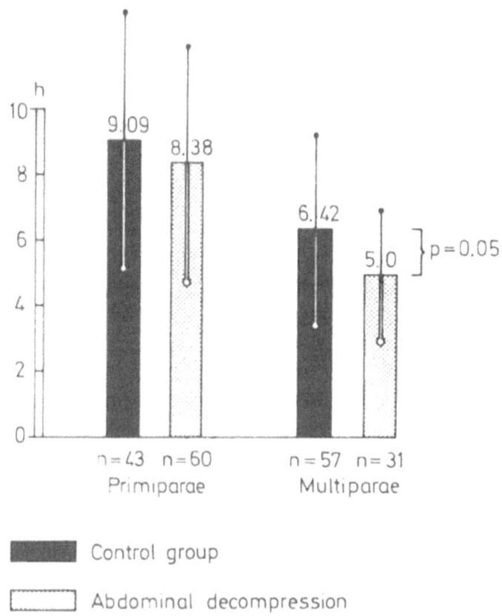

Fig. 3. Duration of delivery

The Use of Intermittent Abdominal Decompression and Oestriol Monitoring in the Treatment of Feto-Placental Insufficiency

D. J. MacRae and S. M. Mohamedally

Intermittent abdominal decompression has been shown to lower prematurity and perinatal mortality rates in cases of pre-eclampsia (1) and also in retardation of foetal growth and development (dysmaturity) in which serial oestriol assays monitored placental metabolism and foetal viability (2, 3). In both these pregnancy complications foeto-placental insufficiency is found.

Decompression was given by the HEYN'S suit at a negative pressure of 70 mm Hg 15 seconds in every minute for half an hour; treatment sessions were repeated according to oestriol levels. Urinary oestriol assays were made by gas chromatography from 24-hour specimens of urine and plasma oestriol was estimated after NACHTIGALL et al.

In a series of 46 patients with pre-eclampsia or essential hypertension serial oestriol levels were found to be an important guide to the severity of the condition and an index of foetal well-being (Fgs. 1, 2). Abdominal decompression therapy increased oestriol output in the cases of pre-eclampsia (Fgs. 3, 4) and resulted in a more favourable outlook with lower prematurity rate than in untreated cases; the one perinatal death, caused by accidental haemorrhage, occurred in the untreated pre-eclamptic cases. There was no increase, however, in plasma or urinary oestriol in cases of essential hypertension treated by decompression.

In a group of 65 cases of dysmaturity (assessed clinically and with two initial oestriol levels below the normal range) 35 patients were given decompression treatment resulting in a prematurity rate of 11.4 per cent with only one perinatal death due to a severe heart lesion; in 30 dysmature cases with serial oestriol monitoring but no decompression treatment there were two neonatal deaths, one from congenital heart disease and one from anoxia originating in a congenitally short cord (20 cm), but the prematurity rate was 54.4 per cent. Decompression treatment of dysmaturity is compared in Figs. 5, 6; and Fig. 7 shows the significant oestriol rise compared with untreated cases. In a separate series of 200 dysmature cases without oestriol monitoring or decompression therapy, the prematurity rate was 77 per cent and the neonatal death rate 14 per cent.

It is considered that intermittent abdominal decompression has the effect of enhancing utero-placental blood flow, an action confirmed experimentally by the use of radio isotopes (4) and this therapy is, therefore, of particular value in cases of foeto-placental insufficiency. The decompression haemodialysis may be thought to be analogous in its action to the physiological hyperventilation of pregnancy by increasing the functional capacity of the placenta. More villi are brought into vital activity thus creating not only improved foeto-placental metabolism of oestriol but, it may reasonably be assumed, better synthesis and transport of nutrients to the benefit of the foetus.

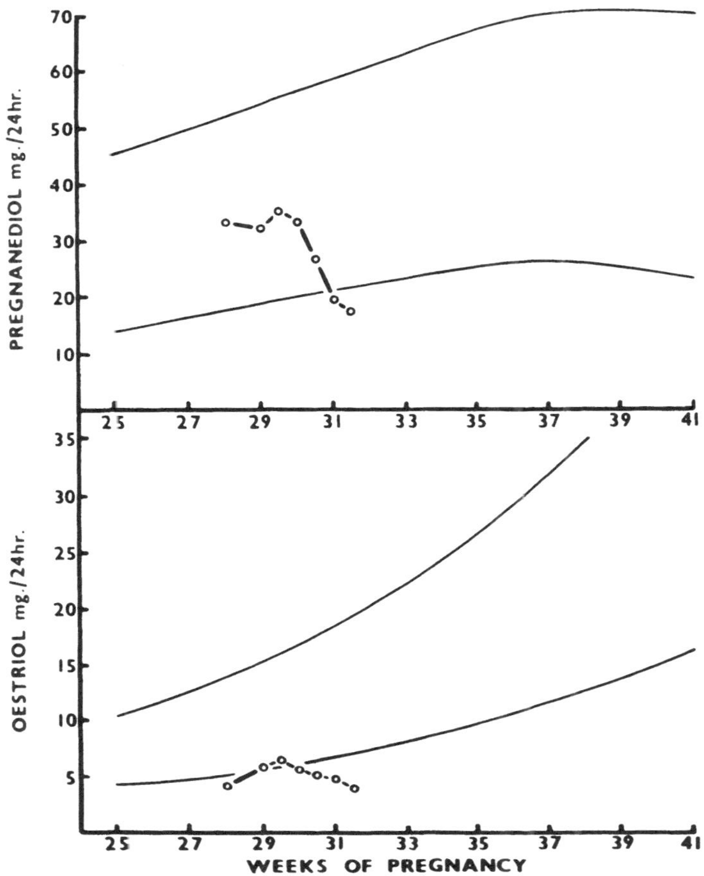

Fig. 1. Pre-eclampsia: falling hormone levels preceded worsening clinical condition

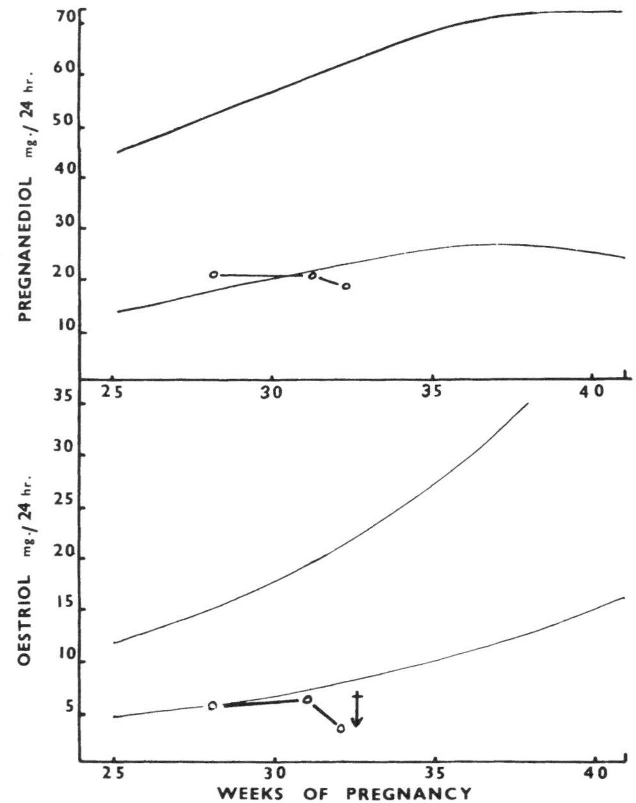

Fig. 2. Pre-eclampsia: hormone level fall preceded concealed A. P. H.

D = commencement of decompression

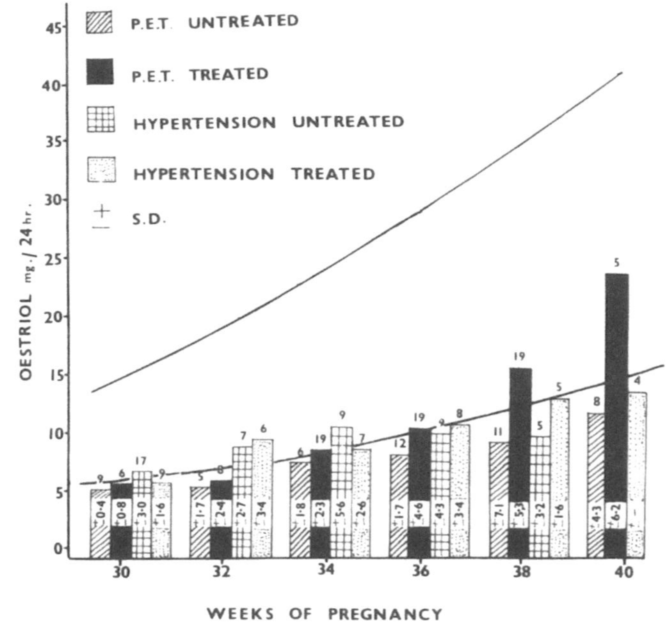

Fig. 4. Significant rise in oestriol levels in given abdominal decompression pre-eclampsia cases

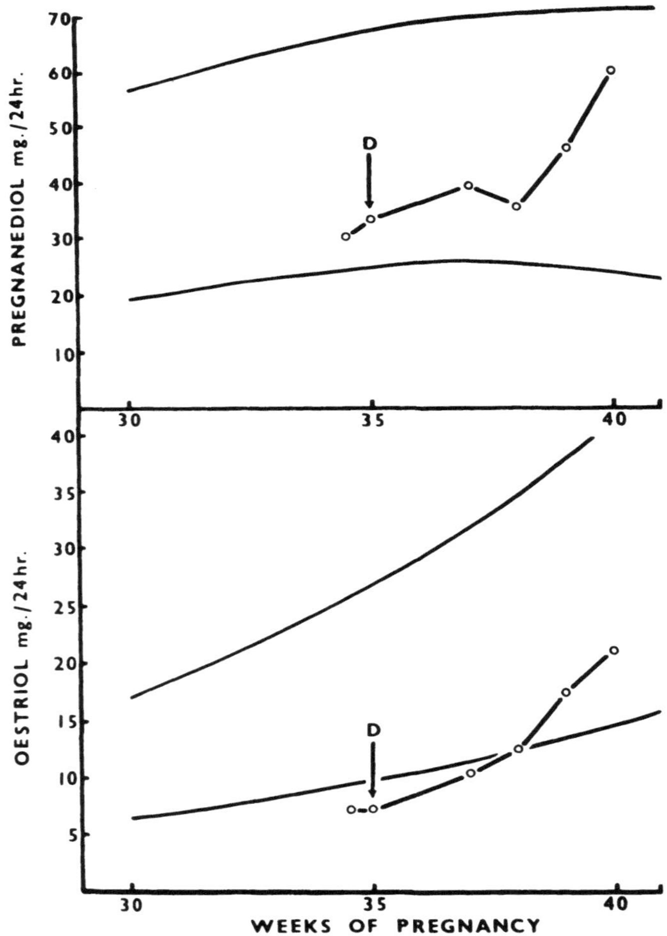

Fig. 3. Pre-eclampsia: oestriol rise with abdominal decompression

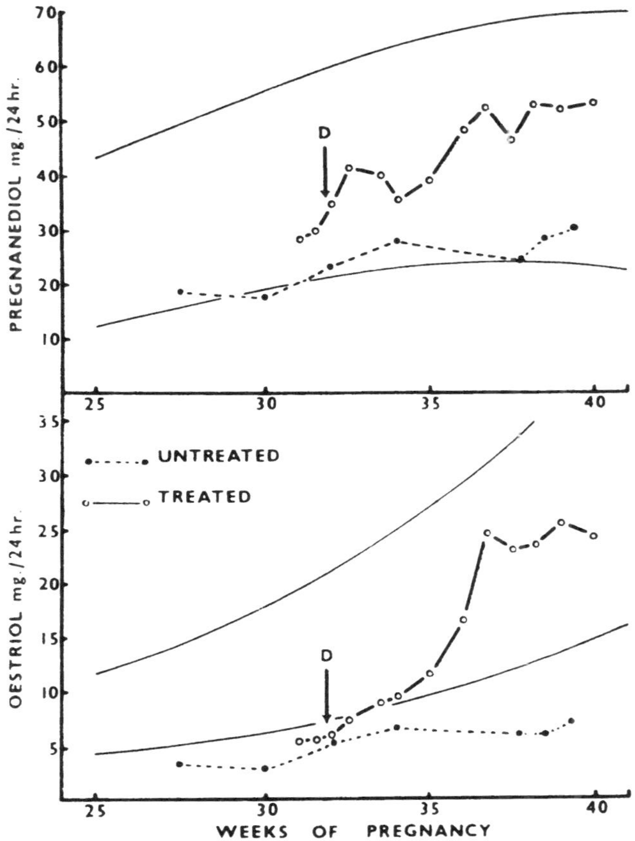

Fig. 5. Dysmaturity: comparison between untreated and treated cases

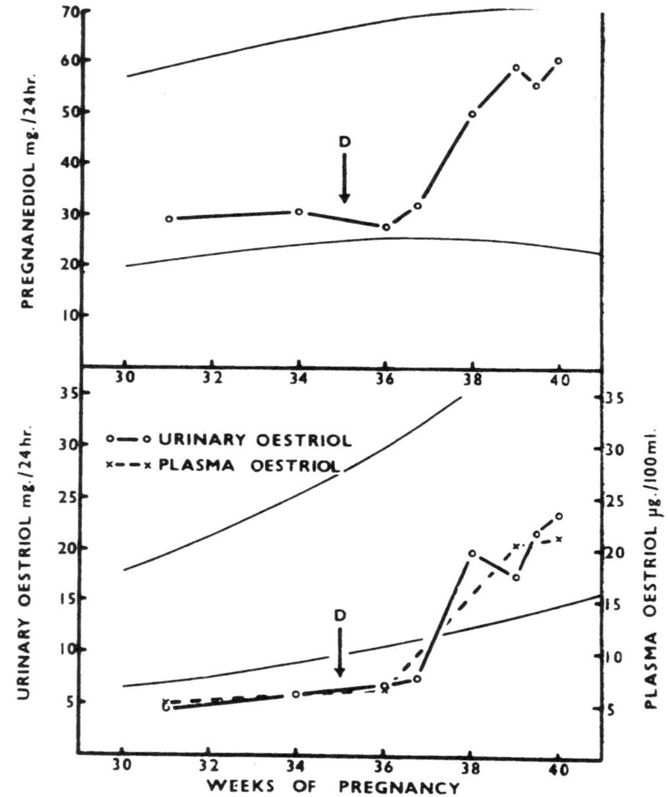

Fig. 6. Dysmaturity: rise in plasma and urinary oestriol with decompression

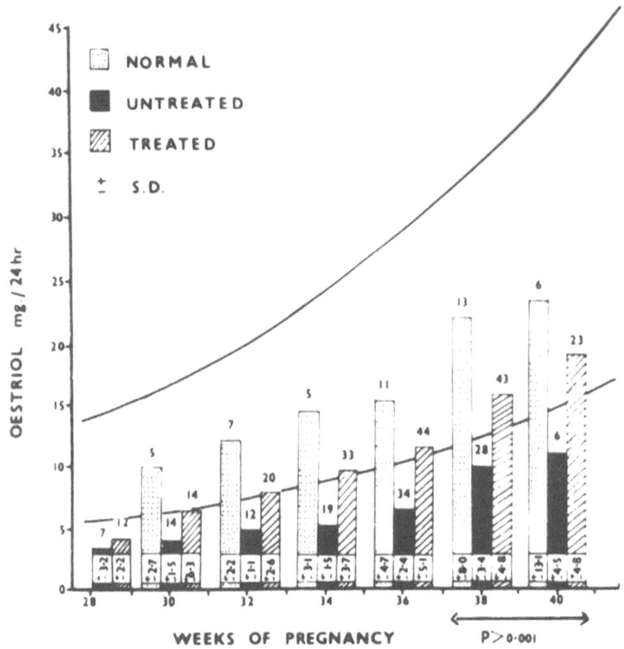

Fig. 7. Dysmaturity: chart shows significant oestriol rise in cases given decompression treatment

References

1. BLECHER, J. A., HEYNS, O. S.: Lancet 2, 621 (1967).
2. MC RAE, D. J., MOHAMEDALLY, S. M.: Proc. Roy. Soc. Med. 63, 502 (1970).
3. MC RAE, D. J., MOHAMEDALLY, S. M., WILLMOTT, M. P.: S. Afr. Med. J. 46, 1027 (1972).
4. COXON, A., HAGGITH, J. W.: J. Obstet. Gynaec. Brit. Cwlth. 78, 49 (1971).

Intra-Amniotic Amino-Acid Injections

R. Renaud, L. Kirstetter, C. Koehl, G. Boog, J. P. Brettes,
J. C. Schumacher, G. Vincendon, D. Willard, and R. Gandar

Energy yielding substances (carbohydrates, amino acids, fatty acids) are mainly transferred through the placenta to the fetus. M. YOUNG (25) did a series of animal experiments which showed that the transfer of amino acids from the mother to the fetus was an active transport mechanism depending essentially on the maternal blood flow to the placenta. Fetal malnutrition may result from maternal disease such as hypertension, renal disease, toxemia or vascular insufficiency. (1, 10, 14) that can reduce this flow. Intra-uterine growth retardation follows and is more severe because the disease has occurred very early during pregnancy, and there is often a permanent decrease in cell division and the cellular protein content (24, 23). In serious cases, the brain, though protected for a long time, does not escape.

Ritodrine, given to the mother under certain conditions seem to increase the uterine and placental flow (4, 19). One would expect this effect to be reduced in cases of vascular lesions, and, if so, other ways of nourishing the fetus would be justified in order to compensate for the lack of placental amino-acid transfer.

SUGAWA et al.(21) demonstrated that the amino acids of the amniotic fluid are used in rodents for the protein synthesis of the fetus. KERR and KENNAN's work (7) with rhesus monkeys demonstrates that the amniotic fluid may have food value. Indeed, the fetus swallows between 220 and 750 ml of amniotic fluid per day (11, 15). There might be also some exchange through the membranes covering the placenta and the umbilical cord.

It was thus logical to investigate under what conditions the fetus might be fed amniotically when the placenta is deficient (2, 6, 9, 16, 17, 18, 20). It is indeed essential to make certain that intra-amniotic injections of amino acids do not adversely affect the uterine activity, the fetus and the newborn infant, and that they have a beneficial effect on the fetus in cases of malnutrition. We need to know what happens to the amino acids that have been injected, and more particularly what quantity of them is absorbed by the fetus. It is almost impossible to reply to this last question: metabolism of amino acids in the amniotic fluid, the placenta and the human fetus is not yet determined. Experimental studies in animals do not give reliable information concerning human protein metabolism.

We have studied, to date, 67 cases that we divided into 3 groups according to the methods of study adopted and parameters we wished to measure (Table 1).

Group 1 is composed of 40 women who had no intra-amniotic injections of amino acids. We have measured the levels of 18 amino acids in the mother's blood taken between 3 and 15 minutes after delivery, in the cord blood and in the placental tissue.

Pregnancy and vaginal delivery were quite normal in 25 women (subgroup Ia). All the newborn infants of this sub-group were of normal

Table 1

Group	Subgroup	Characteristics	Infusion	Amino-acid concentrations measured in	Studies
I	I a (25 cases)	Normal	O	Maternal blood	Control
	I b (15 cases)	Pathological 6 Toxaemia 4 Premature labor 5 Growth retardation			
II	II a (5 cases)	Normal	1 - 2 intra-amniot. infusion (36 - 40 weeks)	Maternal blood	Uterine activity and fetal side effects
	II b (5 cases)	Fetal growth retardation	4 - 14 intra-amniot. infusion (30 - 38 weeks)	Umbilical blood Placenta	Therapeutic effect
	II c (6 cases)	Elective caesarean section	1 intra-amniot. infusion (38 - 42 weeks)	Amniotic fluid	Variations of Concentrations
III	III a (11 cases)	Normal mother	I. V. infusion	Maternal blood	

weight and had an Apgar score at 1 and 5 minutes between 8 and 10. The placenta did not show any macroscopic or microscopic anomaly.

Sub-group Ib is composed at 15 women who had shown various pathological conditions in pregnancy or delivery. Among these women, six showed signs of toxemia but gave birth to a full term baby of appropriate weight and vitality. Three of the placentae were abnormal. Four other women were delivered prematurely between the 30th and 36th week. The newborn infant's weight was between 1300 and 2500 g, but their Apgar scores were normal. The last five women gave birth to hypotrophic term newborn infants whose weight was between 2200 and 2600 g (more than two standard deviations below the normal weight range for our department).

Group II (Table 2) is composed of 16 women who all had intra-amniotic injections of amino acids. It is subdivided into 3 sub-groups.

Sub-group IIa (Table 2, cases 1 to 5) comprises our first 5 cases. In each of these cases one or two injections were given at the end of pregnancy to make sure that the method was innocuous.

Sub-group IIb (Table 2, cases 6 to 10) comprises 5 other patients who had clinically obvious fetal hypotrophy. Each of these 5 patients had between 4 and 14 intra-amniotic injections of amino acids between the 30th and the 41st week of pregnancy. Various parameters were studied (urinary oestriol, HCS, biparietal diameter, FHR) to see if there was therapeutic effect.

Finally, sub-group IIc (Table 2, cases 11 to 16) comprises 6 cases (5 full term elective Caesarean sections before the onset of labor and a therapeutic interruption of pregnancy, in the 19th week) who had one intra-amniotic injection of amino acids 45 minutes before the extraction of the fetus in order to study the early variations of amino acids in the maternal blood taken from the cubital vein at the time of extraction, the umbilical blood, amniotic fluid, and placenta.

Group III is composed of 11 normal pregnant patients between the 30th and 38th week of their pregnancy. These 11 women had a quantity of amino acids injected intravenously. This quantity was determined from the results obtained with group II and the variations in the blood amino acid pattern were recorded. We shall come back to the technical methods of administration of amino acids in this group, when we discuss the results.

The amino-acid solution used is Aminosol 100 sold by Vitrum Laboratories. It is a caseine hydrolysate in which the amino-acid content varies very little from one bottle to another (Fig. 1). In case (No. 2 Table 2) we used simple Aminosol supplied by the same firm.

We injected 50 ml of Ambisol into the amniotic cavity each time except in the first 2 cases of group II. These patients had an injection of 250 and 350 ml over a period of 3 hours. All injections were given under sterile conditions after ultra-sound localization of the placenta.

The samples of amniotic fluid and blood were immediately centrifuged at 1500 r.p.m. and the supernatent was frozen at -18° C. A few hours before chromatography, the samples were thawed, homogenized and deproteinized with sulphosalicylic acid. Acter centrifugation the analysis was carried out on the de-proteinized supernatant.

Table 2

Group	Cases	History	Date of injections (weeks)	Volume	Date and Mode of delivery	Apgar score 1 - 5
II a	1	Toxemia Placental biopsy	39	250 ml^{++} (3 h)	40 weeks - normal ♀ 3000/50	10 - 10
	2	Psych. history Urinary infection Growth retardation	38	300 ml^{++} (3 h)	39 weeks-bradycardia cesarean section ♂ 2100/45	5 - 10
	3	3 Abort. 1 caesarean 2 growth retardation 1 prem. labor threatened	33 33	50 ml^{+} 50 ml^{+}	Ritodrine I. V. 34 weeks - normal ♀ 1600/40	8 - 10
	4	Contracted pelvis Breech - Oligohydramnios	40	50 ml	40 weeks - cesarean section, ♂ 3300/50	10 - 10
	5	Hypertension 1 intra-uterine death	36 38	50 ml^{+} 50 ml^{+}	39 weeks - normal ♀ 3300/50	9 - 10
II b	6	1 Abortion - 1 prem. deliv. - Premat. Labor threat, Growth retard.	35 → 38	50 ml X 9^{+}	38 weeks - normal ♀ 2750/50	9 - 10
	7	Twins - Premature labor threatened Macrocyt. Anemia	30 → 33 34	50 ml X 8^{+} 50 ml^{+}	35 weeks - cord procid. cesarean section ♂ 1800/43, ♀ 1500/41	9 - 10 9 - 10
	8	Growth retard.	31 → 35	50 ml X 14^{+}	36 weeks - breech ♀ 2400/43	8 - 10
	9	1 intra-uterine death 2 normal delivery Growth retard.	37 → 41	50 ml X 8^{+}	41 weeks - normal ♀ 2700/46	9 - 10
	10	First pregnancy Prem. labor threatened Growth retardation	29 → 30	50 ml X 4^{+} Premat. lab. threat 30wks.	41 weeks - fetal distress - cesarean section, ♀ 2950/48	3 - 8 ✝ 3rd day Ivemark synd.

Table 2 - continued -

Group	Cases	History	Date of injections (weeks)	Volume	Date and Mode of delivery	Apgar score 1 - 5
	11	Third pregnancy Two cesarean sections	38	50 ml +	38 weeks - elective cesarean section ♀ 2700/49	6 - 9
	12	One intra-uterine death Pre-diabetes Urinary infection	37	50 ml +	37 weeks - elective cesarean section ♀ 3100/50	8 - 10
II c	13	1 Abortion - bleeding at third month - Growth retard. - Breech	39	50 ml +	39 weeks - elective cesarean section ♂ 2050/45	7 - 10
	14	4 normal deliveries 1 Abortion Cervical agglutination	41	50 ml +	41 weeks - elective cesarean section + sterilization ♀ 3550/49	6 - 8
	15	2 Normal delivery 1 Abortion Placenta praevia	37	50 ml +	37 weeks - cesarean section ♀ 2750/47	7 - 10
	16	Cervical Epithelioma	19	50 ml +	19 weeks - hysterotomy Hysterectomy	

\+ Aminosol 100
++ Aminosol simple

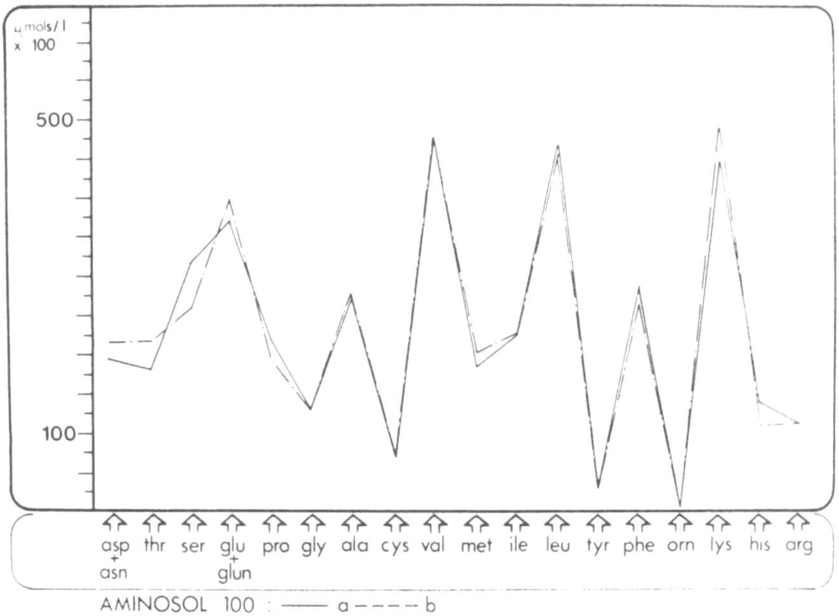

Fig. 1. Amino-acid concentration in two Aminosol 100 bottles

After cutting the cord at the placenta and removing the membranes, the placentae were weighed and divided into two parts, one for anatomo-pathological examination, the other for measurement of amino acids; the latter was immediately frozen at -18° C. 24 hours before chromatography, it was thawed in a container at +4° C and then homogenized in twice its volume of TRIS - phosphate buffer (5 mm) pH 7.2. The homogenate was then centrifuged at 30.000 g in a Beckman ultra-centrifuge (roter 19) and refrigerated at +4° C for four hours. The chromatography was carried out with the supernatant from ultra-centrifugation after deproteinization.

Chromatography was conducted in cathion exchange columns by a technique modified from the STEIN and MOORE method using a TSMI automatic apparatus (Technicon Instruments Corporation, Ardaley, Chauncey, New York, USA).

The amino acids were subsequently treated with a ninhydrine base reagent and read at two wavelengts (570 mm and 440 mm) transposed into peaks with a standard of known concentration (norleucine solution, 2.5 micromoles/ml of chlorhydric acid N/100). With this treatment the glutamine and asparagine are hydrolized which explains why we grouped these compounds with the glutamate and aspartate, respectively.

We shall now consider the following:
1. the aminoacidogram of the mother's plasma after delivery, the umbilical plasma and the placenta in normal and pathological cases (group I).
2. the variations in the amino acidograms of the maternal and umbilical plasma, the amniotic fluid and the placenta after intra-amniotic injection of amino acids.
3. the effect of intra-amniotic injections on uterine activity, the fetus, and the newborn infant.

I. Aminocidograms of Maternal and Umbilical Plasma, of Placenta Immediately after Delivery

1. Normal Cases (Group I a)

From the 25 cases of group I a we have made averages and deviations of the concentrations of 18 amino acids in maternal and umbilical plasma and from the placenta taken a few minutes after delivery. These values are given in Table 3.

Table 3. Amino-acid concentrations in maternal venous plasma, umbilical plasma, and placenta (group I a)

Amino acid	Maternal blood+		Umbilical blood+		Placenta++	
	N	Mean ± SD	N	Mean ± SD	N	Mean ± SD
{Aspartate Asparagine	11	10,2 ± 3,5	12	15,8 ± 5,3	25	107 ± 43
Threonine	18	22,5 ± 5,4	24	29,6 ± 7,3	25	80 ± 36
Serine	17	21,1 ± 3,8	22	26,2 ± 9,3	25	98 ± 45
{Glutamate Glutamine	25	43,6 ± 21,6	22	68,1 ± 22,0	26	343 ± 104
Proline	18	14,6 ± 6,0	18	14,8 ± 3,1	23	71 ± 38
Glycine	22	28,4 ± 8,7	23	40,2 ± 9,1	25	209 ± 82
Alanine	21	38,4 ± 9,0	19	40,4 ± 10,0	25	121 ± 52
Cystine	19	3,9 ± 1,8	20	4,1 ± 2,0	25	25 ± 19
Valine	21	19,7 ± 5,3	21	24,0 ± 7,3	25	50 ± 21
Methionine	21	3,0 ± 1,6	25	4,4 ± 2,0	25	17 ± 8
Isoleucine	20	6,5 ± 2,5	23	7,6 ± 2,3	25	19 ± 10
Leucine	19	14,4 ± 4,3	23	16,0 ± 4,1	25	72 ± 30
Tyrosine	23	6,2 ± 1,9	22	8,0 ± 1,9	25	34 ± 15
Phenylalanine	19	10,0 ± 3,2	19	9,7 ± 1,8	25	38 ± 17
Ornithine	12	13,6 ± 4,8	9	17,1 ± 4,5	24	42 ± 19
Lysine	10	20,3 ± 5,5	8	31,2 ± 6,7	24	92 ± 35
Histidine	21	12,1 ± 5,5	24	15,1 ± 2,9	25	31 ± 13
Arginine	12	8,1 ± 3,7	17	6,3 ± 1,9	23	43 ± 16

\+ μ moles / 100 ml plasma

++ μ moles / 100 g wet weight

We found much higher concentrations of amino acids than other authors (8, 26). For some of those acids, differences in measurement and techniques may explain some of these discrepancies. For example, serine and threonine are not always entirely separated and this might explain the high levels of serine with out technique and we have noted that we regularly have high levels of methionine and ornithine. These technical differences in methods of sampling and storage do not account for all the variations, we think since the amino acids did not all increase in the same proportion. In our opinion these variations are due to the period of time between sampling and delivery and may also be due to our selection of patients. LINDBLAD states (8) that the amino-acid levels in maternal plasma may be modified by: hepatic and renal disease, stress, hormonal changes, the mother's age, number of previous pregnancies, placental anomalies, or interruption of the umbilical circulation. There is, at present, very little published data on the subject.

The levels of amino acids in the umbilical plasma are approximately those given by LINDBLAD (8) except for the serine, glycine, methionine, and ornithine, which are higher in this study. Our methods of conservation and analysis are identical with those used for maternal plasma.

The comparison of the amino-acid levels of placental tissue with those described by other authors is more difficult. The methods of sampling and preparation before homogenization are extremely important particularly for the quantities of maternal and fetal blood expelled from the placenta before homogenization. PAGE (12) emphasizes that the quantity of fluid lost during freezing and thawing may be rich in amino acids.

Our results show, as some authors (4,8,26) have already emphasized that there are less amino acids in maternal blood compared with fetal blood, and there are less amino acids in both bloods than in placental tissue (Table 3) in which they could be stored before they are transferred to the fetus.

2. Pathological Cases (Toxaemia, Premature Deliveries, Intra-uterine Growth Retardation - Tables 4, 5, 6)

The examination of amino acidograms in these cases is extremely important so as to select cases and interpret variations of aminoacidograms after intra-amniotic injections of amino-acids.

The aminoacidogram of maternal venous plasma does not show great variations (I a) in the group of deliveries with intra-uterine growth retardation and in the group of premature deliveries when compared with that of normal group (Table 4). In the premature delivery group we have noticed significant increase of serine glycine and phenylalanine (Fig.2, Table 4) but this was not found by YOUNG and PRENTON. On the contrary, glutamate-glutamine, glycine, cystine and phenylalanine are significantly increased in the toxemic patients of our series (Fig. 3, Table 4).

Compared with the normal group, the aminoacidogram of umbilical blood reveals a significant increase in alanine and phenylalanine in toxemic women's children (Fig. 4, Table 5) together with an increase in proline and phenylalanine and decrease in aspartate-asparagine in the group of premature deliveries as well as a decrease in cystine, isoleucine, arginine in the newborn infants with intra-uterine growth retardation (Fig. 5, Table 5).

As for the placental tissue, we found no difference in amino-acid concentrations between normal group I a and those of toxemic women and intra-uterine growth retardation I b(Figs.6, 7, Table 6). However, serine, glutamate-glutamine, proline, glycine, alanine, valine, methionine, leucine, tyrosine and arginine are significantly increased in the premature delivery group I b (Fig. 7, Table 6).

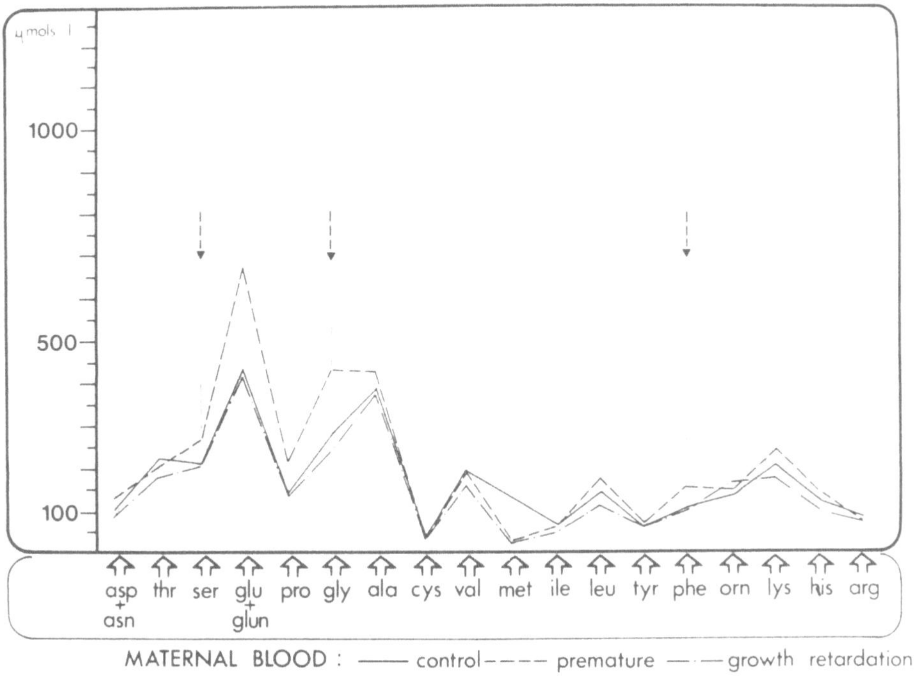

Fig. 2. Amino-acid concentration in maternal venous plasma (micromoles/l). Control group (I a), premature delivery group and growth retardation group (II b). The figure ↓ indicates some amino acids having a significant difference of concentration in the premature group compared with the control one. But there is not such a significant difference in the growth retardation group

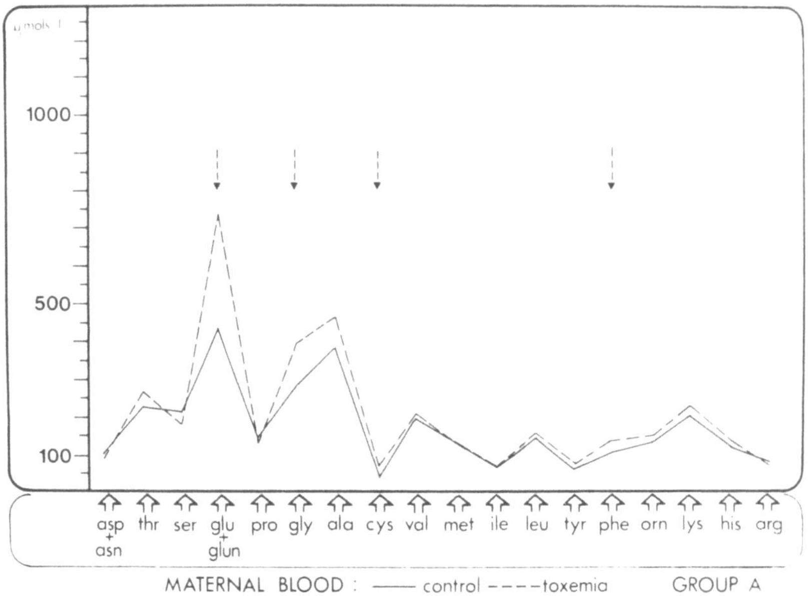

Fig. 3. Amino-acid concentration in maternal venous plasma (micromoles/l). Control (I a) and toxaemia (I b) groups. This figure↓indicates some amino acids that have a significantly different concentration in the toxemia group from the control one

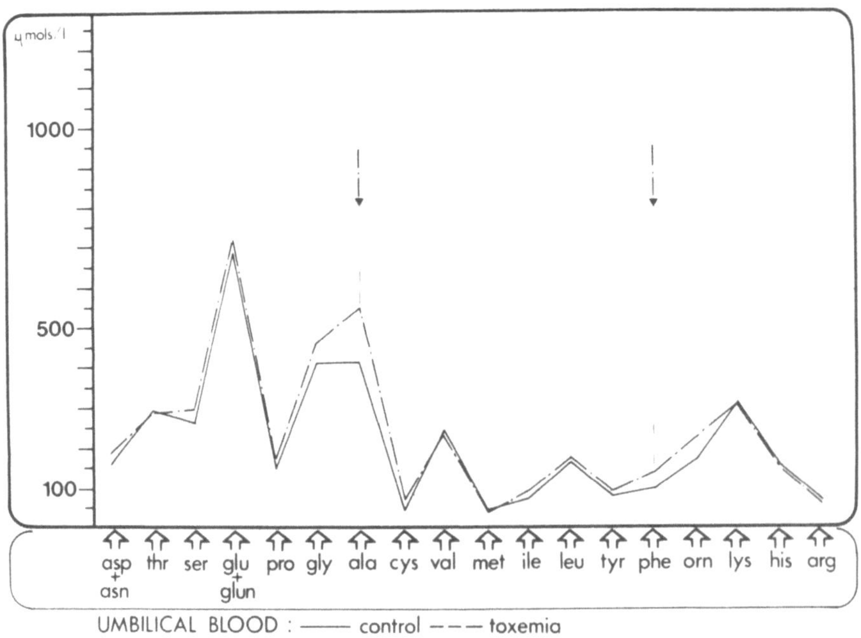

Fig. 4. Amino-acid concentration in umbilical plasma (micromoles/l) Control (I a) and toxemia (I b) groups. This figure↓points out some amino-acids that have a significantly different concentration in the toxemia and control groups

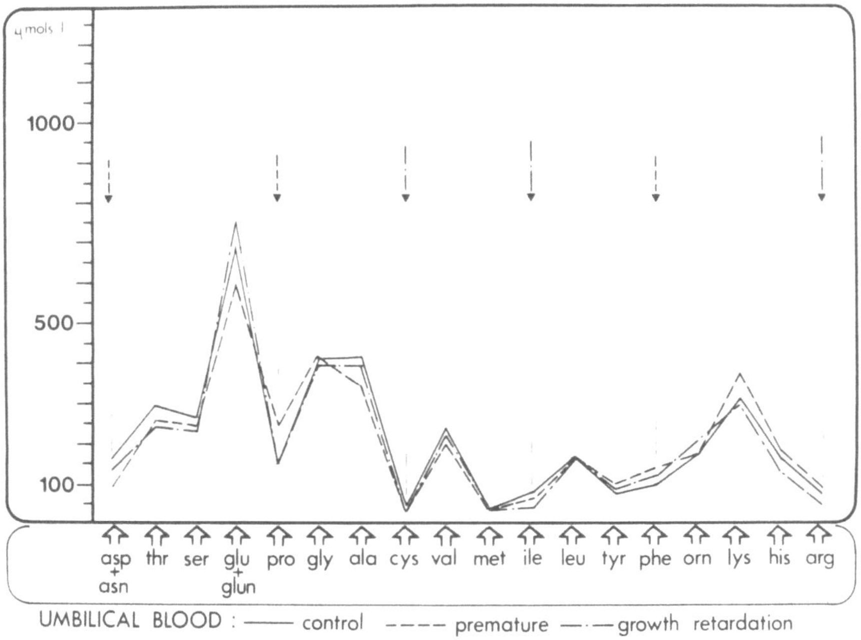

Fig. 5. Amino-acid concentration (micromoles/l) in umbilical plasma. Control group (I a) and premature delivery and growth retardation group (I b). The figure ↓ and ↓ shows some amino acids having a significantly different concentration in the premature group and in the growth retardation one compared with controls

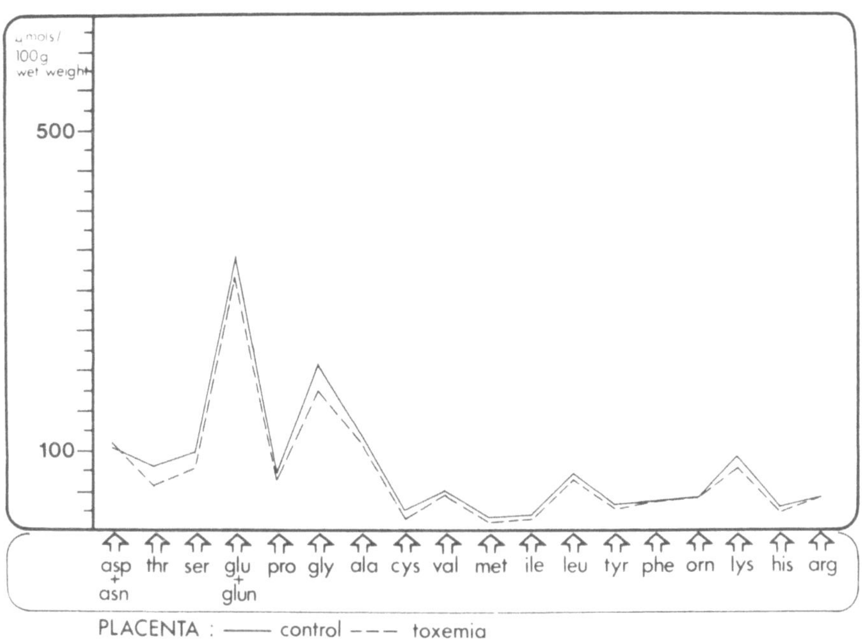

Fig. 6. Amino-acid concentration in placenta (micromoles/100 g wet weight) in control and toxemia groups (I a, I b)

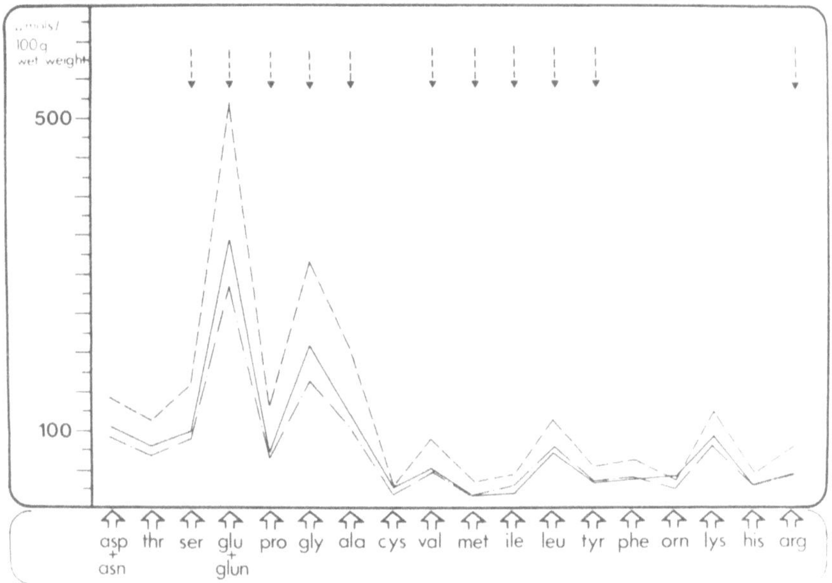

Fig. 7. Amino-acid concentration in placenta (micromoles/100 g wet weight) in control, premature delivery and growth retardation groups (I a, I b). This figure ↓ indicates some amino-acids having a significantly different concentration in the premature group compared with controls. There is not such a significant difference in the growth retardation group

II. Variations of Amino-acidograms in Amniotic Fluid, Maternal Venous Plasma, Umbilical Plasma and Placental Tissue after Intra-amniotic Injections of Amino Acids

1. Amniotic Fluid (Figs. 8, 9)

Immediately after 50 ml of Aminosol 100 had been injected, the total amino-acid concentration ranges from 20.000 up to 65.000 micromoles/l according to the quantity of amniotic fluid. For a few hours after injection we were unable to detect variations in amniotic volume clinically or by means of ultra-sound. An hour after the injection, the amino-acid concentration has decreased lying between 6.000 and 15.000 micromoles/l (Fig. 8) in patients with a normal amniotic volume. This implies that between a third and two thirds of the injected amino-acids have left the amniotic cavity. The plasma amino-acids appear to diminish in the following hours but we failed to make many measurements between 24 and 48 hours. At 48 hours the plasma amino-acid concentratio returned to normal levels but at 72 hours the level falls slightly (Fig. 9).

These observations are similar to those of DUDDENHAUSEN (2) and HELLER (5) who showed that to maintain elevated plasma levels the injections should be repeated between 24 and 48 hours.

Table 4. Amino-acid concentrations in maternal venous (Control, Toxaemia, Premature, Growth retardation and after intra-amniotic inspection of amino-acid) (The statistically significant figures are underlined)

Group	I a (Control)		I b Toxemia			I b Premature			I b Growth retardation			II c 45 min after injection (caesarean)		
Amino-acid	N	M ± S. D.	N	M ± S. D.	P	N	M ± S. D.	P	N	M ± S. D.	P	N	M ± S. D.	P
Aspartate + Asparagine	11	102 ± 35	5	88 ± 24	NS	3	127 ± 48	NS	4	86 ± 38	NS	4	153 ± 94	NS
Threonine	18	225 ± 54	6	263 ± 188	NS	3	199 ± 48	NS	4	179 ± 91	NS	4	279 ± 91	NS
Serine	17	211 ± 38	5	179 ± 48	NS	3	264 ± 23	S 0.05	4	206 ± 103	NS	4	236 ± 74	NS
Glutamate + Glutamine	25	436 ± 216	6	737 ± 318	S 0.01	3	672 ± 297	NS	4	422 ± 214	NS	4	522 ± 146	NS
Proline	18	146 ± 60	6	133 ± 29	NS	3	213 ± 192	NS	4	132 ± 23	NS	4	217 ± 68	S 0.05
Glycine	22	284 ± 87	6	392 ± 151	S 0.05	3	436 ± 112	S 0.01	4	246 ± 39	NS	4	373 ± 103	NS
Alanine	21	384 ± 90	6	463 ± 224	NS	3	423 ± 161	NS	4	371 ± 145	NS	4	306 ± 83	NS
Cystine	19	39 ± 18	6	70 ± 51	S 0.01	3	27 ± 12	NS	4	31 ± 26	NS	4	14 ± 6	S 0.05
Valine	21	197 ± 53	6	204 ± 48	NS	3	192 ± 36	NS	4	153 ± 52	NS	4	195 ± 63	NS
Methionine	21	30 ± 16	6	29 ± 11	NS	3	29 ± 4	NS	4	21 + 17	NS	4	44 ± 22	S 0.05
Isoleucine	20	65 ± 25	6	67 ± 16	NS	3	60 ± 15	NS	4	47 ± 19	NS	4	52 ± 23	NS
Leucine	19	144 ± 43	6	153 ± 16	NS	3	176 ± 56	NS	4	119 ± 22	NS	4	189 ± 65	NS
Tyrosine	23	62 ± 19	6	76 ± 18	NS	3	74 ± 20	NS	4	59 ± 19	NS	4	77 ± 20	NS
Phenylalanine	19	100 ± 32	6	137 ± 50	S 0.05	3	149 ± 11	S 0.05	4	103 ± 36	NS	4	131 ± 47	NS
Ornithine	12	136 ± 48	6	152 ± 31	NS	3	146 ± 80	NS	3	161 ± 69	NS	4	165 ± 32	NS
Lysine	10	203 ± 55	5	232 ± 42	NS	3	241 ± 48	NS	4	175 ± 53	NS	4	324 ± 109	S 0.01
Histidine	21	121 ± 55	6	137 ± 43	NS	3	141 ± 43	NS	4	101 ± 30	NS	4	144 ± 28	NS
Arginine	12	81 ± 37	5	72 ± 21	NS	3	84 ± 48	NS	4	72 ± 52	NS	4	117 ± 65	NS

Table 5. Amino-acid concentration in umbilical plasma (µ mol/l) (Control, Toxemia, Premature, Growth retardation and after intra-amniotic injection of amino-acids) (The statistically significant figures are underlined)

Group	I a (Control)		I b Toxemia			I b Premature			I b Growth retardation			II c 45 min after injection (caesarean)		
Amino-acid	N	M ± S. D.	N	M ± S. D.	P	N	M ± S. D.	P	N	M ± S. D.	P	N	M ± S. D.	P
Aspartate + Asparagine	12	158 ± 53	5	188 ± 227	NS	4	96 ± 30	S 0.05	5	136 ± 70	NS	3	81 ± 27	S 0.01
Threonine	24	296 ± 73	5	291 ± 100	NS	4	260 ± 61	NS	5	250 ± 58	NS	3	371 ± 58	NS
Serine	22	262 ± 93	5	298 ± 153	NS	4	245 ± 36	NS	5	232 ± 89	NS	3	243 ± 75	NS
Glutamate + Glutamine	22	681 ± 220	5	707 ± 173	NS	4	598 ± 159	NS	5	753 ± 301	NS	3	618 ± 292	NS
Proline	18	148 ± 31	5	175 ± 58	NS	4	242 ± 42	S 0.01	5	155 ± 29	NS	3	219 ± 84	S 0.05
Glycine	23	402 ± 91	5	455 ± 94	NS	4	414 ± 130	NS	5	394 ± 82	NS	3	432 ± 169	NS
Alanine	19	404 ± 100	5	546 ± 140	S 0.01	4	343 ± 119	NS	5	393 ± 102	NS	3	330 ± 67	NS
Cystine	20	41 ± 20	5	65 ± 37	NS	4	20 ± 10	NS	5	20 ± 10	S 0.05	3	31 ± 16	NS
Valine	21	240 ± 73	5	235 ± 34	NS	4	199 ± 36	NS	5	219 ± 53	NS	3	257 ± 74	NS
Methionine	25	44 ± 20	5	30 ± 13	NS	4	31 ± 14	NS	5	39 ± 13	NS	3	53 ± 26	NS
Isoleucine	23	76 ± 23	5	94 ± 24	NS	4	61 ± 22	NS	5	40 ± 21	S 0.05	3	76 ± 37	NS
Leucine	23	160 ± 41	5	173 ± 51	NS	4	157 ± 22	NS	5	154 ± 30	NS	3	196 ± 46	NS
Tyrosine	22	80 ± 19	5	92 ± 14	NS	4	100 ± 19	NS	5	92 ± 12	NS	3	89 ± 23	NS
Phenylalanine	19	97 ± 18	5	129 ± 34	S 0.05	4	139 ± 40	S 0.01	5	121 ± 31	NS	3	149 ± 76	S 0.05
Ornithine	9	171 ± 45	4	227 ± 76	NS	4	169 ± 49	NS	5	201 ± 96	NS	3	218 ± 63	NS
Lycine	8	312 ± 67	5	308 ± 51	NS	4	371 ± 79	NS	5	296 ± 42	NS	3	449 ± 94	S 0.05
Histidine	24	151 ± 29	5	143 ± 32	NS	4	180 ± 14	NS	5	128 ± 10	NS	3	154 ± 52	NS
Arginine	17	63 ± 19	3	51 ± 14	NS	3	84 ± 30	NS	5	43 ± 17	S 0.05	3	117 ± 122	NS

Table 6. Amino-acid concentration in placenta (μ mol/100 g) wet weight (Control, Toxemia, Premature, Growth retardation and after intra-amniotic injection of amino-acid) (The statistically significant figures are underlined)

Group	I a (Control)		I b Toxemia			I b Premature			I b Growth retard.			II b			II c 45 min after injection (caesarean)		
Amino-acid	N	M ± S. D.	N	M ± S. D.	P	N	M ± S. D.	P	N	M ± S. D.	P	N	M ± S. D.	P	N	M ± S. D.	P
Aspartate + Asparagine	25	107 ± 43	6	111 ± 29	NS	4	143 ± 10	NS	5	92 ± 52	NS	3	422 ± 336	0.01 S	4	165 ± 28	0.01
Threonine	25	80 ± 36	6	58 ± 24	NS	4	114 ± 31	NS	5	70 ± 42	NS	3	213 ± 199	0.01	4	129 ± 23	0.01
Serine	25	98 ± 45	6	77 ± 28	NS	4	158 ± 58	0.01 S	5	89 ± 57	NS	3	185 ± 114	0.01	4	174 ± 34	0.01
Glutamate + Glutamine	26	343 ± 104	6	320 ± 96	NS	4	519 ± 191	0.05 S	5	285 ± 134	NS	3	742 ± 438	0.01	4	487 ± 71	0.01
Proline	23	71 ± 38	6	66 ± 14	NS	4	133 ± 40	0.01 S	5	66 ± 55	NS	3	86 ± 3	NS	4	143 ± 47	0.01
Glycine	25	209 ± 82	6	175 ± 57	NS	4	317 ± 38	0.01 S	5	163 ± 74	NS	3	691 ± 753	0.01	4	311 ± 33	0.01
Alanine	25	121 ± 52	6	111 ± 33	NS	4	204 ± 58	0.01 S	5	106 ± 65	NS	3	316 ± 260	0.01	4	200 ± 74	0.01
Cystine	26	25 ± 19	6	11 ± 5	NS	3	28 ± 17	NS	5	18 ± 22	NS	3	126 ± 129	0.01	4	27 ± 15	NS
Valine	26	50 ± 21	6	46 ± 11	NS	4	88 ± 23	0.05 S	5	48 ± 32	NS	3	126 ± 134	0.01	4	94 ± 19	0.01
Methionine	26	17 ± 8	6	13 ± 9	NS	4	35 ± 16	0.05 S	5	18 ± 13	NS	3	82 ± 73	0.01	4	39 ± 7	0.01
Isoleucine	26	19 ± 10	6	15 ± 7	NS	4	43 ± 17	0.05 S	5	28 ± 23	NS	3	111 ± 125	0.01	4	48 ± 13	0.01
Leucine	26	72 ± 30	6	66 ± 18	NS	4	116 ± 32	0.05 S	5	77 ± 46	NS	3	273 ± 277	0.01	4	129 ± 22	0.01
Tyrosine	26	34 ± 15	6	30 ± 9	NS	4	56 ± 15	0.05 S	5	35 ± 22	NS	3	126 ± 89	0.01	4	61 ± 11	0.01
Phenylalanine	26	38 ± 17	6	38 ± 7	NS	4	67 ± 19	NS	5	40 ± 24	NS	3	174 ± 160	0.01	4	69 ± 14	0.01
Ornithine	24	42 ± 19	6	43 ± 14	NS	4	37 ± 14	NS	5	24 ± 10	NS				4	38 ± 5	NS
Lycine	24	92 ± 35	6	78 ± 19	NS	4	126 ± 28	NS	5	79 ± 61	NS	3	449 ± 320	0.01	4	144 ± 35	0.01
Histidine	26	31 ± 13	6	23 ± 7	NS	4	47 ± 9	NS	5	28 ± 20	NS	3	125 ± 152	0.01	4	54 ± 13	0.01
Arginine	23	43 ± 16	6	44 ± 20	NS	4	79 ± 22	0.01 S	5	46 ± 29	NS	3	69 ± 54	NS	4	74 ± 32	0.01

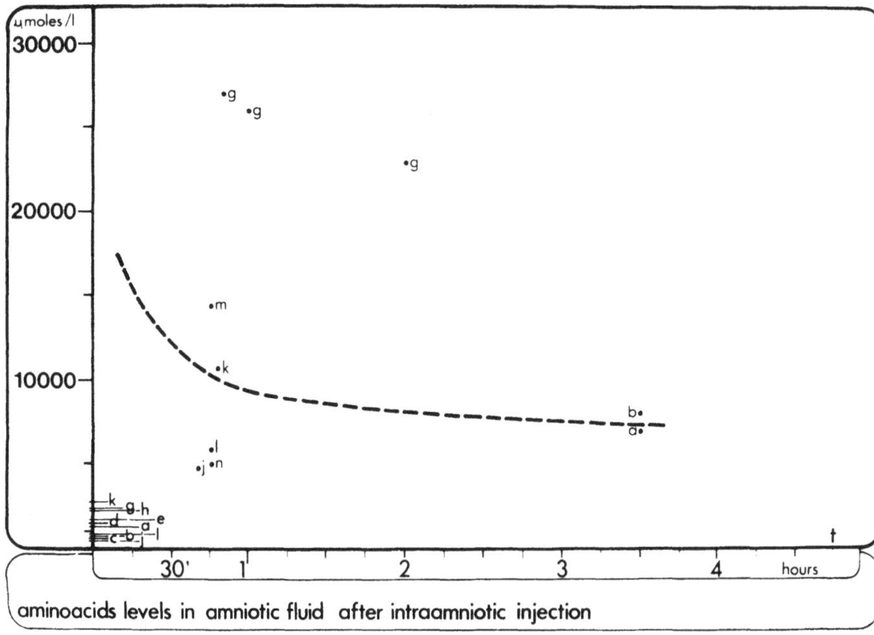

Fig. 8. Amino-acid concentrations (micromoles/l) in amniotic fluid the 4 hours following the intra-amniotic injection

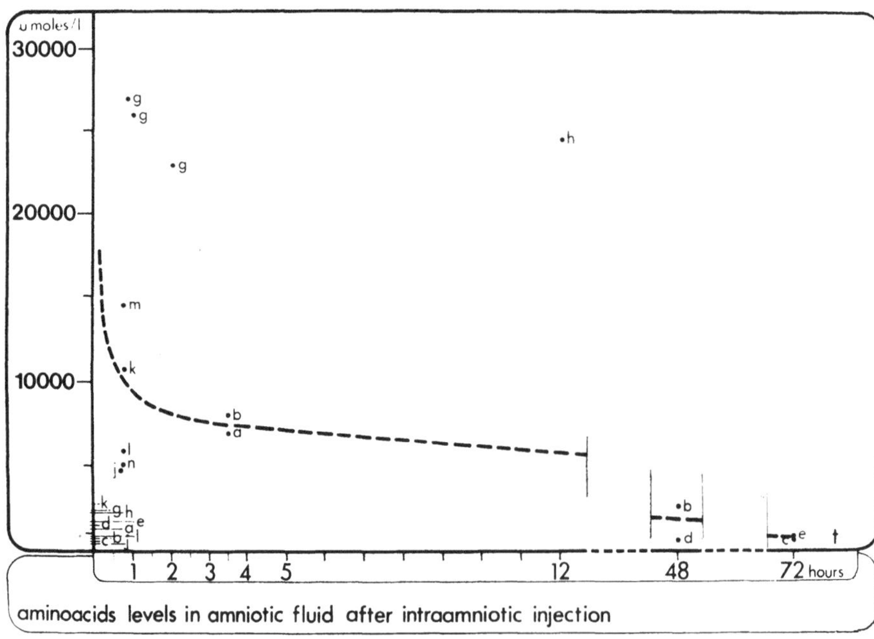

Fig. 9. Amino-acid concentration in amniotic fluid in the 72 hours following the intra-amniotic injection

The high concentrations of plasma amino-acids in cases 9 and 16 are very likely due to the small volume of amniotic fluid (Fig. 9).

The selective examination of each amino acid of the amniotic fluid in the group of elective caesarean sections carried out 45 minutes after intra-amniotic injection reveals that the rate of loss varies. The amino acids that have the highest rate of loss are aspartate-asparagine (86 %), lysine (86 %), valine (84 %), methionine (82 %), isoleucine (81 %), leucine (74 %), alanine (74 %), phenylalanine (73 %), tyrosine (73 %) and threonine (70 %) (Table 7). There is no parallel between these rates of loss of amniotic fluid and the amino-acid concentration in the injected solution. If one takes into account the amino-acid concentration in the Aminosol 100 solution, and the rate of loss of amniotic fluid, amino acids can be classified in decreasing order, according to the quantity lost in the amniotic compartment: valine, lysine, leucine, glutamate-glutamine, alanine, tyrosine, aspartate-asparagine, serine, threonine.

Because of the quantity of amino-acid that have disappeared from the amniotic compartment in an hour and of the different loss rates for each of them, we suggest that phenomena other than fetal deglutition occur leading to a fall in the plasma amino-acid concentration.

Table 7. Amino-acid concentration in Aminosol 100 (micromoles/50 ml) and percentages of amino acids lost from amniotic fluid 45 minutes after intra-amniotic injections. Amino-acids are in decreasing order according to their concentration in Aminosol 100

Amino-acid	Micromoles/50 ml Aminosol 100	% AF loss	Amino-acid	Micromoles/50 ml Aminosol 100	% AF loss
LYS	2444	86	ASP + ASN	1082	86
VAL	2369	84	MET	1014	82
LEU	2275	74	PRO	973	43
GLU	1990	55	GLY	635	58
ALA	1365	74	ARG	632	65
PHE	1326	73	HIS	553	67
SER	1299	68	CYS	348	69
ILEU	1141	81	TYR	148	73
THR	1087	70	ORN	-	-

2. Maternal Venous Plasma

Amino-acidograms of maternal venous plasma taken in the hours following the repeated intra-amniotic injections of group II b (1, 1/2, 2, and 3 hours after injection) are approximately those of the sample preceeding the injection, except case 1 (Table 2) who had received 250 ml of Aminosol 100 and in whom we had carried out a placental biopsy 2 days before the injection. In group II c (elective caesarean section) the venous maternal plasma taken when the fetus was extracted, 45 minutes after intra-amniotic injection has a significantly higher concentration of proline, methionine and lysine and a lower concentration of cystine (Fig. 10, Table 4) than the control group (I a). YOUNG and PRENTO (26) have noticed a decrease in plasma cystine in anesthetized women. The lack of changes in maternal venous aminoacidogram suggests that amino-acids are transferred only in a very small quantities into maternal blood or that their dilution in the maternal blood is considerable.

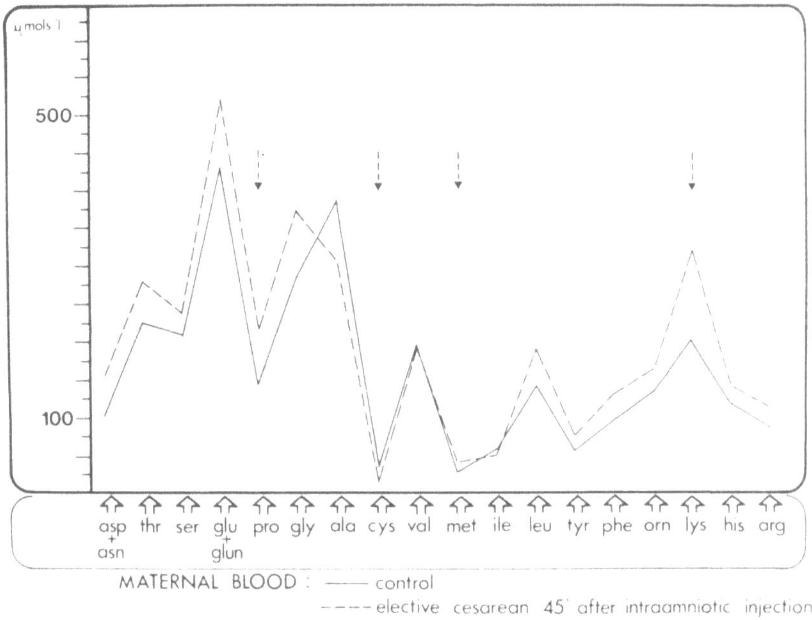

Fig. 10. Amino-acid concentrations (micromoles/l) in maternal plasma. Control and elective caesarean groups (I a, II c). This figure ↓ indicates the amino-acids that have a significantly different concentration in the elective caesarean group compared with the controls

To answer this last question we have calculated in one case from group II c (elective cesarean section) the quantity of amino acids which had left the amniotic cavity after 45 minutes and which were not stored in the placenta by giving it by intravenous infusion at a constant rate. Before and after the infusion maternal blood was sampled from the antecubital vein of the opposite side. These was seen in this group on elevation of proline, alanine, valine, isoleucine, leucine, phenylalanine and lysine after the infusion (Fig. 11 , Table 8). These results seen to confirm that if a significant quantity of amino acids had passed from the amniotic cavity to the maternal circulation we would have been able to observe clear changes in the amino-acidogram 45 minutes after intra-amniotic injection.

3. Umbilical Plasma

In cases of repeated intra-amniotic injections we were not able to show any difference in the amino-acidogram of umbilical plasma from the control group. However, none of the samples of umbilical blood were taken until at least 85 hours after the last intra-amniotic injection and it is probable that after this duration the variations in the amino-acidogram are inperceptible.

The amino-acidogram of umbilical plasma taken 45 minutes after intra-amniotic infection in the group II c cases (elective caesarean section) when compared with the control group I shows a significant increase in proline, phenylalanine and lysine with a decrease in aspartate-asparagine (Fig. 12, Table 5). The concentration of the other amino-acids did not change noticeably. The absence of any large increase in fetal plas-

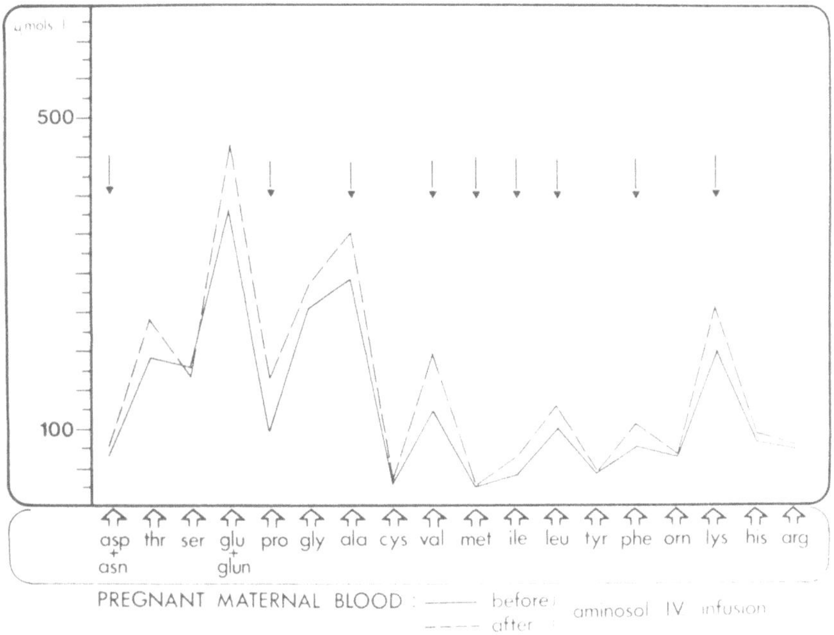

Fig. 11. Amino-acid concentrations (micromoles/l) in pregnant maternal plasma before and after Aminosol intravenous infusion. The figure ↓ indicates the amino-acids that have a significantly different concentration before and after intravenous infusion of Aminosol

Table 8. Amino-acid concentration in maternal plasma before and after intravenous infusion of Aminosol 100

	Before intravanous amino-acid infusion		After intravenous amino-acid infusion		
	mean	S. D.	mean	S. D.	P
ASP + ASN	63,9	12,0	76,0	13,1	NS
THR	192,18	53,20	239,0	70,6	NS
SER	179,9	106,9	167,0	40,8	NS
GLU + GLUN	377,5	86,5	465,0	76,6	S
PRO	98,5	23,3	166,3	20,6	S
GLY	252,7	62,6	285,4	44,0	NS
ALA	290,3	41,2	349,4	50,0	S
CYS	26,6	14,7	28,8	8,6	NS
VAL	120,0	29,2	197,2	63,0	S
MET	22,7	4,1	27,9	4,5	S
ILEU	39,7	7,8	62,6	16,4	S
LEU	102,8	24,3	127,8	29,0	S
TYR	42,2	13,7	44,7	14,8	NS
PHE	75,2	19,0	105,5	30,9	S
ORN	65,0	21,4	68,8	25,0	NS
LYS	198,5	35,9	253,6	40,4	S
HIS	81,6	19,5	91,6	22,15	NS
ARG	73,4	22,5	77,0	12,9	NS

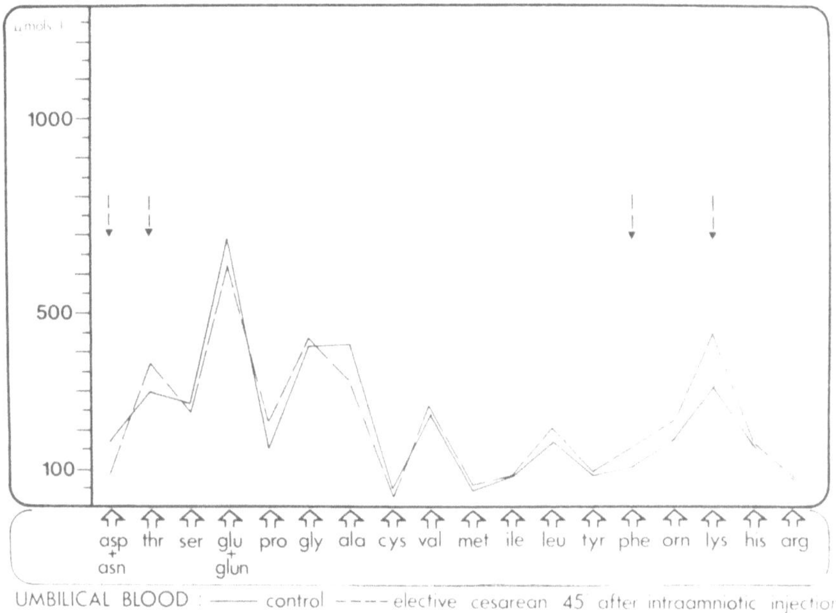

Fig. 12. Amino-acid concentrations (micromoles/l) in umbilical blood control and elective caesarean groups (I a, II c). The figure↓shows those amino-acids that have significantly different concentrations in the elective caesarean group and in the controls

ma amino-acid concentrations does not necessarily mean that the amino acids did not pass into the fetus in quantity. They may have been stored or rapidly assimilated and the blood pool in such conditions would only represent a small fraction of the amino-acids absorbed by the fetus.

4. Placenta

We noticed an increase in the amount of amino acids extracted from several placentae in cases of repeated intra-amniotic injection. We put forward the hypothesis of storage of amino-acids in the placenta when injections were repeated (18). This was less evident when there was only one injection, but we had only two placental aminograms in this group. Placental amino-acidograms were made on 26 normal placentas and were used as controls.

The amino-acidograms of the placentae from group II c (elective caesarean section patients) show a significant increase in all amino acids except cystine and ornithine (Fig . 13, Table 5). In cases of normal amniotic volume, the amount of amino-acids stored in placental tissue, 45 minutes after intra-amniotic injection, is close to 1/2 or 1/3 of the quantity of amino-acids that left the amniotic compartment.

The amino-acids stored in greatest quantity in the placenta are, in decreasing order of concentration: glutamate-glutamine, glycine, alanine, serine, proline, aspartate-asparagine, leucine, lysine. These amino acids, except lysine and leucine, are not essential ones. The lack of increase in cystine and ornithine is due to a low concentration in the

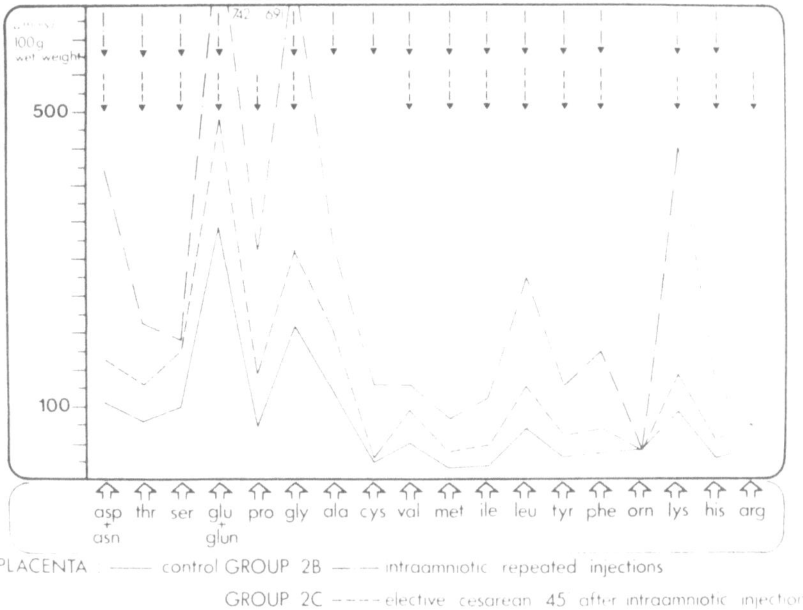

Fig. 13. Amino-acid concentrations in placenta (micromoles/100 g wet weight). The figure ↓ and ↓ shows those amino-acids that have a significantly different concentration in the intra-amniotic repeated injection group and in the intra-amniotic injection before elective caesarean section group compared with the controls

Aminosol 100, and another phenomenon which may explain the low concentration is the absence of the enzyme cystinase which is not present in the human liver before birth (22). Cystine may therefore be rapidly taken up.

These results suggest that the placenta rapidly stores a great proportion of injected amino-acids. The fetus may transfer these amino acids to the placenta after having absorbed some of them after deglutition and the remainder by unknown processes. These amino-acids may also reach the placenta directly through surrounding membranes and through the cord that would be permeable to these substances (2). The two processes may coexist.

III. Effect of Intra-amniotic Injections on Uterine Activity on the Fetus and Newborn Child

1. Uterine Activity

In our first 2 cases which had an Aminosol infusion, one of 250 ml, the other of 300 ml in 3 hours, uterine concentrations occurred while the perfusion was being carried out but they stopped once the catheters were removed. We abandoned this technique substituting repeated and slow injections of 50 ml.

In the four cases (3, 7, 8, 10) of group II a and II b (Table 2) the Aminosol infusion is possibly unrelated to the premature deliveries. In 3 cases hospital admission was due to the threat of premature delivery and the fourth was due to twin pregnancy (No. 7).

The onset of labor may have been due either repeated intra-amniotic punctures or to the hypertonicity and quantity of the fluid injected. Amniotic punctures do not seem to induce labor (13), but the quantity of fluid injected may play some part. We noticed this with infusion between 200 and 300 ml. The strong osmolarity of the solution does not seem to have any effect since the amino-acids leave the amniotic compartment rapidly and we have never noticed any great clinical or ultrasonic variations in amniotic volume.

2. Effects on the Fetus

We have not noted alterations in the fetal heart rate during the first hours or days following the infusions. Moreover, HELLER (5) noted improved oscillations and disappearance of late decelerations during the oxytocin test in a case treated by intra-amniotic injections of amino acid.

The urinary oestriol levels rose to normal values in 4 (6, 7, 8, 9, Table 2) out of 5 cases of growth retardation treated by us, (Figs. 14, 15). This rise is unlikely to be explained by other factors - rest, for example - since injections began two weeks after admission and the patients received no other therapy. HELLER (5) made the same observations following this treatment.

Human chorionicsomatrophin (HCS) measurements were made in two cases (6 and 10 Table 2) as we have only had the assay for a year. In case 6, the abnormally low levels rose to normal values after the third injection. In case 10, levels were normal before treatment and remained unchanged. The effects of the treatment are less clear as regards increased in biparietal diameter. In 4 of the 5 cases of intrauterine growth retardation treated, it remained within normal limits. In case 8 (Table 2) the biparietal diameter curve seemed to fall below the second standard deviation at about the 31st week. A week after injections commenced, the measurement became normal again (Fig. 16).

3. Effects on Delivery and Newborn infant

The treatment does not appear to affect delivery. In 4 cases of group I a and I b a caesarean section has been carried out. The indications were: contracted pelvis with breech presentation of the cord after rupture of the membranes and two cases of fetal distress. In these last two cases the final injection was made 8 days and 11 weeks before delivery.

Except for the last two fetuses, all had a normal heart rate during delivery and all the Apgar scores were between 8 and 10 at the first and fifth minutes. Only one newborn child died on the third day. There was fetal distress and he had a very severe malformation (IVEMARK's syndrome).

Among the 10 cases of group I a and I b, 8 of them have been reexamined a year later. They all had a satisfactory psychomotor.

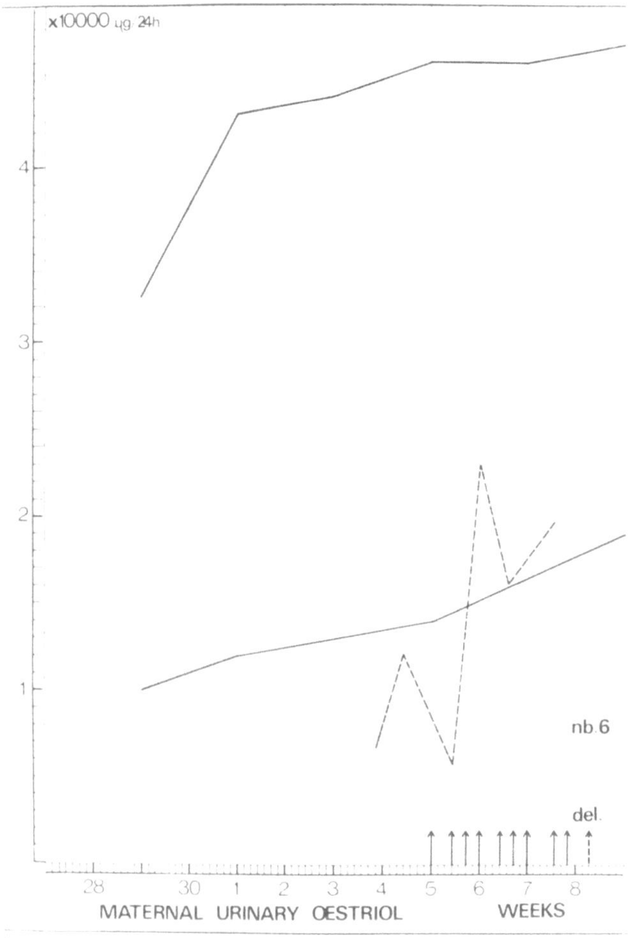

Fig. 14. Maternal urinary oestriol in case 6

Conclusions

We have treated too few cases to form a firm conclusion. More work is necessary. However, some tentative conclusions can be drawn from our results. The amino-acids leave the amniotic cavity very rapidly. For a therapeutic effect, the injections must be repeated every 24 and 48 hours. Amino-acids do not pass in great quantity to the maternal blood. After injections the amino-acids are rapidly removed to the placenta where they are stored. Repeated intra-amniotic injections have no apparent side effects on uterine activity, fetus, or newborn child. In some cases of intra-uterine growth retardation we have seen a rise in maternal urinary oestriol excretion and plasma HCS.

However, such treatment if shown to be of value, should be kept, because of its potential dangers, for cases in which the placental blood flow fell seriously and could not be improved by other means.

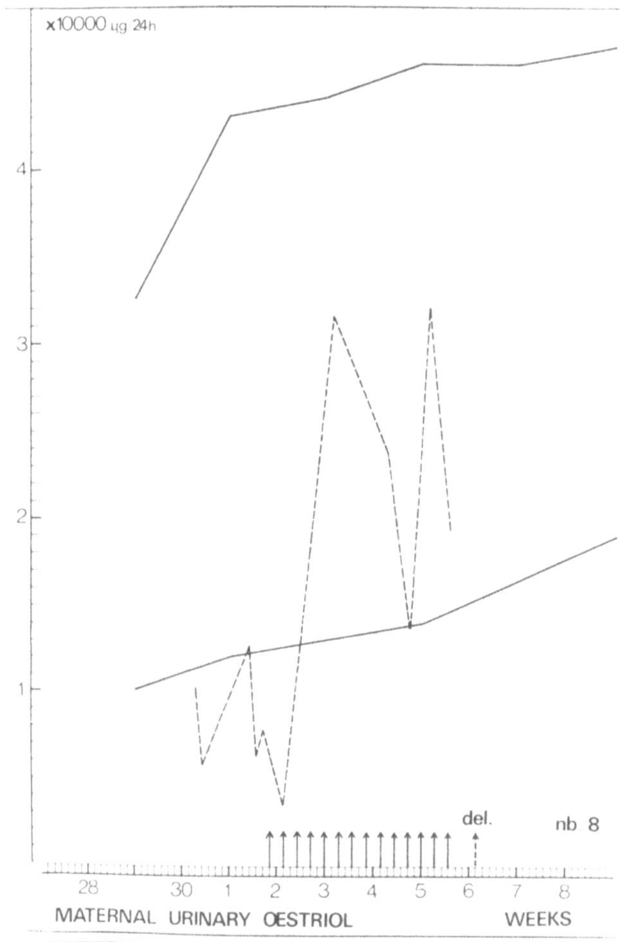

Fig. 15. Maternal urinary oestriol in case 8

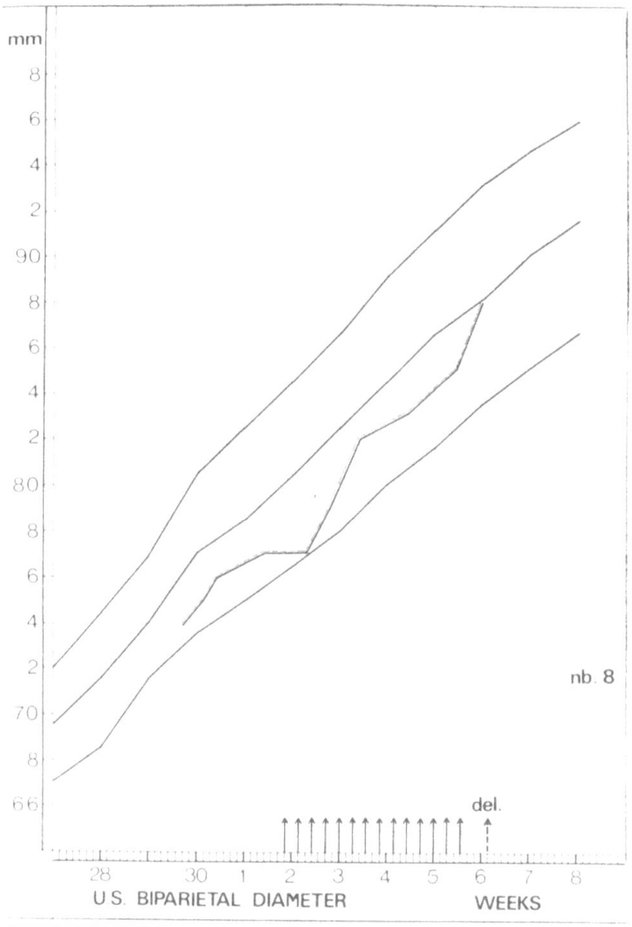

Fig. 16. Ultra-sound biparietal diameter in case 8

References

1. BROWNE, J. C. M., VEALL, N.: The maternal placental blood flow in normotensive and hypertensive women. J. Obstet. Gynaec. Brit. Emp. 60, 141 - 147 (1953).
2. DUDDENHAUSEN, J.W., KYNAST, G., SALING, E.: Kompensatorische Nutrition des mangelversorgten Feten. 4. Deutscher Kongreß für Perninatale Medizin, Berlin, 4 - 6, November 1971.
3. GAUDIER, B., PONTE, C., LACOMBE, A., CALLENS, G., CALLENS, M., BLANC-GARIN, A. P.: Etudes des acides aminés sanguins dans le sang du cordon et dans le sang maternel. Ann. Pediat. 19, 277 - 284 (1972).
4. HELLER, L.: Arteriovenöse Differenzen im Aminosäurenmuster bei Mutter und Kind. Arch. Gynäk. 211, 304 - 305 (1971).
5. HELLER, L.: Intra-uterine Aminoacid feeding of the fetus. IX. International Congress of Nutrition, Mexico-City, 1972.

6. JANISCH, H., LEODOLTER, S., REINOLD, E.: Der Effekt von Ritodrine auf die Plazentadurchblutung. International symposium on the treatment of fetal risks, Baden, Austria, May 1972 (in press).
7. KERR, G., KENNAN, A. L.: Free amino-acids of amniotic fluid during pregnancy of the rhesus monkey. Amer. J. Obstet. Gynec. 105, 363 - 367 (1969).
8. LINDBLAD, B. S.: The plasma aminogram in "small for dates" newborn infants. In JONXIS, S. H. P. et coll. Metabolic process in the foetus and newborn infant. H. E. Stenfert Kroese, Ed. Leider, 111 - 126 (1971).
9. MANZANILLA, S. R., SUAREZ, C. M., CASANOVA, A. N., MAASS, E. R.: Intra-uterine fetal oral feeding: basic research using intra-amniotic albumin I^{131}. VI. World Congress of Gynecology and Obstetrics, New York, 1970. Internat. J. Gynaec. Obstet. 8, 238 - 239 (1970).
10. MORRIS, N., OSBORN, S. B., WRIGHT, H. P., HART, A.: Effective uterine blood-flow during excroine in normal and pre-eclamptic pregnancies. Lancet 2, 481-484 (1956).
11. OSTERGARD, D. R.: The physiology and clinical importance of amniotic fluid. A review. Obstet. Gynec. Surv. 25, 297 - 319 (1970).
12. PAGE, E. W.: Discussion in: PEARSE, H. W., SORNSON, H.: Free amino-acids of normal and abnormal human placenta. Amer. J. Obstet. Gynec. 105, 696 - 701 (1969).
13. PEREZ, M. A., ALONSO, J. L., BELITZKY, R.: La puncion amniótica transparietoabdominal (P. A. T.) efectas immediatos sobre la contractilidad uterina y su relación con el comienzo del parto espontâneo. Rev. Argent. Ginec. Obstet. II, 153 - 159 (1971).
14. PONTONNIER, G., DELMAS, H., LAGORCE, J. C., JOSSERAND, P.: Mesure du débit placentaire par le Xenon 133 dans la grossesse humaine normale et pathologique. Bull. Fed. Soc. Gynéc. Obstét. lang. franc. 22, 97 - 127 (1970).
15. PRITCHARD, J. A.: Deglutition by normal and anencephalic fetuses. Obstet. Gynec. 25, 289 - 297 (1965).
16. RENAUD, R., VINCENDON, G., BOOG, G., BRETTES, J. P., KOEHL, C., SCHUMACHER, J. C., KIRSCHTETTER, L., GANDAR, R.: Premiers résultats de perfusions et d'injections d'acides aminés intra-amniotiques dans les malnutritions foetales. 1ères Journées Nationales de la Société Francaise de Médicine Périnatale, Paris 1971.
17. RENAUD, R., BOOG, G., BRETTES, J. P., IRRMANN, M., DE MOT, E., SCHUMACHER, J. C., GANDAR, R.: Souffrance foetale - Aspects thérapeutiques. XXIIème Congrès National d'Anesthésie - Réanimation - Paris, 1972; Arnetter éd., Paris, 851 - 1125, 1972.
18. RENAUD, R., VINCENDON, G., BOOG, G., BRETTES, J. P., SCHUMACHER, J. C., KOEHL, C., KIRSCHTETTER, L., GANDAR, R.: Injections intra-amniotiques d'acides aminés dans les cas de malnutrition foetale. Premiers résultats. J. Gyn. Obst. Biol. Repr. 1, 231 - 244 (1972).
19. RENAUD, R., BRETTES, J. P., IRRMANN, M., BOOG, G., SCHUMACHER, J. C., GANDAR, R.: A double blind cross-over trial to assess the effect of Ritodrine on uterine blood in normal and pathologic pregnancies. International symposium on the treatment of fetal risks, Baden, Austria, May 1972 (in press).
20. SALING, E., SALCHOW, P., DUDDENHAUSEN, J. W.: Intra-uterine Ernährung des Feten - Erste Untersuchungen. III. Deutscher Kongreß für Perinatale Medizin, Berlin, Stuttgart. Georg Thieme Verlag 1968.
21. SUGAWA, T., NAKAMURA, K., OZAKI, M.: Studies on the amino-acids and protein metabolism in foetal growth. Dynamics of free

amino-acids in the amniotic fluid and its nutritive role in the foetus. J. Jap. Obstet. Gynec. So. 10, 1 (1963).
22. STURMAN, J. A., GAULL, G., RAIHA, N. C. R.: Absence of Cystathionase in human fetal liver: is cystine essential? Science 169, 74 - 75 (1970).
23. WIDDOWSON, E. M.: Protein status of "small for date" animals. In JONXIS, S. H. P. et coll. Metabolic process in the foetus and newborn infant. H. E. Stenfert Kroese, Ed. Leiden, 165 - 174 (1971).
24. WINICK, M.: Fetal malnutrition. Klin. Obstet. Gynec. 13, 526 - 541 (1970).
25. YOUNG, M.: Placental transport of free amino-acids. In JONXIS, S. H. P. and coll. Metabolic process in the foetus and newborn infant. H. E. Stenfert Kroese, Ed. Leiden, 97 - 108 (1971).
26. YOUNG, M., PRENTON, M. A.: Maternal and fetal plasma amino-acid concentrations during gestation and in retarded fetal growth. J. Obstet. Gynaec. Brit. Cwlth. 76, 333 - 344 (1969).

The Effects of Maternal Infusions of L-Amino Acids as a Treatment of Chronic Fetal-Placental Insufficiency

F. E. Mansani, E. Cavatorta, M. Ceruti, and E. Vadora

'Small for dates' neonates are sub-nourished with particular reference to protein: It is important to feed these neonates parenterally with emphasis upon the amino-acid content of their infusion. Such amino-acids may be obtained from hydrolysates of fibrin or caseine, or by using synthetic mixture similar to that of human lactoalbumin or a solution containing amino-acids in concentrations similar to that of plasma.

In pregnancies where 'small for dates' infants are suspected, oral or intravenous amino-acid supplements have been suggested. We have infused some pregnant patients with L-amino-acids together with progesterone and beta-mimetic drugs to increase placental blood flow and perhaps encourage amino-acids to reach the fetal circulation. The mother was also given dihydroepiandrosterone to assess placental function.

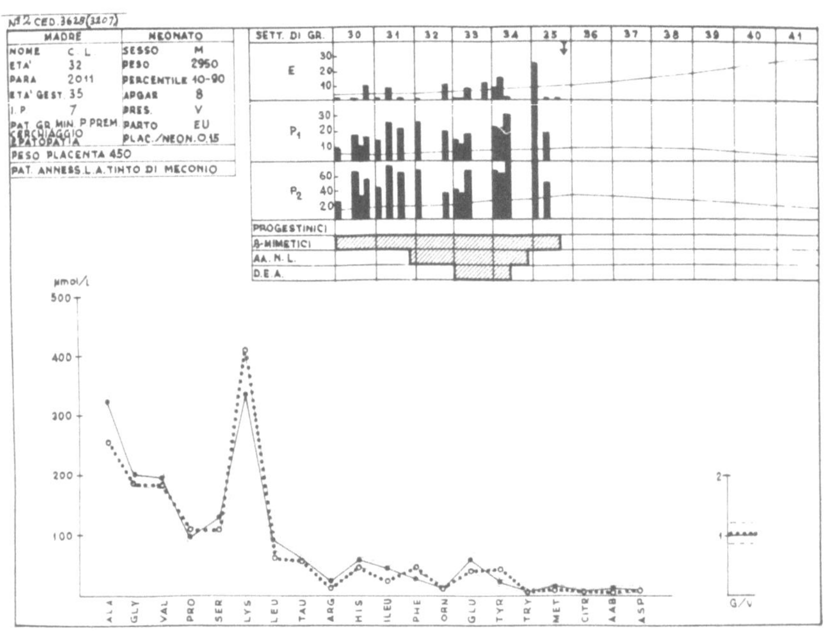

Fig. 1

We treated five patients suspected to be carrying 'small for dates' babies. The mothers also had one of the following: jaundice of pregnancy, threatened premature labour or premature rupturing of the membranes. The patient was given L-amino-acids by daily infusion of 500 ml of solution containing 18 amino-acids (3.5 g/100 ml) for a minimum period of two weeks. The length of each infant was measured and we have also measured certain hormones, the amino-acid concentration of the umbilical venous blood and the glycine/valine ratio from this blood.

One of the most interesting cases is shown in Table 1. The continuous and the broken lines respectively indicate mean and standard deviation for each amino-acid in the umbilical venous plasma of a normal new-born infant, while the dotted line represents the amino-acids in the umbilical venous plasma of the new-born infant. Of the five pregnancies investigated, four resulted in normal neonates and one was a 'small for dates' infant. Four patients delivered at term and one prematurely. All neonates were in good condition at birth (Apgar 8 to 10). In four of the five, amino-acid concentrations were normal; in all the glycine/valine ratios were normal.

Because we used a mixture of drugs with the L-amino-acids it is impossible to know whether the amino-acid infusions were of any benefit. The amino-acid concentrations were normal in four of the neonates and the glycine/valine ratio normal in all.

Plasma Amino-Acids in "Small for Date" Newborn Infants

F. E. Mansani, E. Cavatorta, M. Ceruti, and F. Coppola

The authors have measured the plasma amino-acids in 'small for date' newborn infants and compared these figures with others obtained from a control group of neonates of normal weight and of a full-term pregnancy.

The plasma amino-acids were measured in 10 normal neonates and in 9 'small for dates', some from abnormal pregnancies and others from apparently normal pregnancies.

Fig. 1 shows the plasma amino-acids measured in blood from the umbilical vein and the glycine/valine ratio of the normal neonates. The mean (continuous line) and the standard deviation (dashed line) have

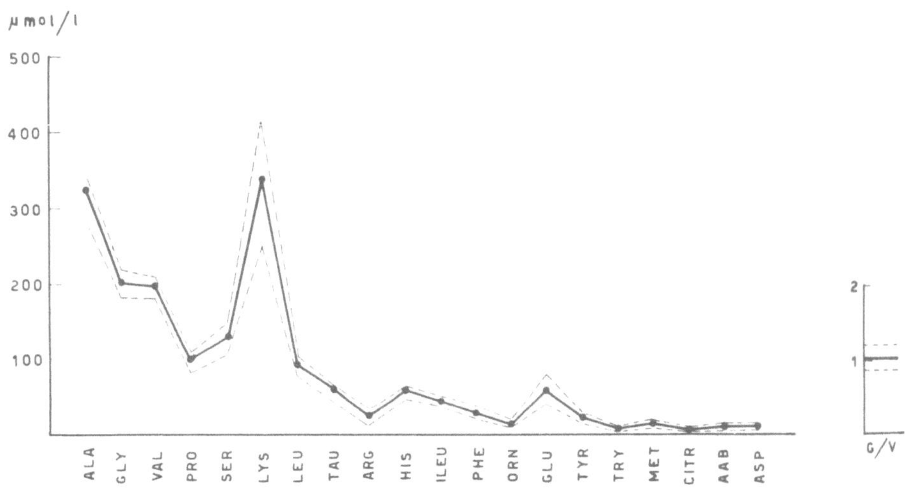

Fig. 1

been plotted. The total mean concentration of the amino-acids is 32.0 mg/100 ml of plasma, which is higher than that found in a normal adult. In particular, the healthy neonate has a higher concentration of alanine and lysine; all the other amino-acids are increased in a smaller proportion and proline is a little reduced. The glycine/valine ratio has an average of 1.01, with a standard deviation of 0.85 to 1.21.

Fig. 2. shows the plasma amino-acids measured in blood from the umbilical vein and the glycine/valine ratio of the small for dates neonates, (vertical lines: mean and standard deviation) compared with those of normal neonates (continuous line: mean; dashed lines: standard deviation). The total mean concentration of the amino-acids is 36.2 mg/100 ml

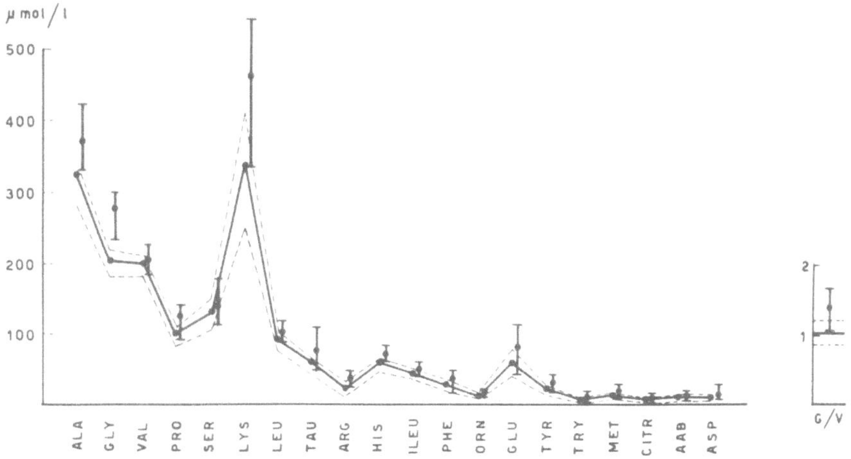

Fig. 2

of plasma, 13 % greater than the average for normal newborn babies. In the 'small for dates' babies most of the amino-acids have increased compared with those of a normal new-born baby. In particular alanine, glycine, proline and lysine, and to a lesser extract taurine, histidine and glutamic acid are increased. The glycine/valine ratio is increased with a mean of 1.37 and a standard deviation of 1.03 to 1.63.

In 'small for dates' neonates, the fetal/maternal ratio of amino-acids falls, (the maternal concentration increases more than the fetal), in particular the essential amino-acids valine, leucine and isoleucine. This increase in the plasma in "small for dates" neonates is at variance with their small sizes. Perhaps the increased concentration represents a lack of incorporation of these amino-acids and hence the small size of the infant. This is similar to the findings in an adult with protein starvation. We suggest that the increase in the glycine/valine ratio found in the 'small for dates' babies, but not in the controls, is of value in differentiating between a 'small for dates' infant and one born prematurely with a weight proportional to the gestational age.

Treatment of Severe Feto-Placental Insufficiency by Means of Intraamniotic Injection of Amino-Acids

M. Massobrio, E. Margaria, M. Campogrande, F. Badini Confalonieri, and A. Bocci

The fetus uses for the protein synthesis the amino-acids of the labelled albumin injected into the amniotic fluid (2); he is also able to swallow and to exploit for his nutrition the amino-acids directly injected into the amniotic cavity (1, 4, 5). This is the assumption for the use of the intra-amniotic injection of amino-acids in order to nourish the fetus in case of placental insufficiency (1, 4, 5).

For the moment our experience in this field is still limited to five cases in which the conditions of the feto-placental unit, mainly evaluated through the biparietal diameter (BPD) and the mother urinary estriol and pregnanediol, were severely affected.

The clinical characteristics of the cases treated are synthetized in Table 1.

Our method, after ultrasonic localization of the placenta, consists in transabdominal injection into the amniotic cavity of 50 ml of an amino-acid solution of recent synthesis (Protinutril-Roger Bellon Co.), after having drawn an equal quantity of amniotic fluid. The injections were repeated with an interval from 24 up to 72 hours.

Among these five cases, the case No. 1 and No. 3 are those in which the few intra-amniotic injections of the amino-acids effected were unsuccessful. In both cases, the former complicated by a serious trisymptomatic toxemia, the latter with three previous intra-uterine deaths due to placental insufficiency, the mother's urinary estriol dropped, before the beginning of the treatment, below 4 mg/24 hours, suggesting the imminent death of the fetus, whose BPD and amniotic creatinine showed a serious delay of maturity, confirmed by the weight at birth (1330 and 700 g).

The success obtained with case 4 is obviously not to be ascribed only to the single intra-amniotic injection of amino-acids, but to the collateral therapy directed to lower the arterial pressure (190/130 at the start of the therapy), to promote the diuresis (contracted at the start of the therapy), to improve the uterine blood flow through vasodilators and macromolecules.

Particulary interesting are, on the contrary, cases 2 and 5, where it was possible to do the greatest number of intra-amniotic injections (eight and five respectively) and to observe the spontaneous birth of living and viable fetuses, which at the long term control are in very good health conditions.

Case 2 refers to a patient who had 6 previous pregnancies, 3 with spontaneous abortions between the second and fifth month, and 3 with premature births before the 33rd week of stillborn fetuses weighing less than 1050 g.

The patient with a brachytypical-megalosplanchnic constitution (height: 1,41 m; weight: 86 kilos) showed also a rather high degree of hypo-

Table 1. Case of severe placental insufficiency treated with intra-amniotic injection of amino-acids

Case	Age	Parity	Associated pathology	Pregnancy week at the beginning of the therapy	Number of intra-amniotic injections	Delivery	Newborn		Further control
							Weight (g)	Apgar score	
1 FA	34	2012	Severe toxemia	32	3	Spontaneous 34 weeks	1330	1 (died after 15 min)	-
2 GL	33	0330	Primitive infertility Hypothyroidism	30	8	Spontaneous 34 weeks	1750	9	very good conditions after 3 months
3 TS	31	0300	Primitive infertility Albuminuria	27	2	Spontaneous 29 weeks	700	0 (still born)	-
4 CA	30	0000	Multiple fibromyomas Renal insufficiency Nefrectomy	35	1	Cesarian section and hysterectomy 36 weeks	1350	8	very good conditions after 2 months
5 DV	30	0100	Infertility	35	5	Spontaneous 37 weeks	2700	10	very good conditions after 1 month

thyroidism (thyroxinic iodine = 2.8 μg/100 ml with N. V. = 5,6 ± 0,8; percentage of insaturated TBG = 72 % with N. V. = 47 - 58 %) treated with thyroid (1 tablet pro die) and triodotyronine (40 mg pro die for short periods of time). The patient presented a considerable edema at the ankles and a slight increase of the pressor values, which rapidly regressed duing to the use of vasodilators (theophyllinics and isossi-suprine) and diuretics (furosemide).

The mother's urinary estriol was below the lower normal limit, whereas the pregnanediol showed a normal value; the BPD, measured by ultrasonic method, during the two weeks before the beginning of the therapy showed only a modest increase, near the lower limits of the physiological range.

During the four weeks of treatment with intra-amniotic injections of amino-acids, the pregnanediol fell to a rather low level; the estriol did not change at first, but soon before the delivery it increased joining the physiological range, and the BPD increased much more evidently, approaching the average normal values (Figs. 1, 2, 3).

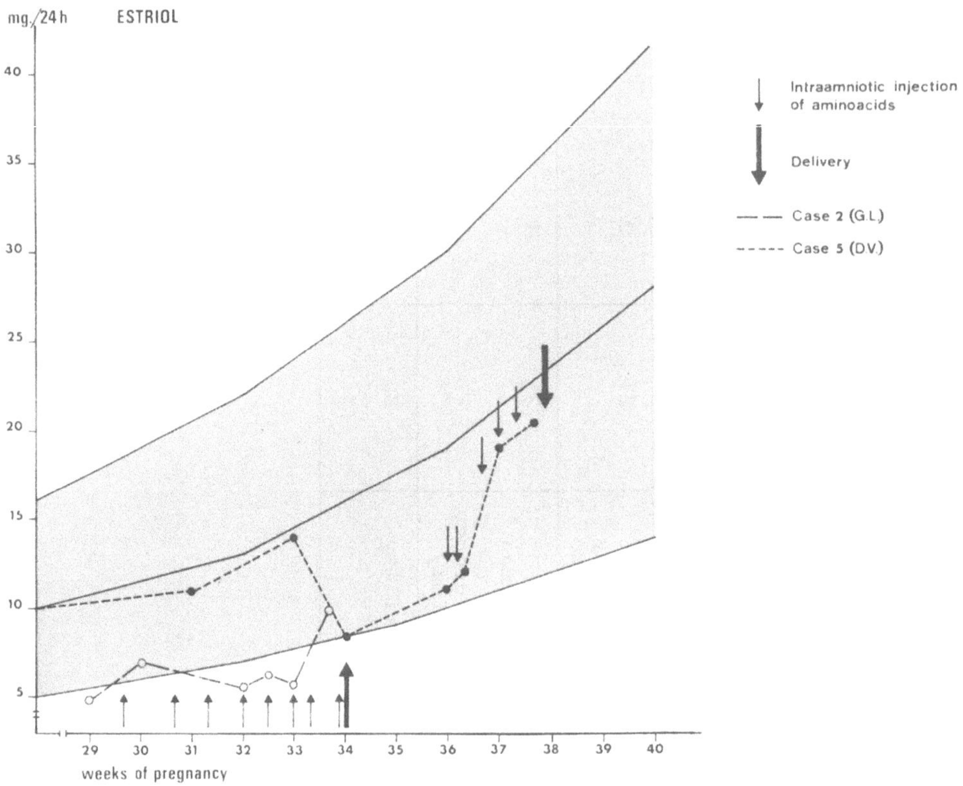

Fig. 1

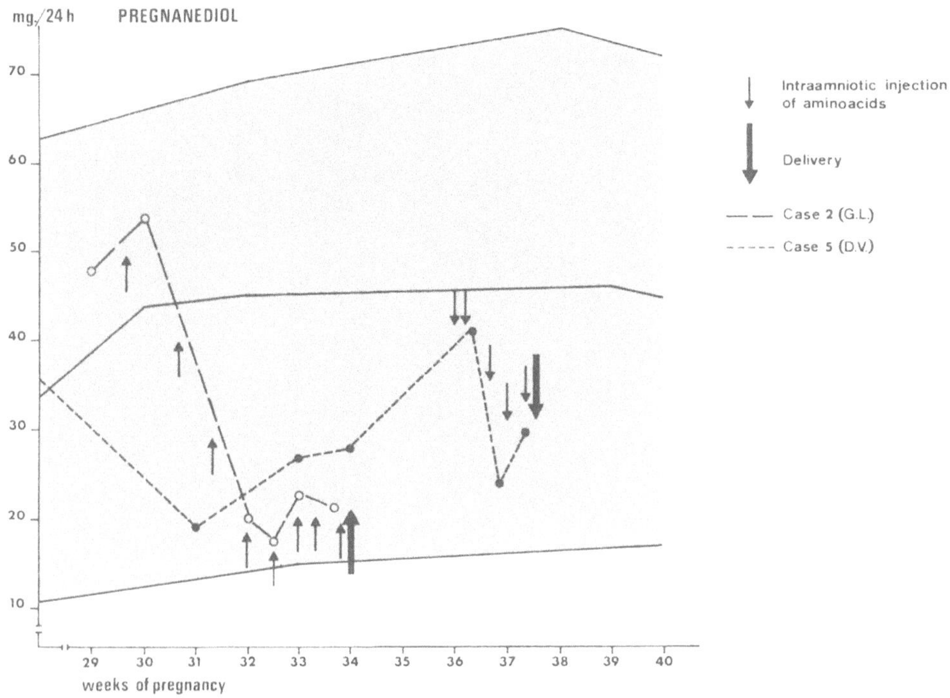

Fig. 2

After 8 intra-amniotic injections, during the 34th week, the patient was delivered of a fetus of 1750 g with Apgar score of 9; after three months from the delivery he was still in perfect health conditions.

Case 5 refers to a patient unipara who had a previous pregnancy with intra-uterine death of the fetus due to placental insufficiency (the delivery occurred at the 38th week, the fetus weighed 1850 g). The patient did not show any sign of toxemia and the laboratory data were normal, with the exception of the hormonal values showing a fall of estriol between 33 and 34 weeks and of the pregnanediol around 31 weeks. At the beginning of the therapy the estriol was still near the lower normal limit, whereas the pregnanediol was already returned to normal. During the treatment the estriol increased up to 20 mg/24 hours; the pregnanediol decreased again, and increased slightly before delivery (Figs. 1, 2).

In the same case the BPD was below the physiological range and approached the limit of this range with a rather rapid increase only after the fetal intra-amniotic nutrition (Fig. 3). At the 37th week the patient was delivered of a fetus of 2700 g with an Apgar score of 10, which was in very good health conditions a month later.

During the treatment in both cases the concentration of the nitrogenous compounds in the amniotic fluid was evaluated. An increase in urea (from 60 to 100 mg/100 ml) was observed in case 2, together with a

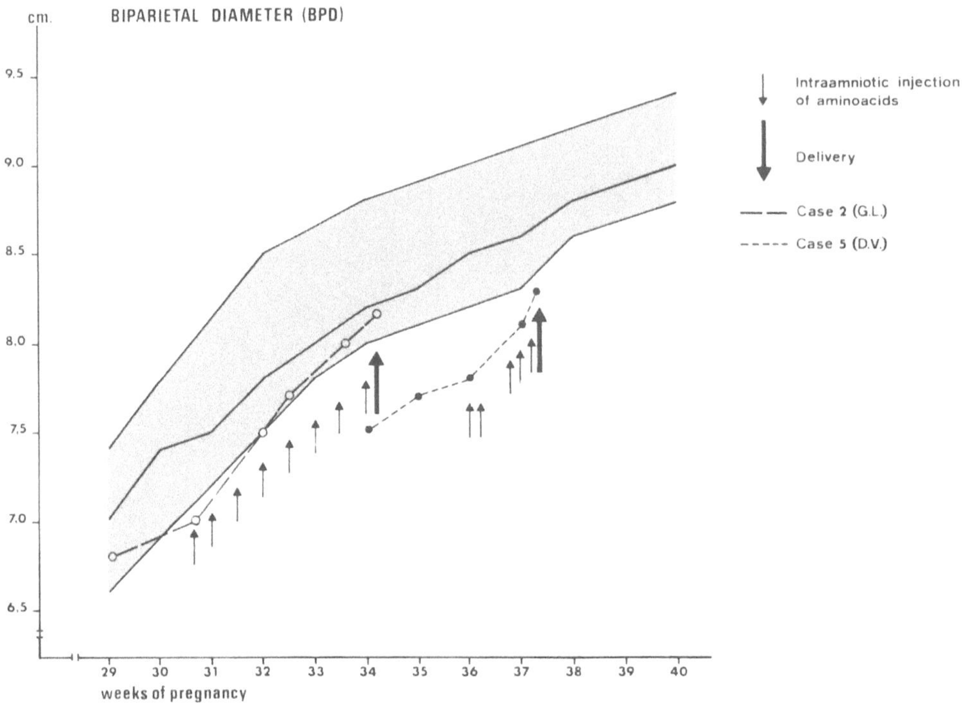

Fig. 3

decrease of proteins (from 350 to 150 mg/100 ml), whereas the creatinine increased from 1,2 to 2,6 mg %, decreasing then to 1,6 soon before delivery.

A decrease of the total proteins was confirmed with case 5 (from 120 to 95 mg/100 ml) whereas urea and creatinine did not remarkably change (50 - 55 mg/100 ml, and 1,2 - 1,3 mg/100 ml respectively). A wider experience is necessary to establish a cause-effect relationship between the treatment and the changes of the BPD and the hormonal values; however it is clear that in cases 2 and 5 after the intra-amniotic injections of amino-acids we observed a remarkable increase of estriol and a decrease of pregnanediol, which suggest that the fetal conditions improved, despite an aggravation or, at least, an instability of the placental function. The BPD has increased much more evidently after the beginning of the therapy than before, as pointed out be RENAUD and coll. (4).

The fall of the amniotic fluid proteins was more evident that the decrease commonly observed in the same period of pregnancy; this suggest, in agreement with QUEENAN's hypothesis (3), that the fetal swallowing should increase as a consequence of the improvement of the fetal conditions. The highly evident increase of urea in the amniotic fluid in case 2 is an indirect demonstration of the fetal swallowing, absorption and metabolization of the injected amino-acids.

In the same case it is not possible, for the time being at least, to explain the behaviour of the amniotic creatinine, which mainly depends on the fetal renal function.

In conclusion, although it is difficult to demonstrate the actual efficiency of any treatment directed to correct the feto-placental insufficiency, we have the impression that in two of the treated cases the repeated intra-amniotic injections of amino-acids have prolonged the fetal life up to a sufficient degree of maturity allowing the survival of the newborn child.

In any of the treated cases no complications were observed, either for the mother or for the fetus.

We found some difficulty when the placenta was inserted on the anterior uterine wall (case 3), or when the amniotic fluid quantity was very poor (case 4). Under such circumstances and particularly, if repeated injections are necessary to find the amniotic cavity, it is possible to cause a bleeding of uterine or placental origin; we feel that this may stimulate uterine contractions, which are easier in placental insufficiency.

Despite its harmlessness, the prescription of the fetal intra-amniotic nutrition with amino-acids is still limited to cases of serious feto-placental insufficiency with previous reproductive failures, possibly without significant associated toxemia and, in any case, before the fetus has reached a sufficient degree of maturity. The therapy must also consider the possible causal symptomatic treatment of placental insufficiency.

References

1. DUDENHAUSEN, J. W., KYNAST, G., SALING, E.: Kompensatorische Nutrition des mangelversorgten Feten. 4. Deutscher Kongreß für Perinatale Medizin, Berlin 1971.
2. MANZANILLA, J. R., SUAREZ, C. M., CASANOVA, A. N., MAAS, E. R.: Intra-uterine fetal oral feeding: basic research using intra-amniotic albumin I. Internat. J. Gynaec. Obstet. 8, 238 (1970).
3. QUEENAN, Y. T., GADOW, E. C., BACHNER, P., RUBARYCH, S. F.: Amniotic fluid proteins in normal and Rh sensitized pregnancies. Am. J. Obstet. Gynec. 108, 406 (1970).
4. RENAUD, R., VINCENDON, G., BOOG, C., BRETTES, J. P., SCHUMACHER, J. C., KOEL, C., KIRSCHSTETTER, L., GANDAR, R.: Injections intra-amniotiques d'acides aminés dans les cas de malnutrition foetale. Premiers résultats. J. Gynec. Obstet. Biol. Repr. 1, 231 (1972).
5. SALING, E., SALCHOW, P., DUDENHAUSEN, J. W.: Intra-uterine Ernährung des Feten. Erste Untersuchungen. In: Saling E., Schulte F. J.: Perinatale Medizin. Band II. 3. Deutscher Kongreß für Perinatale Medizin, 26. - 28. November 1970, Berlin. Stuttgart; Thieme 1972.

Fetal and Maternal Uptake of S_e 75 Methionine after Intra-Amniotic Injection in Rabbits

E. Margaria, M. Massobrio, G. V. D'Arcangelo, and
F. Badini Confalonieri

The impossibility of providing sufficient nutrition to the fetus through the mother because of the presence of a hindrance at the level of the placental filter and the demonstration that the fetus is able to swallow the amniotic fluid (5), and utilize, for its own alimentation, both proteins and amino-acids contained in it (2, 4, 6, 7), justifie the treatment of fetal hypotrophy due to the placental insufficiency by means of intra-amniotic injection of amino-acids.

In order to analyze the fate of the amino-acids introduced into the amniotic fluid, we have carried out an experiment by injecting $S_e{}^{75}$ selenomethionine into the amniotic sac of 4 rabbits on their 24th day of pregnancy. There are many reasons why we choose this labelled amino-acid, i, e.:

1. the replacement of the S atom of the methionine by a $S_e{}^{75}$ one does not alter the biochemical properties, including incorporation into proteins (1);
2. the $S_e{}^{75}$ is a gamma radiating isotope and consequently a more easily measurable one, when compared with the beta radiating isotopes; its halflife is 128 days;
3. the methionine has a basic importance not only in the protein metabolism, but also in the lipid one; it represents a lipotropic factor contributing to the synthesis of the choline (3).

For our study we have chosen 4 female rabbits from New Zealand of an average weight of 3800 g, whose fecundation day was known with no possibility of mistake.

After laparotomy we injected into five amniotic sacs of each rabbit 0,25 mC of $S_e{}^{75}$ methionine diluted in 0.5 ml of saline solution in five parts. For each rabbit an amniotic sac was kept for control. The operation was carried out with ether anesthesia, trying to avoid every possible contamination. After 24 hours the animals were killed, their fetus were extracted and samples of amniotic fluid from each sac collected. From each fetus we took away the following organs: placenta, liver, blood, bowel and kidney. A sample of liver, blood, uterus and urine was drawn from the mother. The incorporation of the $S_e{}^{75}$ methionine was tested with a "gamma-camera" properly adjusted.

The average values of the radioactivity founded in the 20 fetuses treated, in the 4 control fetuses and in the 4 mothers, are shown in the Table 1 in cpm/g (counts x minute x gram) of tissue.

The comparison of the radioactivity of the tissues from the fetuses injected with those of the control fetuses shows a highly significant difference. The radioacitivity in the latter can be ascribed not only to the unavoidable contamination due to contiguity, but also to the reabsorption of the amino-acid in the mother plasma and to its redistribution also to the non injected fetus.

Table 1. Uptake of S_e^{75} methionine after intra-amniotic injection in rabbits on their 24th day of pregnancy

Average values cpm / g	Fetuses treated (20)	Control fetuses (4)	Mothers (4)
Placenta	301.118	128.308	-
Amniotic fluid	153.328	103.748	-
Blood	169.050	31.880	48.112
Liver	949.574	184.662	190.344
Kidney	275.420	51.400	328.868
Bowel	521.018	82.660	-
Uterus	-	-	615.214
Urine	-	-	80.780

It is interesting to note that blood and liver both of control fetuses and mothers have similar values of radioactivity. In the mothers only the kidney, beside the uterus of course, presents a high incorporation, as the emunctory organ of the whole isotope injected.

A remarkable concentration is also present in the placenta as amino-acid storing organ (6) and in the kidney as excretory organ.

The level of labelled methionine in the amniotic fluid and in the fetal blood is much lower as a consequence of the swallowing occurred after 24 hours and of the amino-acid uptake by the fetal liver and placenta.

In the final analysis, we may conclude that the S_e^{75} methionine, when injected into the amniotic fluid is swallowed by the rabbit's fetus and electively incorporated in the liver, where it will be presumably utilized for the protein synthesis.

References

1. BLAU, M., BENDER, M. A.: S_e^{75} - Selenomethionine for visualization of the pancreas by isotope scanning. Radiology 78, 974 (1962).
2. DUDENHAUSEN, J. W., KYNAST, G., SALING, E.: Kompensatorische Nutrition des mangelversorgten Feten. 4. Deutscher Kongreß für Perinatale Medizin, Berlin 1971.
3. HARPER, H. A.: Chimica fisiologica e patologica. Piccin ed., 1970 (2^ed.).
4. MANZANILLA, J. R., SUAREZ, C. M., CASANOVA, A. N., MAAS, E. R.: Intra-uterine fetal oral feeding; basic research using intra-amniotic albumin I^{131}. Internat. J. Gynec. Obstet. 8, 238 (1970).
5. PRITCHARD, J. A.: Fetal swallowing and amniotic fluid volume. Obstet. Gynec. 28, 606 (1966).
6. RENAUD, R., VINCENDON, G., BOOG, G., BRETTES, J. P., SCHUMACHER, J. C., KOEL, C., KIRSCHSTETTER, L., GANDAR, R.: Injections intra-amniotiques d'acides aminês dans les cas de malnutrition foetale. Premiers rêsultats. J. Gynec. Obstet. Biol. Repr. 1, 231 (1972).
7. SALING, E., SALCHOW, P., DUDENHAUSEN, J. W.: Intra-uterine Ernährung des Feten. Erste Untersuchungen. In: Saling, E., Schulte, F.J.: Perinatale Medizin. Band II. 3. Deutscher Kongreß für Perinatale Medizin, 26. - 28. November 1970, Berlin. Stuttgart; Thieme 1972.

Exogenous Progesterone and Feto-Placental Function

B. Salvadori

Progesterone is regarded by definition as the gestagen hormone. Behind this apparently exhaustive statement, however, lies the profound uncertainty as to its metabolic fate and in particular its utilization and degradation by the foetus.

We have examined the effects of progesterone by assessing the parameters of the efficiency of foeto-placental function, such as the total estrogens and the urinary estriol in conjunction with the study of the behaviour of the pregnandiol and pregnenolone secretion levels, which reflect the progesterone metabolism.

The results of this research, covering observations on 117 cases over a period of two years, may be summarized as follows. The administration of progesterone (200 mg/d) causes in pregnancy with a low estrogen secretion a percentage increase in the basic values (estrogen gain) of 48.34 % for the total urinary estrogens and of 43.49 % for the urinary estriol.

Urinary estrogen gain after progesteron (200 mg daily)

	% Estrogen gain (average value)	% Estriol gain (average value)
After progesteron	48.34	43.49
Controls	10.48	t 9.1254 $p < 0.001$

The difference between two groups is statistically significant.

In the control group (bed rest + traditional therapy) the estrogen gain was 10.48 % for the total estrogens. The difference in the estrogen gain between the progesterone cases and the controls is highly significant ($t = 9.1254$, $p < 0.001$). This increase in the level is a real increase and is independent of the factors of bed rest, traditional therapy and physiological increment.

Analysing the behaviour of the curves of the estrogen secretion levels after treatment with progesterone, we can distinguish the three following groups (Fig. 1):
A = persistent increase
B = retarded or transitory increase
C = no increase

Taking into account the perinatal prognosis for each individual group of estrogen response, we then obtain:

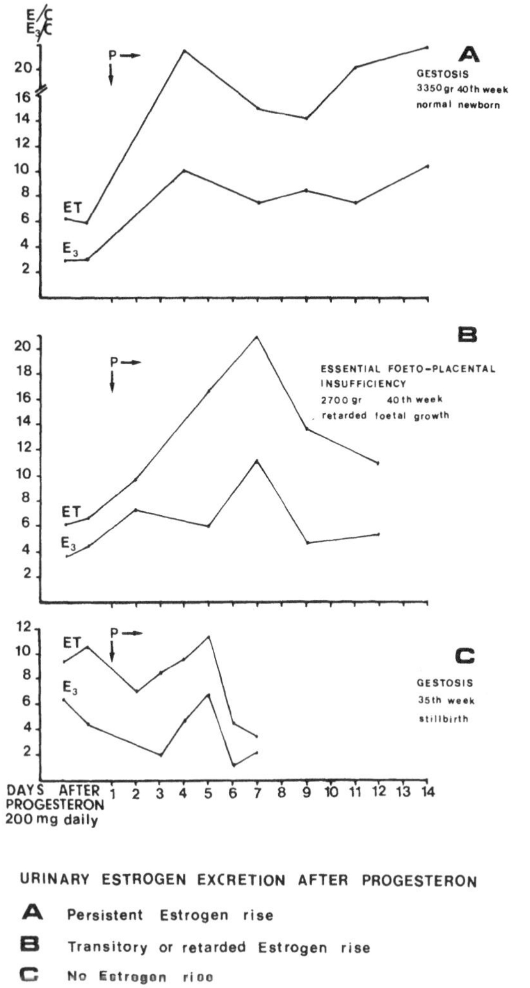

Fig. 1. A Persistent estrogen rise
B Transitory or retarded estrogen rise
C No estrogen rise

Estrogen response and neonatal outcome

Group	No. of cases	Normal newborns	Perinatal° morbidity	Perinatal mortality
A	32	23	9	-
B	15	8	6	-
C	19	7	9	3

° Small for gestation age
Respiratory distress syndrome
Diabetic's baby syndrome

Group A vs group B $\kappa^2 = 0.460$ $p < 0.05$
Group A vs group C $\kappa^2 = 7.177$ $p < 0.05$

The difference in the behaviour between the two groups A and B is not statistically significant ($\kappa^2 = 0.460$), whereas that between groups A and C is statistically significant ($\kappa^2 = 7.17$, $p < 0.05$).
Duration of pregnancy: not significant.
The study of the placental conditions in this patient material is not yet complete.

In six cases with a type C estrogen curve we carried out the oral DHA-S test with a daily administration of 75 mg DHA-S over a period of 10 days. An increase in the estrogen secretion of more than 25 % over the basic values was observed in four cases, while in two cases there was no such increase in the estrogen secretion.

The findings of a more detailed analysis of the case histories according to the different pathological conditions were as follows:

Gestosis

37 cases were observed in all, including 21 following progesterone treatment and 16 controls.

Gestosis No. 37 cases, 21 cases with Progesteron, 16 controls

Urinary estrogen gain after progesteron (200 mg daily)

	% Estrogen gain (average value)	S. D.
After Progesteron	37.51	83.47
Controls	9.85	43.58

The difference between two groups is statistically significant ($t = 1.9632$ $p < 0.05$)

The estrogen gain after progesterone was a mean 37.51 % with a standard deviation of 83.47, as against 9.85 % with a standard deviation of 43.58 in the controls. The difference between the two mean values is statistically significant ($t = 1.9632$, $p < 0.05$). This shows that after progesterone administration there was a real estrogen gain of greater duration than that produced by the factors of bed rest and traditional therapy in the controls. Examination of the perinatal prognosis for each individual group of estrogen response gave the following results:

Gestosis

Estrogen response and neonatal outcome

Group	No. of cases	Normal newborns	Perinatal morbidity	Perinatal mortality
A	7	4	3	-
B	3	1	2	-
C	6	3	2	1

No significance

The difference between the various groups is not statistically significant.

Diabetes

27 cases in all were kept under observation, including 18 following progesterone treatment and 9 controls.

Diabetes No. 27 cases, 18 cases with progesteron, 9 controls

Urinary estrogen gain after progesteron (200 mg daily)

	Average % estrogen gain	S. D.
After progesteron	48.05	81.50
Controls	16.19	45.02

The difference between two groups is statistically significant ($t = 1.7252 \quad p < 0.1$)

The estrogen gain after progesterone was a mean 48.05 % with a standard deviation of 81.50 as against 16.19 % with a standard deviation of 45.02 in the controls. The difference between the mean values in the two groups is statistically significant ($t = 1.7252$, $p < 0.1$).

From the clinical point of view we observed for the three groups A, B and C the following perinatal prognose in regard to the estrogen response.

Diabetes
Estrogen response and neonatal outcome

Group	No. of cases	Normal newborns	Perinatal morbidity	Perinatal mortality
A	8	6	2	-
B	5	2	3	-
C	5	2	2	1

No significance

The difference between the various groups was not statistically significant.

Threatened Premature Delivery

24 cases in all were kept under observation, including 14 following progesterone and 10 controls.

Urinary estrogen gain after progesteron (200 mg daily)

	Average % Estrogen gain	S. D.
After progesteron	54.20	80.35
Controls	2.64	58.47

The difference between two groups is statistically significant ($t = 2.2353 \quad P < 0.01$)

The estrogen gain following progesterone was a mean 54.20 % with a standard deviation of 80.35 as against 2.64 % with a standard deviation of 58.47 in the controls. The difference between the two groups is statistically significant ($t = 2.2353$, $p < 0.01$).

This shows that after the administration of progesterone a true rise in the total estrogen secretion values occurs, independently of the factors of bed rest and traditional therapy.

Examination of the perinatal prognoses for each individual group of estrogen responses gives the following picture:

Threatened premature labor
Estrogen response and neonatal outcome

Group	No. of cases	Normal newborns	Perinatal morbidity	Perinatal mortality
A	6	4	2	-
B	3	3	-	-
C	5	2	2	1

No significance

The difference between the various groups is not statistically significant.

Essential Foeto-Placental Insufficiency

18 cases were kept under observation after administration of progesterone.

Essential foeto-placental insufficiency 18 cases with progesterone
% estrogen gain 51.08 % $\pm$ 68.20
Average value $\pm$ standard deviation

The mean value for the estrogen gain was 51.08 % with a standard deviation of 68.20. The increase is statistically significant. Over an observation period of three weeks the quota due to the physiological increment does not in fact exceed 10 - 15 %.

Examination of the perinatal prognoses for each individual group of estrogen response gives the following finding

Essential foeto-placental insufficiency
Estrogen response and neonatal outcome

Group	No. of cases	Normal newborns	Perinatal morbidity	Perinatal mortality
A	11	9	2	-
B	4	2	2	-
C	3	-	3	-

No significance

Principles of the Test

Influence of Bed Rest and Any Traditional Therapy

In order to exclude any possible influence of the bed rest factor, the administration of progesterone was started on the third morning after admission, when at least two basic values for the urinary estrogen had already been recorded. It has in fact been found that the effects of bed rest on estrogen secretion is maximal during the first three days.

The controls, without progesterone, who were placed under the same bed rest conditions and received a traditional therapy, exhibited estrogen gain values appreciably lower than those obtained after the administration of progesterone.

All this was aimed at excluding any decisive influence of bed rest and other factors in the estrogen gain values, recorded after progesterone.

Influence of diuresis

Our research on the estrogen secretion values, using the SPEARMAN index, have led us to the conclusion that the urinary levels are independent of the diuresis volume. This is shown also in the figure 2.

Influence of Absorption

We have to consider in connection with an intramuscular administration the factor of absorption, in particular in relation to the type of estrogen response obtained and also the specific intolerance which occurs in some cases in relation to the oily vehicle (sesame oil).

Nevertheless the consistent relationship between the level of estrogen gain, on the one hand, and the perinatal prognoses and clinical evolution of the pregnancy, on the other, gives reason to suppose that the influence of the absorption factor is not of great importance in a fairly wide range of patient material.

The lack of estrogen response in group C, moreover, cannot be attributed to an inadequate progesterone absorption in view of the increase in the elimination of urinary pregnandiol.

Possible Metabolism of Progesterone

We have not been able, using labelled progesterone (^{14}C-4-progesterone), to demonstrate any progesterone-estrone in pregnancy. This conversion has only been proved in cases of metastatic carcinoma of the chorion (DAVIS, PLOTZ, 1958).

On the other hand, the perfusion of the foetus with progesterone and the injection of labelled progesterone in the umbilical vein has always revealed a clear metabolism of Δ4-androstenedione (SOLOMON, BIRD, LING, YWAMIYA, YOUNG, 1967).

The foetus is not believed to possess any metabolic capacity which would give rise to the formation of 19-carbon steroids based on progesterone, thus leading to the conclusion that, whereas (always in

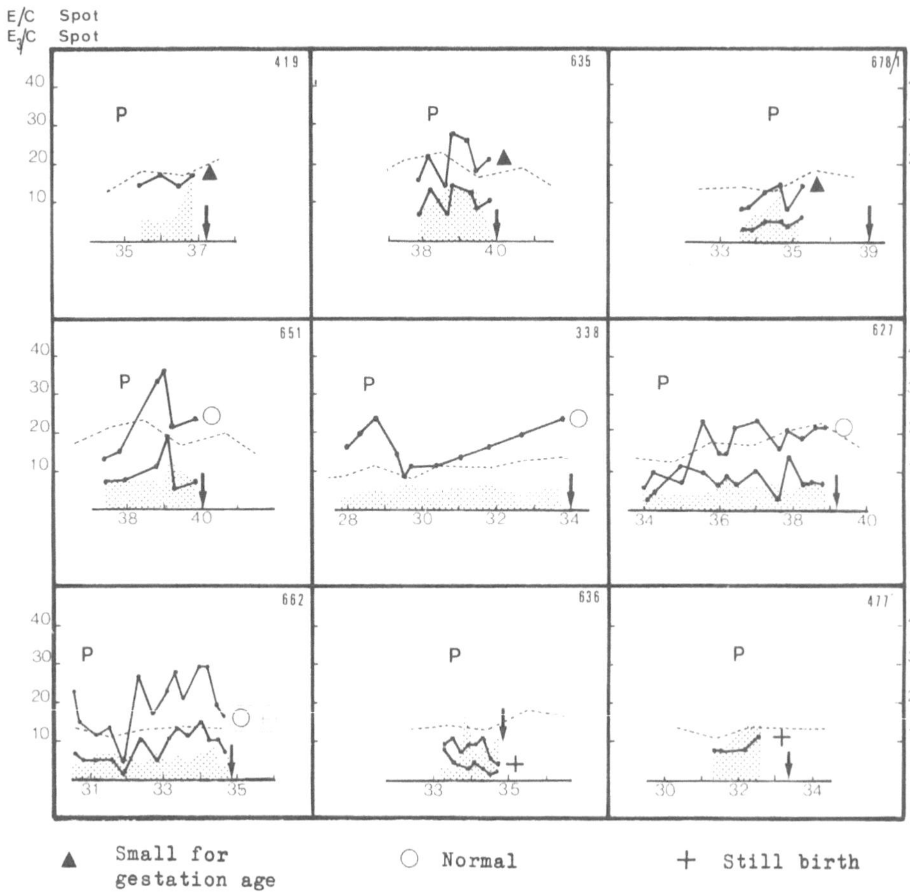

Fig. 2

the foetus) pregnenolone is used for the production of the whole steroid series (21, 19 and 18 carbon atoms), progesterone is predominantly destined for metabolism in connection with the 21-carbon steroids; it is still true that, in order to discover the origin of androstenedione and foetal testosterone, recourse must be had to the hypothesis of other metabolic pathways (the conversion of 17 OH progesterone in the foetal testicle is hardly probable; derivation from maternal DHAS or derivation from the foetal DHAS).

Although in some experiments with the incubation of foetal adrenals gland in vitro androstenedione has been obtained from progesterone (JOHANNISSON 1968, MILNER, MILLS 1970), this may have been due either to artificial changes in the enzyme composition of the parenchyma (homogenate) or to a real metabolic possibility.

The main function of progesterone in the foetus appears to be corticosteroid synthesis (DICZFALUSY, 1969, KLEIN, GIROUD 1966, KLEIN, GIROUD 1967). In comparison with the pregnandiol compounds (SOBREVILLA, HAGERMAN, VILLEE 1964; PION, JAFFE, ERIKSSON, WIGVIST, DICZFALUSY 1965; SINGH 1969) no 17-hydroxylase, 17-20-desmolase or sulphoquinase activity is believed to occur in the placenta.

Considerable research, using perfusion and incubation methods, has not revealed any valid metabolic process for the reduction of progesterone by the human placenta (DICZFALUSY 1966; PALMER, BLAIR, ERIKSSON, DICZFALUSY 1966; PALMER, ERIKSSON, WIQUIST, DICZFALUSY 1966; RYAN, MEIGS, PETRO 1966).

Possible mechanism of action

The only valid hypothesis with which we are left is to regard the estrogen gain as independent of any form of metabolism of estrogen taken as a precursor, at least in regard to the foeto-placental function, accepting the possible but hardly credible metabolism within the maternal ovary.

It is therefore necessary to revert to a hypothesis, based on an indirect effect of the progesterone, leading in some way to an improved efficiency of the foeto-placental unit and reflected in a greater utilization of the endogenous precursors and thus in an estrogen gain in the urine. This treatment test will, in consequence, be regarded in a totally different light from the tests of the pregnenolone and DHAS contributions.

It is frankly impossible to define the mechanisms of action of progesterone on the foeto-placental unit in this direction and it is hardly possible even to guess at an effect on the level of the myometrium, or even of the myometrium in the area of the placenta. At the same time it is difficult to specify any effect on the enzyme equilibrium of the foeto-placental unit itself.

Summary

1. A statistically significant increase ($p < 0.001$) occurs in the total estrogens and the urinary estriol after progesterone administration (200 mg/d) in pregnancies with a low level of estrogen secretion. The mean estrogen gain is 48.34 % for total estrogen and 43.49 % for estriol in relation to the basic values.
2. The perinatal prognosis in regard to the estrogen response exhibits a variation between types A, B and C, that between groups A and C being statistically significant.
3. The absence of estrogen response to progesterone does not exclude the possibility of an increase in the estrogen secretion after the oral administration of DHAS.
4. Regarding the connection between the estrogen gain and the various types of pathological conditions, it would appear that the risk of premature delivery shows the clearest response (estrogen gain: 54.20 %), while the lowest response occurs with the gestoses (estrogen gain: 37.51 %).
5. The absence of estrogen response in the cases in group C cannot be ascribed to a defective progesterone absorption, since an increased elimination of urinary pregnandiol is observed and the correlation coefficient between the total estrogen and pregnandiol values is negative ($r = -0.146$), whereas in groups A and B the respective correlation coefficients were positive ($r = 0.381$ and $r = 0.435$).
6. The failure to demonstrate a metabolism of labelled progesterone into estrogens during pregnancy, the failure to recover Δ-4-androstenedione after the injection of labelled progesterone in the umbilical vein and after perfusion of the foetus and above all the insufficient metabolic capacity of the desmolase in comparisons of progesterone in placental function exclude any possibility of regarding progesterone as a precursor.

The possible mechanism of action of progesterone is therefore regarded as being an effect on the foeto-placental level, leading to a better utilization of natural precursors.

Human Placental Lactogen Production in Vitro 1. Dynamic Studies on Normal-Term Placentas after Stimulation with 17-β-Oestradiol

E. Desole, E. Springolo, F. Di Chiara, L. Franzolini, and G. C. Tosolini

Introduction

Human placental lactogen (HPL), which is produced by the human placenta and whose prominent biological activities are prolactine-like and growth hormone-like activity is considered to be an important metabolic hormone of pregnancy regulating and modifying many of the metabolic adjustment which take place during pregnancy. We have no precise knowledge of the mechanisms controlling the synthesis and secretion of HPL. In our present study, we have attempted to elucidate the dynamic aspects of synthesis and release of HPL in-vitro under normal conditions and after stimulation with 17-beta oestradiol.

Materials and Methods

Synthesis and release of HPL by human placenta in-vitro has been studied. Seven normal placentas were obtained immediately after delivery. Fragments from the middle-central area of about 1 mm^3 each were cultivated in flasks. The culture medium consisted of 10 % calf serum and 90 % Eagle Basal Medium together with antibiotics. The bottles were filled every 12 hours with 95 % air and 5 % CO_2. The cultures were incubated at 37° C for 96 hours. In two experiments the cultures were stimulated with increasing doses of 17 beta-oestradiol (from 0.1 to 5 gamma). In the following experiments the stimulated and non-stimulated cultures were blocked every 24 hours. For every culture the wet weight of the fragments was determined and they were microscopically examined. The HPL in the medium was assayed at intervals. We used the double antibody method followed by centrifugation of the precipitate. The results are expressed in micrograms/ml with reference to the Scavo standard. The kits used were provided by Sorin company.

Results

In our culture method, the dose of 3 gamma of 17 beta-oestradiol seems to give a maximal increase in the release of HPL (Fig. 1). The increase in concentration of HPL rises rapidly during the first 24 hours, and there is a slower synthesis during the following hours. Stimulation with 17-beta-oestradiol at the 24th, 48th, 72nd hour showed variable increase in the synthesis of HPL, proving the integrity of structures which synthesize it (Fig. 2).

The curve perhaps suggests the existence of two pools of HPL, one which rapidly and the other one which slowly releases HPL, which may be of great metabolic importance. The relations between oestrogens and HPL have to be further investigated.

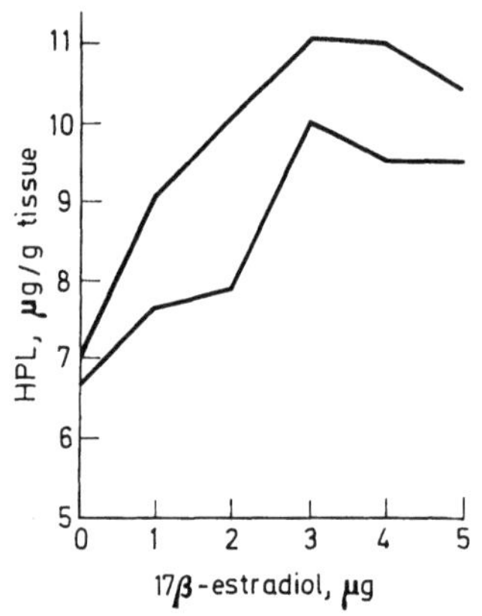

Fig. 1. Amount of HPL in medium in two different placentas. Incubation for 48 hours. Stimulation after 24 hours with increasing doses of 17 beta-oestradiol

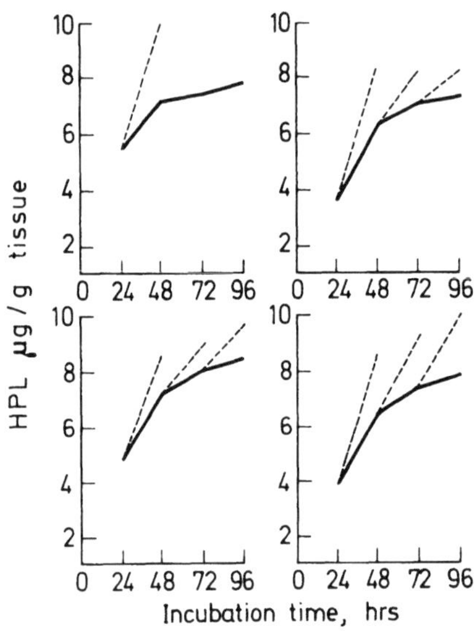

Fig. 2. Amount of HPL in medium in 4 different placentas. Outlines showed changes after stimulation with 17 beta-oestradiol (3 gamma)

References

CATT, K. J., MOFFAT, B., NIALL, H. D.: Science 157, 321 (1967).

FRIESEN, H. G.: Endocrinology 83, 774 (1968).

GENAZZANI, A. R., BENUZZI-BANDONI, M., FELBER, J. P.: Metabolism 18, 593 (1969).

GRUNBACH, M. M., KAPLAN, S. L., SCIARA, J. J., BURR, J. M.: Ann. N. Y. Acad. Sci. 148, 501 (1968).

LASCAR, G.: J. Gyn. Obst. Biol. Repr. 1, 509 (1972).

SAMAAN, N., YEN, S. C., GONZALES, D., PEARSON, O. H.: J. Clin. Endocr. 28, 485 (1968).

TURTLE, J. R., KIPNIS, D. M.: Biochem. Biophis. Acta 144, 583 (1967).

TURKINGTON, R. W.: Endocrinology 82, 575 (1968).

Daily Urinary Hormonal Pattern Following 17 ß-Oestradiol Treatment of Prolonged Pregnancies

J. Jakowicki, W. Szymański, M. Krauze, and M. Dankiewicz

Urinary oestriol excretion is an index of fetal status (1, 3, 5). Placental function can be assessed by urinary pregnanediol excretion (1, 2, 5). In the third trimester of pregnancy human chorionic gonadotrophin reaches a mean value of about 20.000 I. u./l (1, 7, 8, 11). Abnormal prolongation of pregnancy is frequently associated with decreasing placental efficiency (1, 5, 9).

Material and Methods

Twenty pregnant women, aged from 21 to 37 years, all with prolonged pregnancies received twice daily 10 mg intramuscular injections of 17 β-oestradiol to stimulate uterine contractions. The prolongation of pregnancy was confirmed by the birth weight and length of the neonates each with high one-minute Apgar scores.

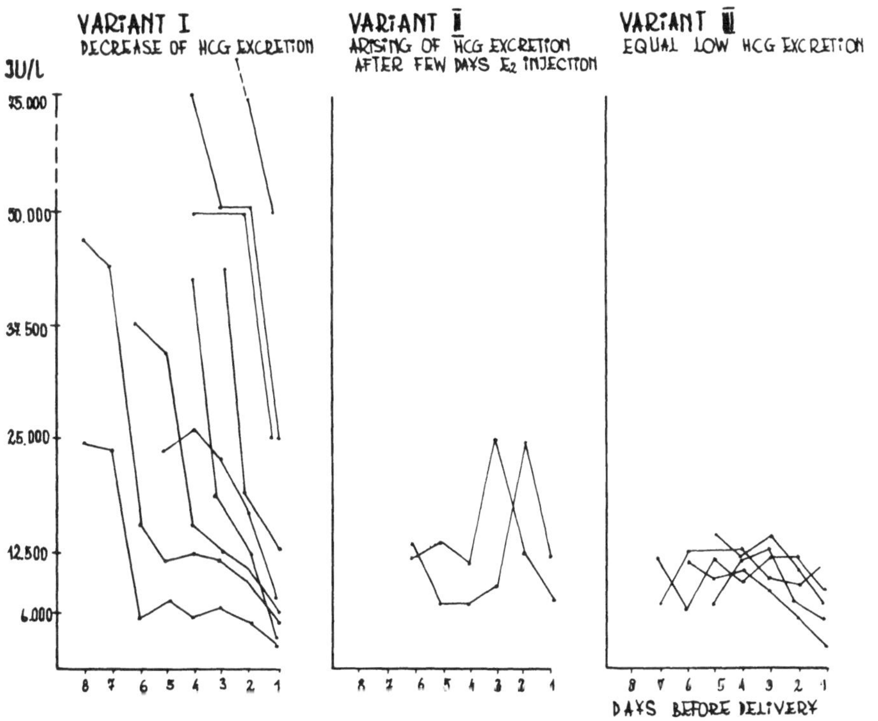

Fig. 1. Mean values of urinary estriol (E_3) and pregnanediol (PD) in prolonged pregnancy after estradiol - 17β administration

Urinary excretion of oestriol was determined by the method of FRANDSER (3) and pregnanediol by the method KLOPPER and COWORK (6). HCG was measured daily in 16 pregnant women using the agglutination-inhibition assay described by WIDE and GEMZELL (11), and SWIERCZYNSKA and SAMOCHOWIEC (10).

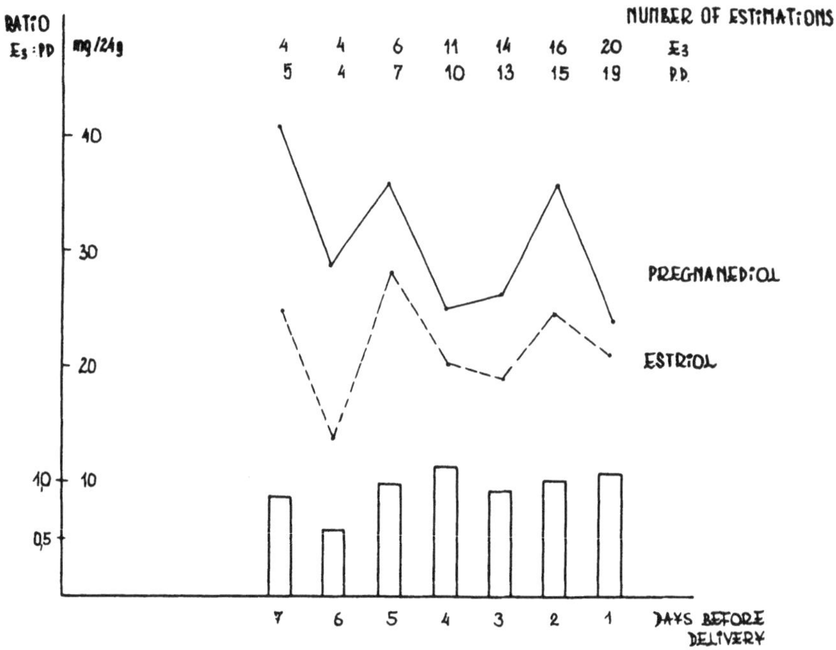

Fig. 2. Urinary of HCG excretion in prolonged pregnancy after estradiol - 17 β administration

Results

Mean values of urinary oestriol and pregnanediol excretion were roughly parallel. The average oestriol/pregnanediol ratio showed generally lower values of oestriol. The ratio did not fluctuate markedly during observation.

The results of urinary HCG were divided in three patterns. The largest group consists of nine patients with elevated titres of urinary HCG which decreased to normal during treatment. A few patients had a low level of urinary HCG. A short-lived increase in HCG excretion a few days before parturition was noted in the urine of two patients.

Comments

Mean values of oestriol and pregnanediol excretion decreased rapidly in the first day of 17 β-oestradiol administration in a few patients treated for one week. The differences between mean values of the steroids in days following a short course of oestrogen treatment were small, in particular the oestriol concentrations. Although the normal pattern of steroid excretion in prolonged pregnancy was not estimated, the findings of this investigation indicate that treatment with 17β-oestradiol did not depress pregnanediol and oestriol excretion. There was a decline of HCG towards the end of prolonged pregnancies in the urine of patients with Variant I and to a smaller extent with Variant III. It is of interest that the level of HCG dropped sharply during the second or third day after oestrogen treatment.

Two of 16 patients showed an increase in HCG values after a few days of treatment but they declined just before parturition. It is difficult to explain the growth of chorionic gonadotrophin in above cases. That 17β-oestradiol directly depress HCG excretion may well be a group over-simplification. Perhaps placental vascular impairment is of some importance in leading to a decrease in HCG excretion in our patients with over-long pregnancies.

References

1. BEISCHER, N. A., BROWN, J. B., SMITH, M. A., TOWNSEND, L.: Amer. J. Obst. Gynec. 103, 483 (1969).
2. COYLE, M. G., GREIG, M., WALKER, J.: Lancet 2, 275 (1962).
3. FRANDSEN, V. A.: The excretion of oestriol in normal human pregnancy, Munksgaard, Copenhagen 1963.
4. FRANDSEN, V. A., STAKEMANN, G.: Acta Endocr. 44, 183 (1963).
5. GREENE, J. W., Jr., DUHRING, J. L., SMITH, K.: Amer. J. Obstet. Gynec. 92, 1030 (1965).
6. KLOPPER, A., MICHIE, E. A., BROWN, J. B.: Endocr. 12, 209 (1955).
7. McCARTHY, C., PENNINGTON, G., CRAWFORD, W.: J. Obst. Gynaec. Brit. Cwlth. 71, 85 (1964).
8. SAMOCHOWIEC, E.: Wartość kliniczna badań serologicznych nad gonadotropina kosmówkowa w przebiegu ciazy prawidlowej oraz niektórych jej powiklaniach. Katowice 1966.
9. SMITH, K., GREENE, J. W., Jr., TOUCHSTONE, J. C.: Amer. J. Obst. Gynec. 96, 901 (1966).
10. SWIERCZYNSKA, Z., SAMOCHOWIEC, E.: Pol. Tyg. Lek. 15, 1217 (1960).
11. WIDE, L., GEMZELL, C. A.: Acta Endocr. 35, 261 (1960).

Experiences with Administration of Dehydroepiandrosterone-Sulfate and Pregnenolone in Cases of Feto-Placental Insufficiency

Ch. Lauritzen

Dehydroepiandrosterone-Sulfate (DHEA-S) is the most important fetal and maternal adrenocortical precursor for the placental production of oestrogens. Pregnenolone-sulfate (PS) is one of the precursors for the placental production of progesterone and, via dehydroepiandrosterone, also of oestrogens. On the bases of these physiological facts we have developped a test of fetoplacental function: 50 mg DHEA-S are injected intravenously to the mother and the transformation of the steroid administered into oestrogens is measured by comparing the values before injection with the values following injection in urine or plasma. The % increase is significantly correlated with the placental biosynthetic reserve and the general fetoplacental metabolic capacity. In cases of placental insufficiency the conversion of DHEA-S to eostrogens is low or nil. This has been shown clearly in about 300 own cases (LAURITZEN, 1967 a, b; 1968; 1969; 1971 a, b, c, d; 1972 a, b). There are proved correlations to placental histology , to placental aromatization capacity in vitro, to uteroplacental perfusion, to fetal outcome, fetal weight, pathology of cardiotocogram and Apgar scores of the newborn. The physiologic basis of the test is well founded. The test is more reliable than simple urinary or plasma oestrogen determinations. The diagnostic and prognostic validity of the DHEA-S test was confirmed by several papers of different authors in about 1000 patients (BOKELMANN, 1971; VAN DER CRABBEN et al., 1969; 1970 a, b; 1971; VAN DER CRABBEN and WERNER, 1972; KAISER et al., 1970; KELLER et al., 1971; KNAPSTEIN et al., 1971; STEMBERA and HERZMANN, 1971; 1973; VULLIEMOZ et al., 1970).

In the course of performing the tests and evaluating the test results we noticed that in a greater number of cases following more than one injection of DHEA-S the oestrogen values increased not only temporarily, but permanently. We also noticed that when the oestrogens increased permanently following DHEA-S, a favourable outcome resulted in spite of primarily deficient oestrogen values.

On the ground of this impression, we decided because of the possible practical importance to investigate the problem whether repeated injections of DHEA-S could be considered as a real therapy improving the function of the feto-placental unit or must be merely looked upon as a sort of cosmetics for the oestrogen values only, without really improving the course or outcome of pregnancies at risk.

Some basic metabolic data following administration of different DHEA preparations: Non pregnant women: DHEA-S+ was given in a dose of 30 mg oral for 3 days (HARTMANN and LAURITZEN, 1969). In the urine a small increase in DHEA-excretion (method: PENG et al., 1965) was shown, which amounted to less than total 3 % of the dose administered within 5 days

+ We thank the German Hoffmann - La Roche AG, Grenzach, and the Schering AG, Berlin, for the generous gift of DHEA-S and DHEA-oenanthate.

and which was less than 1 % per day. The increase in excretion of 17-ketosteroids (PETERSON and PIERCE, 1960) was also small and the increase in total oestrogens (ITTRICH, 1960 a) was only 0.048 % of the dose administered. Following injection of 100 mg of DHEA-oenanthate i. m., which has a depot effect of 6 days, the values of additional excretion for DHEA, 17 KS and oestrogen were even lower (Table 1).

Table 1. Oral medication of dehydroepiandrosterone-sulfate
Non-pregnant women (N = 38)

	Control	Following DHEA-S 3 days 30 mg orally/die	Following DHEA-oenanthate 100 mg i. m.+
DHEA mg 24^h urine (range)	0.40 (0.06 - 1.33)	1.94 (0.31 - 1.58)	0.82 (0.13 - 1.50)
Increase	total	2.81	1.12
% of the dose administered	(per day)	(0.87)	(0.19)
17 KS mg 24^h urine (range)	6.32 (4.59 - 7.94)	8.66 (5.00 - 10.85)	11.01 (9.64 - 12.12)
Increase	total	3.52	5.99
% of the dose administered	(per day)	(1.81)	(1.19)
Total oestrogens mg 24^h urine (range)	0.0104 (0.0065 - 0.0201)	0.0139 (0.0031 - 0.0221)	0.0124 (0.0085 - 0.0169)
Increase	total	0.048	0.143
% of the dose administered	(per day)	(0.0044)	(0.0155)

+ Depot effect 6 - 10 days

Pregnant women (IV. - VII. month): Following oral DHEA-S the total % increase was 4.6 % of the dose administered for DHEA, 16.44 % for 17 KS and 5.19 % for total oestrogens.

100 mg of DHEA-oenanthate produced a smaller increase, namely of total 1.56 % for DHEA, 9.92 % for 17 KS and 4.36 for total oestrogens (Table 2).

Pregnant women (VIII. - X. month): In pregnant women between the VIII. and X. month of pregnancy oral DHEA-S medication for three days resulted in a total additional increase of DHEA excretion of 26.4 % within 5 days. The 17 KS increase was total 30 % and the oestrogen increase total 32.8 % and about 6.1 % of the dose administered per day. Following injection of DHEA-oenanthate a somewhat lower additional total excretion of 16.4 % DHEA, 20 % 17 KS and 16.6 % oestrogens was seen (Table 3).

Table 2. Oral medication of dehydroepiandrosterone-sulfate
Pregnant women IV. - VII. month (N = 33)

	Control	Following DHEA-S 3 days 30 mg orally / day	Following DHEA-oenanthate 100 mg i. m.+
DHEA mg 24^h urine	0.60	1.17	0.79
(range)	(0.08 - 1.35)	(0.58 - 2.92)	(0.21 - 2.63)
Increase	total	4.68	1.56
% of the dose administered	(per day)	(0.75)	(0.24)
17 KS mg 24^h urine	8.25	13.60	11.82
(range)	(6.67 - 9.90)	(11.50 - 18.80)	(8.55 - 14.53)
Increase	total	16.44	9.92
% of the dose administered	(per day)	(4.69)	(2.48)
Total oestrogens mg 24^h urine	4.11	5.14	4.83
(range)	(2.18 - 6.70)	(2.23 - 8.15)	(3.55 - 4.85)
Increase	total	5.19	4.26
% of the dose administered	(per day)	(1.04)	(0.73)

+ Depot effect 6 - 10 days

Table 3. Oral medication of dehydroepiandrosterone-sulfate
Pregnant women VII. - X. month (N = 28)

	Control	Following DHEA-S 3 days 30 mg orally / day	Following DHEA-oenanthate 100 mg i. m.+
DHEA mg 24^h urine	0.52	1.81	0.83
(range)	(0.12 - 0.93)	(0.65 - 3.19)	(0.30 - 2.94)
Increase	total	26.44	16.47
% of the dose administered	(per day)	(5.31)	(2.83)
17 KS mg 24^h urine	10.51	15.72	13.36
(range)	(7.43 - 12.88)	(12.13 - 20.50)	(10.40 - 17.27)
Increase	total	30.76	20.13
% of the dose administered	(per day)	(5.20)	(3.44)
Total oestrogens mg 24^h urine	24.20	31.63	27.05
(range)	(12.35 - 35.71)	(18.53 - 44.38)	(15.50 - 39.14)
Increase	total	32.80	16.60
% of the dose administered	(per day)	(6.13)	(2.53)

+ Depot effect 6 - 10 days

Intravenous Injection of DHEA-S

Normal cases: Following one intravenous injection of 50 mg of DHEA-S a significant increase in total oestrogen excretion is not seen before the 14. - 16. week of pregnancy. From this time on a steady increase is registered up to the end of pregnancy where the additional oestrogen excretion may amount to 10 - 50 % of the DHEA-S dose administered.

In the plasma a mean total net increase of the oestrone-oestradiol-17 β-values was seen from the 36. - 40. week between 20 - 40 ng with ITTRICH's (1960) fluorimetric method (Table 4) and in the same range between 21 and 38 μg/100 ml plasma by radioimmunoassay (Table 4) (WU and LUNDY, 1971; EDQUIST and JOHANNSON, 1972; EMMENT and COLLINS, 1972).

Table 4. Normal cases

Plasma oestrogen increase following test: 50 mg DHEA-S i. v. ng/ml

Initials	Week of pregnancy	Control	15'	30'	1^h	2h	3^h	5^h	Mean total net increase[+]
E.Sch.	30	18	55	55	43	43	37	17	21.9
I.K.	31	6	25	37	37	35	35	35	26.8
L.D.	33	30	70	76	70	70	76	54	33.3
A.O.	36	10	43	45	40	40	50	40	30.1
K.Z.	36	28	63	80	70	73	65	56	38.0
A.R.	39	25	59	60	43	73	45	38	22.9

[+] M of the 5 values -20 % for variation (STRECKER and LAURITZEN)

When doses of increasing magnitude were administered, a decrease of the percental conversion to oestrogens was observed. With an injection of 300 mg DHEA-S only 1 - 5 % were excreted as additional oestrogens.

When an infusion of 400 - 500 mg was given for 8 hours, an additional oestrogen-excretion of 0- (between -3 and +3 %) was registered (Table 5). So it can be assumed that the functional capacity of the placenta to split the sulfate conjugate or/and to aromatize the C_{19} steroid reaches its critical level at this dose (see also JEFFERY et al., 1970).

Pathological cases: In pathological pregnancy cases (gestoses) between the 36. - 40. week the additional oestrogen excretion following 50 mg DHEA i. v. was between 0 - 10 % only.

In the plasma only a mean total net increase between 0 and 17 ng/100 ml of oestrone-oestradiol-17β was seen in the first 5 hours in the ITTRICH and also in the radioimmunoassay method (Table 6).

Medication of β-Mimetica

It should be mentioned here that medication of β-mimetica (Isoxypren and Iproveratril = Th 1165 a[+]+ Isoptin) may prevent the typical oestrogen increase after the 32. week of pregnancy. The oestrogen excretion may even be depressed by Th 1165 a and the increase of oestrogens following DHEA-S injection is also abolished in our case presented here. The cause for this depression of aromatization is not known at present.

[+] Boehringer, Ingelheim

Table 5. % Conversion of increasing doses of DHEA-S to oestrogens in urine of normal pregnancies (34. - 40. week)

Dose administered mg		Conversion into oestrogens in % of the dose administered+ Pat. 1	2	3	4	5
<u>i. v.</u>	50	26	37	19	27	16
	100	18	36	21	25	18
	150	14	31	15	20	11
	200	10	17	11	14	6
	250	6	7	5	9	4
	300	3	5	2	3	1
<u>Infusion</u>						
	300	4	3	2	2	1
	400	3	0	-1	-1	0
	500	2	0	-2	-3	0

+rounded off values

Table 6. Pathological cases (gestoses)

Plasma oestrogen increase following test: 50 mg DHEA-S i. v. ng/ml

Initials	Week of pregnancy	Control	15'	30'	1^h	2^h	3^h	5^h	Mean total net increase+
A.K.	32	14	32	25	25	26	25	-	9.6
A.M.	32	11	26	28	33	27	36	30	16.6
B.D.	35	30	66	53	58	53	41	36	15.1
M.Sch.	37	27	42	36	34	50	50	29	11.1
M.H.	41	20	39	30	25	35	30	20	5.8
A.Sch.	42	11	25	28	32	36	25	20	14.3

+M of the 5 values -20 % for variation

However, it is very interesting that the levels of glucose and insuline increased significantly. Lactate and pyruvate increased 4 fold and the plasma potassium was decreased significantly (Table 7). <u>In vitro</u> aromatization studies of placentae with added Th 1165 are under way in my clinic (LEHMANN and LAURITZEN).

Table 7. Influence of a β-mimeticum on the oestrogen values in pregnancy urine (30. - 34. week)

	Control	Total oestrogens mg/24^h-urine day 1	2	3	4
Without medication	12.5	13.0	12.5	13.4	13.0
Following DHEA-S 50 mg i. v.	12.1	[19.8] inj.	20.3	18.6	13.5
During Th 1165 a 30 mg/24^h	10.4	8.7	6.3	6.6	7.1
During Th 1165 a + DHEA-S 50 mg i. v. (day 1)	11.4	[11.9] inj.	10.2	10.6	9.8

During Th 1165 a increase of glucose, insulin 5-fold, increase of lactate, pyruvat + 4-fold, decrease potassium < 3 m val/l

Pregnenolone and Pregnenolone-sulfate

In four cases of normal pregnancies at term 100 mg of pregnenolone (Sigma Chemicals) was infused in 500 ml of physiological saline within 8 hours. Plasma progesterone (JOHANNESSON, 1970) and oestrogens were measured by radioimmunoassay, pregnanediol (according to the method of KLOPPER et al., 1968) in 24 hours urine. A relatively small increase in plasma progesterone, oestrone-oestradiol-17β and in urinary pregnanediol (Table 8) was registered. In 12 cases 100 mg of pregnenolone-sulfate (MERCK) were administered intravenously in cases of normal pregnancies at term and a transformation to urinary pregnanediol was seen in 10 - 35 % of the dose administered (LAURITZEN and SCHNEIDER, 1968).

Table 8. Influence of an infusion of 100 mg Δ^5pregnenolone on plasma progesterone, pregnanediol values in urine and plasma oestrogens (4 normal patients, 36. - 40. week of pregnancy)

	Control	Following infusion of 100 mg of pregnenolone i. v.	
		Day 1	Day 2
Plasma Progesterone μg/100 ml	10.8	12.5	13.8
	12.4	13.0	12.7
	13.7	19.8	21.2
	13.9	24.6	23.9
Urine Pregnanediol mg/24^h	36.4	38.7	40.2
	38.7	39.6	39.1
	39.2	46.2	48.0
	44.0	45.9	46.7
Plasma Oestrogens ng/ml	18.0	27.2	26.3
	10.4	23.6	21.0
	14.5	20.3	20.6
	28.3	39.7	36.4

So far only 5 pathological cases (EPH-gestosis) have been investigated with injection of pregnenolone). An increase of urinary pregnanediol between 0 - 10 % was seen, correlating to the gravity of the disease and the state of the fetus.

Therapeutic Use of Repeated Injections of DHEA-S and of Oral DHEA-S:

DHEA-S in a dose of 60 mg oral per day over a time of several weeks was given in 22 patients with an imminent abortion. An increase of total oestrogens from 4 to 9 mg and of pregnanediol from 4 to 11 mg/24 hours urine was seen in cases where the pregnancy could be maintained (Table 9). In cases where abortion did occur, no significant oestrogen increase was seen following DHEA-S. A case where an increase in hormone values occurred is shown in Fig. 1. Also repeated i. v. injections of DHEA-S produced a highly significant increase of total oestrogens in urine and plasma which in cases with a good prognosis proved to become a permanent normalisation of oestrogen values.

The Table 10 demonstrates an interesting case of heavy EPH-gestosis with initially no oestrogen increase following the DHEA-S test. Later on, when the conditions of the patient had somewhat improved by bed

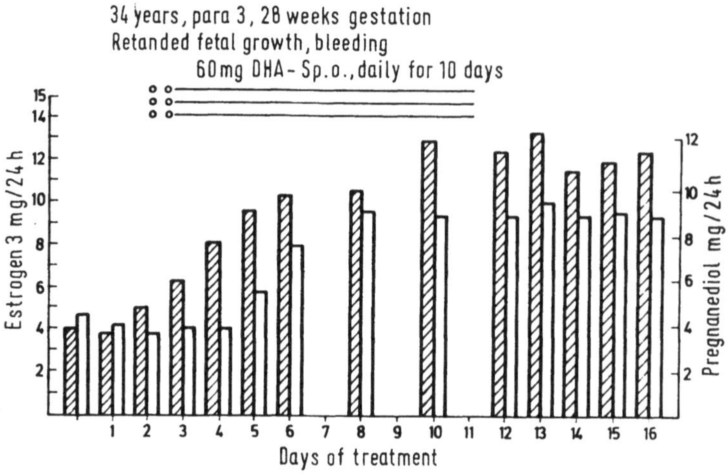

Fig. 1. Increase of estriol and pregnanediol values following a medication of 60 mg DHEA-S orally per day in a case with abortion bleeding

Table 9. Results of therapy of imminent abortion with DHEA-S 60 mg/day orally (N = 22, 16. - 23. week)

	Permanent rise of urinary oestrogens	No or no permanent rise of urinary oestrogens
Pregnancy maintained	18 pat. (4.1→9.5)	-
Pregnancy not maintained	0 pat.	4 pat.
before the 12. - 14. week <u>no</u> oestrogen increase		

rest and sedative and diuretic therapy, an improvement of the conversion rate to oestrogens occurred. Later on a sort of therapy with daily injections of 100 mg of DHEA-S was tried. While the oestrogen values in urine increased at the beginning, a decrease was noted when the conditions of the patient, the proteinuria, the blood pressure, urea and creatinine values finally worsened again. When the conversion rate was at the lowest values, a cesarean section had to be performed because of imminent danger for the mother and the fetus. This table shows that DHEA depressed glucose-6-phosphate dehydrogenase but did apparently not influence significantly total plasma protein, sodium, potassium, urea and creatinine values. The hypothesis might be discussed, whether the DHEA-S medication caused an additional exhaustion of the placental biosynthetic capacity in this special case. A similar case but of a successful DHEA-S injection "therapy" is seen in Fig. 2. The Table 11 summarizes the results in 36 patients following DHEA injection "therapy". Only in cases where the oestrogen excretion in the urine increased permanently a clinical improvement with a favourable outcome was registered or vice versa: only in cases where the pregnancy later on progressed uneventfully a permanent oestrogen increase had been noticed.

The experience with pregnenolone and its sulfate are not yet sufficient to be discussed here in detail (see also LITTLE et al., 1971).

Table 10

M. A., 41 y., 178/63, I. para EPH-gestosis. Index: 11 32. week, therapy: Albumine Lasix, Reserpin, Nepresol		DHEA-S i. v. 50 mg			100 mg		days			100 mg	100 mg	100 mg	100 mg	100 mg	100 mg	100 mg	
	Control	1	2	3	4	5	6	7	8	9	10	11	12	13	14	15	Sectio
																	psychosis
Total oestrogens mg/24h	2,8 3,1	1,1	1,1	2,4	6,2	6,3	6,3	10,8	10,7	30,4	20,8	17,8	8,6	7,4	2,8	2,2	Apgar 4
DHEA urine mg/24h	0,14 0,21	0.04	0,19	0,51	1,29	1,37	0.03	0,16	0,87	2,81	6,27	5,25	6,98	0,41	0,14	0,10	♀
																	1560 g
Urinary volume/spec. weight	440 / 1013	820 / 1020	400 / 019	1460 / 1018	1000 / 1020	1000 / 1020	950 / 1021	900 / 1023	900 / 1018	1480 / 1016	1840 / 1018	2320 / 1016	1760 / 1016	1250 / 1014	820 / 1011	280 / 1007	44 cm
Proteinuria °/oo	3	1	1	0,6	-	0,3	-	0,1	-	0,1	-	-	0,8	1,4	1.9	2,4	
Blood pressure mgHg	240/110	180/95	-	160/90	-	150/90	-	150/90	-	-	150/95	-	150/90	-	180/110	-	
Urea mg % serum	48,2	42,8	-	-	32,8	-	48,2	-	37,5	-	26,7	-	22,8	26,7	42,8	42,8	
Creatinine mg %	1,1	1,2	-	-	1,5	-	0,9	-	1,0	-	1,1	-	0,9	1,9	1,2	1,5	
G6P-DH mU/10^9 Ery	126	104	92	98	77	-	-	-	87	81	75	-	70	63	37	35	
Sodium mäq/L	139	142	-	-	140	-	-	-	139	146	136	-	138	140	134	139	
Potassium mäq/L	4,2	3,9	-	-	4,4	-	-	-	4,6	4,9	3,9	-	4,6	5,0	5,3	4,9	
Total protein	5,7	5,3	-	-	4,9	-	-	-	4,8	4,8	5,0	4,7	4,8	5,5	5,6	5,9	

LDH, GLDH, alk. phosphatase, pO_2 slightly pathological

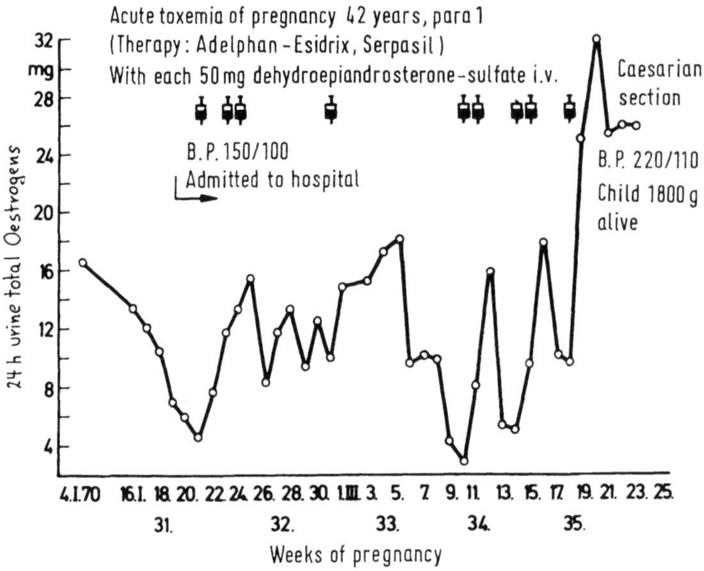

Fig. 2. Final rise of total oestrogens and favourable outcome following repeated i. v. injections of 50 mg DHEA-S

Table 11. Results following DHEA-S injections in pregnancies at risk with low estrogen values (3 - 8 injections à 50 mg i. v.)

No. of patients	Oestriol mg 24^h urine	No. of patients with estrogen increase	Oestriol increase up to mg/24^h urine
36	7,6 (4,2-14,6)	22	19,2 (10,8 - 28,9)

No. of patients without estrogen increase	Oestriol mg/24^h urine	Cases showing clinical improvement+
14	6,1 (4,2 - 9,5)	22

+Gestoses. Criteria: Blood pressure, proteinurea, urinary volume, weight, edema, HCG, HCS, progesterone, pregnanediol. Clinical outcome. After a period of 3 days bed rest.

Discussion and Conclusion

Administration of the oestrogen precursor DHEA-S orally and intravenously and of DHEA-oenantate i. m. increases the plasma level of oestrone-oestradiol-17β and the urinary excretion of total oestrogens in normal pregnancies after the 16. week, besides of effecting a rise of DHEA and 17-ketosteroids in urine. It seems of especially practical interest that DHEA-S is orally resorbed and effective in rising oestrogen values. This finding corresponds to the results of GURPIDE and VANDE WILE (1971), who found a 63 - 80 % resorption of oral DHEA-S and a more than 50 % conversion to oestrogens in pregnant women.

The rate of aromatization of administered DHEA-S has been used and confirmed as a test of fetoplacental function, a high conversion rate suggesting a good condition of the feto-placental unit and a low or failing conversion rate signalizing a risk to the fetus and a danger of infavourable outcome of the pregnancy. The test has been proven to be much more reliable than urinary oestrogen determination, heat stable alkaline phosphatase, cystaminopeptidase and better than HCS determination in plasma. There is no doubt that a prolonged oral medication of DHEA-S and repeated i. v. injections of DHEA-S in pregnancy may induce a rise of depressed oestrogen values in urine and plasma, the plateau of which will also persist after withdrawel of the precursor. Persistent normal values seem however to result only if the state of the pregnancy is improved. In pathological pregnancies with ensuing abortion or placental insufficiency with perinatal pathology no or no significant increase of oestrogen values following DHEA will be seen.

It is not clear at present by what mechanism the improvement of oestrogen production is brought about. It might be suspected that an inducing or inhibiting effect on certain enzyme systems, for instance on the glucose-6-phosphate dehydrogenase might play a role. It is moreover known that an increased offer of oestrogens to the placenta might stimulate the uteroplacental perfusion (LIM and WALTERS, 1970). An acceleration of fetal growth in cases of growth retardation could not be shown so far under DHEA-S medication. Of course, the question whether the oestrogen increase following prolonged DHEA medication effects a real improvement of feto-placental function or is only a sort of oestrogen cosmetics, without real benefit for feto-placental function and bringing along merely the danger of misinterpreting the oestrogen values or exhausting placental capacity is difficult to decide. The small statistics available so far argue for a real improvement of fetoplacental function by DHEA-S. This is also suggested by the posttherapeutic increase of the HCS values in some cases. A further clarification of this critical question of a possible therapeutic effectivity would perhaps be possible by measuring uteroplacental perfusion by the aid of radioactive isotopes and by studying enzmye concentrations (e. g. G-6-PDH and Arylsulfatase) and in vitro aromatizing capacities of the placentas of treated and untreated patients, finally by measuring fetal growth rates and by increasing the number of patients in the statistics. Such investigations will be carried out in the near future in my clinic.

Summary

Oral administration and repeated intravenous injections of DHEA-S cause an increase of lowered oestrogen values in cases of light to moderate placental insufficiency. This rise will persist in cases who thereafter improve clinically and which therefore have a good prognosis. In the few cases of very severe placental insufficiency the rise of oestrogens will not occur or will not persist. Some data are also given for pregnenolone and pregnenolone-sulfate administration. The results of DHEA-S medication so far suggest that a prolonged administration of DHEA-S may be of "therapeutic value" by not only rising the oestrogen values but also improving the basic biosynthetic and metabolic conditions of the feto-placental unit. The mechanism, by which this is effected, is unknown so far.

Further investigation will have to prove further this hypothesis of a real basic improvement of feto-placental function by DHEA-S and will on the other hand have to disprove the possibility that the rise of oestrogens occurs without really altering vital functions of the placenta and the state and prognosis of the underlying disturbance of pregnancy.

References

BOKELMANN, J.: Leistungsfähigkeit verschiedener Methoden zur Überwachung des erhöht gefährdeten Feten in der Spätschwangerschaft. Perinatale Medizin, Bd. III., Berlin: De Gruyter 1971.

CRABBEN, H., van der, HAERING, H., WERNER, CH.: Die Bedeutung des DHEA-Belastungstests für die antenatale Beurteilung des Morbus haemolyticus fetalis. Geburtsh. u. Frauenheilk. 31, 844 (1971).

CRABBEN, H., van der, HAMMACHER, K., SCHMIDT-ELMENDORFF, H., KUNKEL, A., KAISER, E.: The Early Diagnosis of Placental Insufficiency by a New Dehydroepiandrosterone-sulfate Load Test Compared to Cardiotokography, Placental Histology and other Methods Relating Thereto. Acta endocr. (Kbh), Suppl. 138, 244 (1969).

CRABBEN, H., van der, HAMMACHER, K., WERNER, CH., KAISER, E.: Die Beurteilung der Placentafunktion im Vergleich zur Kardiotokographie und Placentahistologie. Geburtsh. u. Frauenheilk. 30, 71 (1970a).

CRABBEN, H., van der, KAISER, E., WERNER, CH.: The placenta function test by Dehydroepiandrosterone-sulfate, an estrogen precursor 2. Internat. Congr. Perinat. Med., Basel: Karger 1970 b.

CRABBEN, H., van der, WERNER, CH.: Vergleichende Untersuchungen über den Aussagewert der Oestriolausscheidung im 24^h-Urin und des Dehydroepiandrosteronsulfat-Belastungstests mit Hinzuziehung der histologischen Plazentabefunde. In: EPH-Gestosis. RIPPMANN, E. T., and RIPPERT, CH., Edit. Berlin: Walter de Gruyter 1972, p. 241.

EDQUIST, L.-E., JOHANNSSON, E. D. B.: Radioimmunoassay of oestrone and oestradiol in human and bovine peripheral plasma. Acta Endocr. 71, 716 - 730 (1972).

EMMENT, Y., COLLINS, W. P., SOMMERVILLE, J. F.: Radioimmunoassay of oestrone and oestradiol in human plasma. Acta Endocr. 69, 567 - 582 (1972).

GURPIDE, E., VANDE WIELE, R. L.: Utilization of Ingested Dehydroepiandrosterone Sulfate for the Production of Estrogens by Normal and Adrenalectomized Pregnant Subjects. Steroid Biochem. 2, 11 (1971).

HARTMANN, D., LAURITZEN, CH.: Ausscheidung und Stoffwechsel von Dehydroepiandrosteron-Sulfat nach oraler und parenteraler Applikation von DHEA-Estern bei schwangeren und nichtschwangeren Frauen. Dissertation Hartmann, Kiel, 1969.

ITTRICH, G.: Eine Methode für die klinische Routinebestimmung der Harnöstrogene. Zbl. Gynäk. 82, 429 (1960 a).

ITTRICH, G.: Eine Methode zur chemischen Bestimmung von oestrogenen Hormonen in Blut, Milch und Colostrum. Hoppe Seylers Z. Physiol. Chem. 320, 103 (1960 b).

JEFFERY, J., SWAPP, G. H., WILSON, G. R.: Studies in vivo on the Control of Oestrogen Secretion in Human Pregnancy. Proc. Roy. Soc. Med. 63, 1088 (1970).

JOHANNESSON, E. D. B.: A simplified Procedure for the Assay of Progesterone Acta endocr. (Kbh), Suppl. 147, 188 (1970).

KAISER, E., WERNER, CH., CRABBEN, H., van der, WERNER, CH.: Neuer Hormon-Belastungstest bei Plazentainsuffizienz. 70. Int. Congr. Clin. Chem., Vol 3: Hormones, Lipids and Miscellaneous p. 6. Basel, München, Paris, New York: Karger 1970.

KELLER, P. J., BADER, P., SCHMID, J., BAERTSCH, U., GERBER, C., SOLTERMANN, R., KOPPER, E.: Biochemical Detection of Fetoplacental Distress in Risk Pregnancies. Lancet I, 729 (1971).

KLOPPER, A., MICHIE, E. M., BROWN, J. B.: A Method for Determination of Urinary Pregnanediol. J. Endocr. 12, 209 (1955).

KNAPSTEIN, R., MARTIN, K., HIRSCHE, H., HEIDENREICH, J., WORTMANN, W., OERTEL, C. M.: Untersuchungen zur Prüfung der Plazentafunktion mit dem DHEA-Sulfat-Belastungstest. Arch. Gynäk. 211, 249 (1970).

LAURITZEN, CH.: A clinical test for placental functional activity using DHEA-sulphate and ACTH injection in pregnant women. Acta Endocr. (Kbh), Suppl. 119, 188 (1967).
LAURITZEN, CH.: Ausscheidung und Stoffwechsel von Dehydroepiandrosteron in der normalen und pathologischen Schwangerschaft. p. 313, 13. Sympos. Dtsch. Ges. Endokrinologie, Berlin, Heidelberg, New York: Springer-Verlag 1967 a.
LAURITZEN, CH.: A Clinical Test for Placental Functional Activity using DHEA-Sulphate and ACTH injections in Pregnant Women. Acta Endocr. (Kbh), Suppl. 119, 188 (1967 b).
LAURITZEN, CH., SCHNEIDER, H. P. G.: Ausscheidung von Pregnandiol nach Injektion von Pregnenolon in der normalen und pathologischen Schwangerschaft. Geburtsh. u. Frauenheilk. 28, 396 (1968).
LAURITZEN, CH.: Conversion of DHEA-Sulfate to Estrogens as a Test of Placental Function. Hormone a. Metab. Res. 1, 96 (1969).
LAURITZEN, CH.: Placental Steroidogenesis. In: Hormonal Steroids, p. 37, Excerpta Medica, Amsterdam 1971 a.
LAURITZEN, CH.: Die hormonelle Diagnostik der Plazentainsuffizienz Fortschritte der perinatalen Medizin, Bd. II, p. 36, Stuttgart: G. Thieme 1971 b.
LAURITZEN, CH.: Therapieversuche mit Dehydroepiandrosteron-Sulfat bei bedrohten Schwangerschaften. Arch. Gynäk. 211, 247 (1971 c).
LAURITZEN, CH., LEHMANN, W. D.: Metabolic Behaviour of Dehydroepiandrosterone and Aromatizing Capacity of the Placenta in Pregnancy Cases of Diabetes Mellitus. Acta endocr. (Kbh), Suppl. 155, 186 (1971 d).
LAURITZEN, CH.: Bedeutung der Oestrogenbestimmung und des Dehydroepiandrosteron-Tests in der Beurteilung und Behandlung von Risikoschwangerschaften. Perinatale Medizin, Bd. II, p. 7, Stuttgart: C. Thieme 1972 a.
LAURITZEN, CH., LEHMANN, W. D.: Untersuchungen über die physiopathologischen Grundlagen des Dehydroepiandrosteron-Belastungstests bei normaler und bedrohter Schwangerschaft. 39. Tagung Dtsch. Ges. Gynäk. /.2.0.9 p. 42 (1972 b).
LIM, Y. L., WALTERS, W. A.: Oestrogens and maternal circulation. Austr. New Zeal. J. Obstet. Gynaec. 10, 61 (1970).
LITTLE, B., BILIAR, R. B., HALLA, M., HEINSONS, A., JASSANI, M., KLINE, J. T., PURDY, R. H.: Pregnenolone production in pregnancy. Amer. J. Obstet. Gynec. 111, 505 (1971).
PENG, T.-CH., VENA, R., OFFNER, P., MUNSON, P. L.: A simple Method for the Determination of Urinary Dehydroepiandrosterone Steroids 6, 571 (1965).
PETERSON, R. S., PIERCE, C. E.: In: Lipids and the Steroid Hormones in Clinical Medicine, p. 158, F. W. SAUNDERS and F. W. SAUNDERS Edit., Lippincott, Philadelphia 1960.
STEMBERA, Z. K., HERZMANN, J.: Oestriol Examination after DHEA-S as a Test of Placental Insufficiency. Cs. Gynek. 36, 10 (1971).
STEMBERA, Z. K., HERZMANN, J.: Index of Fetoplacental Insufficiency In: EPH-Gestosis. RIPPMANN, E. T., and RIPPERT, Edit., Berlin: Walter de Gruyter 1973.
VULLIEMOZ, P., OBOLENSKY, W., VARGA, L.: L'appréciation de l'état fonctionel de l'unité foeto-placentaire par le test au sulfate de déhydroépiandrostérone. Méd. et Hygiène, 917, 774 (1970).
WERNER, CH., SCHNEIDERHAN, W.: Plazentamorphologie und Plazentafunktion in Abhängigkeit von der diabetischen Stoffwechselführung. Geburtsh. u. Frauenheilk. 32, 959 (1972).
WU, CH.-H., LUNDY, E.: Radioimmunoassay of plasma estrogens. Steroids 18, 91 (1971).

Variation in Maternal Urinary Excretion of Total Oestrogens Following ACTH Administration to the Fetus in Utero

W. Bellati, S. Dell' Acqua, G. Plotti, A. Lucisano, and A. Bompiani

There is strong evidence showing that for oestriol synthesis the feto-placental unit chiefly uses dehydroepiandrosterone sulphate (DHAS) from the fetal adrenals and to a lesser extent DHAS from the maternal adrenals (a ratio of about 8 : 2). This is strengthened by the fact that though ACTH stimulation of maternal adrenals results in an increase in the synthesis of DHAS, several investigators have failed to demonstrate a significant increase in urinary oestriol excretion (SCOMMEGNA et al., 1968; DICKEY, THOMPSON, 1969; JEFFERY et al., 1970).

In 8 pregnant women whom we have examined, 50. I. U. of ACTH (Synacten, Ciba), administered intravenously over a 12 hours period did not induce any significant increase in urinary total oestrogen excretion (Fig. 1). The maternal adrenals were fully stimulated, as shown by the increase in the urinary excretion of 17-OH-corticosteroids and 17-keto-steroids in the women studied (Fig. 2). This response is further confirmed by the increase in plasma levels of DHAS and pregnenolone, as shown in Fig. 3. As maternal ACTH cannot cross the placental barrier in physiologically active amounts, (SAMUELS & UCHIKOWA, 1967), we attempted to determine whether fetal adrenals are stimulated by ACTH produced by the hypophysis of the foetus.

Two groups of investigators, BURD et al. (1970) and ARAI et al. (1972) injected ACTH into the foetus in utero but obtained conflicting figures for the maternal urinary oestrogen excretion. While BURD et al. found no significant variations, ARAI et al. demonstrated a gradual and significant increase in the excretion of urinary oestrogens over days 1 to 3 after injecting 40 I. U. of ACTH. To evaluate the maturity of six RH-isoimmunised mothers with Rh+ positive foetuses, at ages ranging from 34 to 39 weeks, we gave ACTH to the foetuses.

The following technique was used. By amniography with liposuluble contrast medium, injected several days before the procedures, we easily demonstrated the foetus. Under image intensification when the foetus was in the most suitable position, an injection of 50 I. U. of ACTH was given. Because of maternal sedation and good image intensification no trauma occurred (Fig. 4). Fig. 5 shows daily urinary total oestrogen excretion before and after ACTH administration. The urinary excretion of total oestrogens increased after ACTH. In most cases the peak increment occurred few days after the ACTH. These results are substantially in agreement with those obtained by ARAI et al. and support the hypothesis that fetal adrenals respond to ACTH produced by the fetal hypophysis.

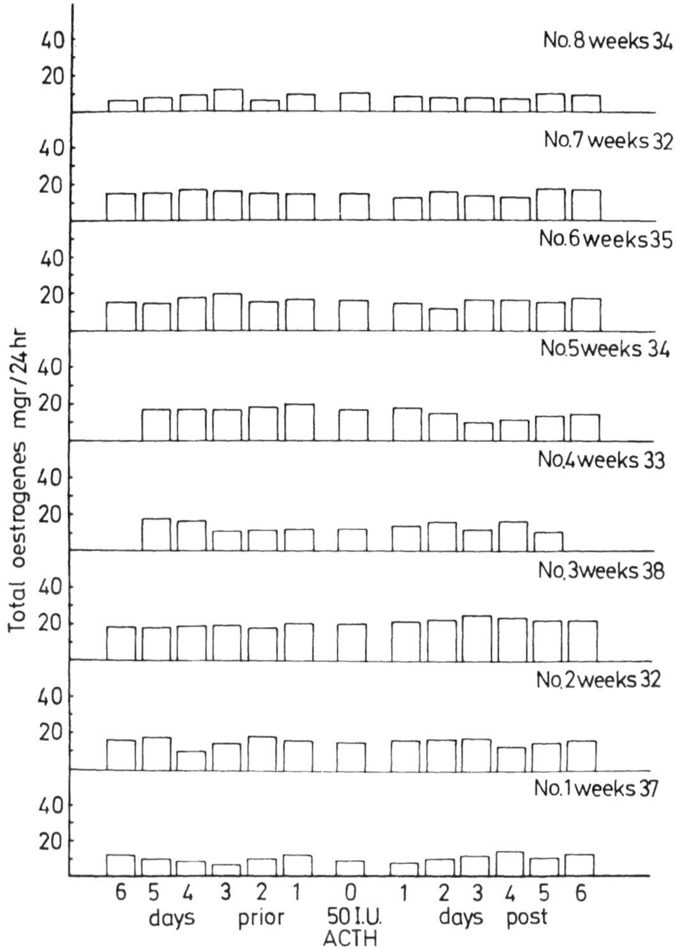

Fig. 1. Urinary excretion of total oestrogens in pregnant patients before and after intravenous administration of ACTH

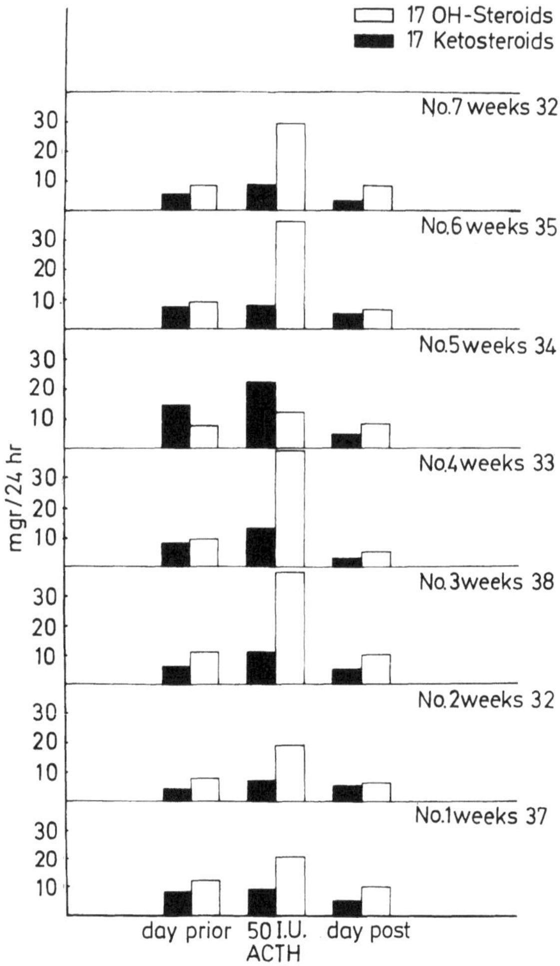

Fig. 2. Urinary excretion of 17-OH-Corticosteroids and 17 keto-steroids in pregnant women before and after intravenous administration of ACTH

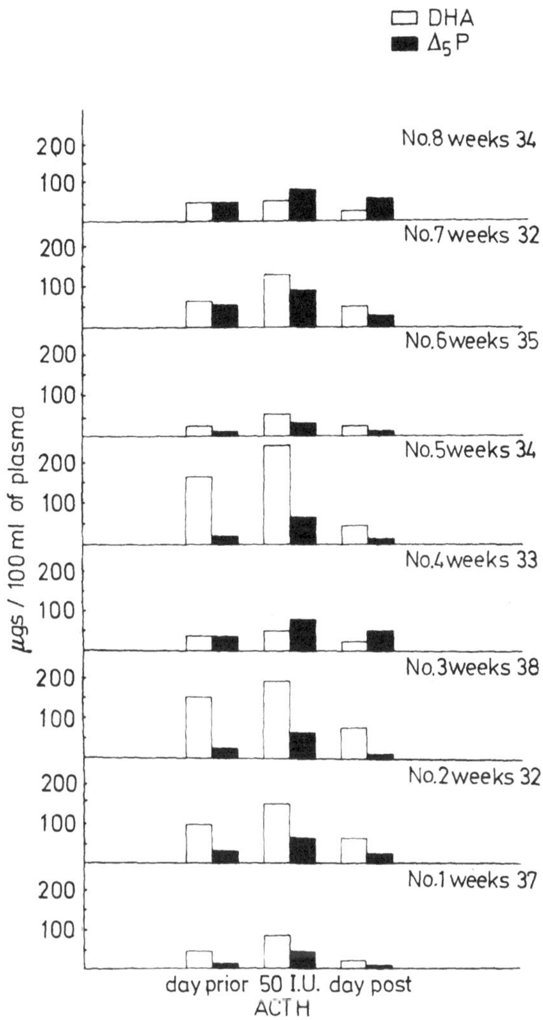

Fig. 3. Plasma levels of dehydroepiandrosterone (DHA) and (Δ_5P) in pregnant women before and after intravenous administration of ACTH

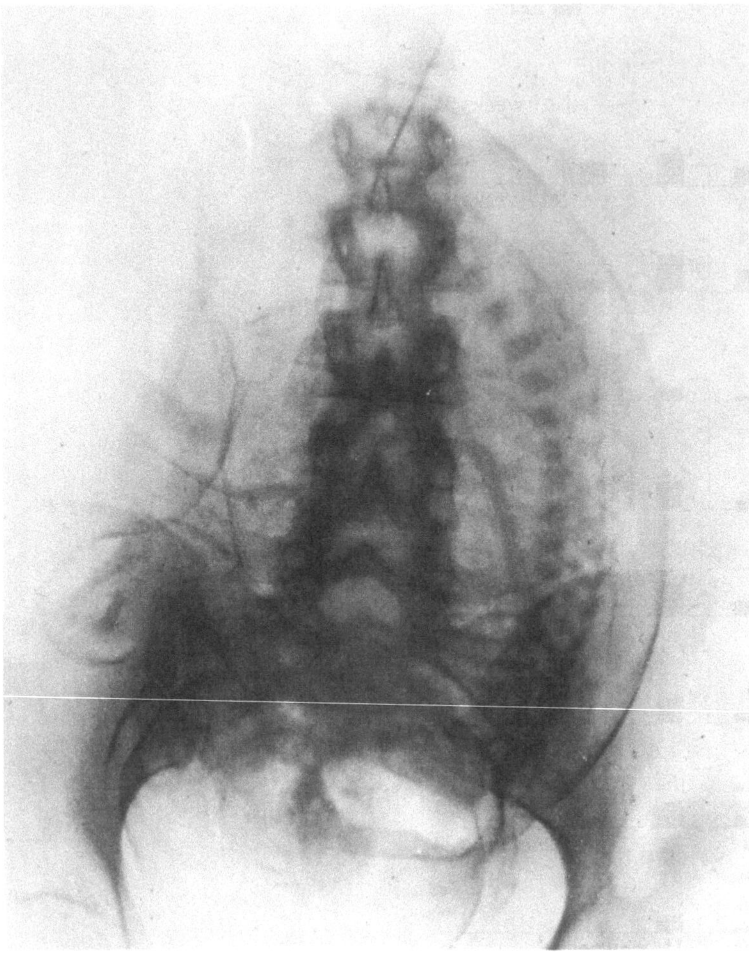

Fig. 4. Image internsification of an intra-uterine injection of ACTH into the foetus

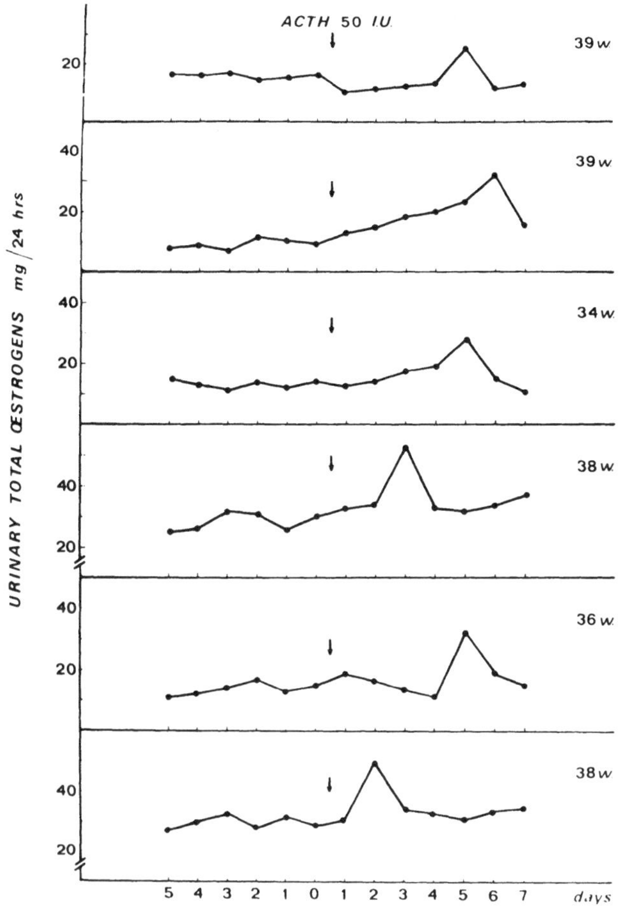

Fig. 5. Urinary excretion of total oestrogens in pregnant women before and after intrauterine injection of ACTH to the foetus

References

ARAI, K., KUWABARA, Y., OKINAGA, S.: Am. J. Obstet. Gynecol. 73, 316 (1972).

BURD, L., BIENIARZ, J., NEDOSS, B., CHARLES, A., SCOMMAGNA, A.: Obstetrics and Gynecology 36, 574 (1970).

DICKEY, R. P., THOMPSON, J. P.: J. Clin. Endocr. Metab. 29, 701 (1969).

JEFFERY, J., SWAPP, G. M., WILSON, G. R., FOTHERBY, K.: J. Endocr. 48, 591 (1970).

SAMUELS, L. T., UCHIKOWA, T.: In Eisenstein A. B., Ed.: The adrenal cortex, Boston: Little, Brown & Company, p. 61, 1967.

SCOMMEGNA, A., NEDOSS, B. R., CHATTORAY, S. C.: Obstetrics and Gynecology 31, 526 (1968).

A Study of Feto-Neonatal Effects of Maternal Administration of Dehydroepiandrosterone Sulphate (DEAS) in Rats

G. Celasco and G. Bruni

Apart from being an established agent in evaluating feto-placental function (1 - 8) DEAS has been recently reported to be of therapeutic value in some forms of at-risk pregnancies (9, 10). DEAS may be injurious to a foetus; the present study aims at providing some insight into the possibility.

Pregnant rats of Wistar strain were divided into three groups of 7 - 10 animals each and, from day 12 to 20 of pregnancy, treated by daily subcutaneous injections of DEAS (sodium salt) at doses of 1 and 25 mg/kg in aqueous suspension. A similar number of rats received "sham" treatment. At delivery newborn rats were counted, weighed, subdivided according to sex, alive or dead, and submitted to a macroscopic inspection involving the external aspects and skeletal morphology. Ano-urethral (females) and ano-phallic (males) distances were measured with a micrometer caliper under optical magnification. The young rats were observed daily up to day 21 to check on their survival, then weighed separately, and killed. Testes, ovaries and adrenals were dissected and weighed; adrenals were also processed histologically and stained with hematoxilin and eosin. Serum corticosterone was measured in animals born from both control and mothers treated with high doses of DEAS.

Table 1 shows that DEAS, even at the higher dose, did not interfere with the normal outcome of pregnancy. The average litter size appeared to be slightly reduced by treatment, the reduction involving only the males (Table 2). Average body weight, number of dead foetuses and postnatal survival were not appreciably affected. Body and skeletal defects were not seen. Ano-urethral and ano-phallic distances, which are good indices of possible abnormalities in urogenital development, did not differ from those in controls (Table 3), which points to the absence of virilizing or feminizing effects of DEAS. On day 21 of life (Table 4) the young born from both treated groups of mothers showed an average weight gain which was slightly greater than that of controls. This finding is similar to that observed in the mothers at the same date but owing to the lack of metabolic data and a dose-response relationship, is of doubtful interpretation. Adrenal, testicular and ovarian weights did not differ from those of controls in the low-dose group, but were somewhat reduced in the high-dose one. The finding of smaller adrenals is in agreement with GOLDMAN's data (11); however, serum corticosterone was not reduced (26.9 ± 2.91 µg/100 ml in high-dose group against 24.3 ± 2.01 in controls) and adrenal histology appeared to be normal; in particular, the ratios between glomerulosa, fasciculata and reticularis zones were not altered. While adrenal behaviour is not easily explainable, the smaller size of gonads could be interpreted as due to conversion of DEAS into oestrogens, and to the consequent depression in gonadotropin secretion.

Table 1. Outcome of pregnancy and weight of mothers

Treatment (from day 12 to 20 of pregnancy, s.c.)	Dose (mg/kg)	No. of animals		Body weight (g)		
		treated	delivered	initial	soon after delivery	on day 21 after delivery
Vehicle	-	9	9	216 ± 5.0	218 ± 4.5	241 ± 4.9
DEAS	1	10	10	213 ± 4.4	214 ± 3.8	243 ± 4.9
	25	7	7	222 ± 3.9	225 ± 2.8	257 ± 6.1

Table 2. Data on newborn rats

Treatment	Dose (mg/kg)	No. of young		Av. body weight (g)	No. of males					No. of females				
		total	per litter		total	per litter	alive	dead	ab-normal	total	per litter	alive	dead	ab-normal
Vehicle	-	98	10.8	5.42	53	5.8	52	1	-	45	5.0	45	-	-
DEAS	1	99	9.9	5.75	41	4.1	41	-	-	58	5.8	57	1	-
	25	66	9.3	5.64	29	4.1	28	1	-	37	5.2	37	-	-

Table 3. Ano-urethral distances at birth

Treatment	Dose (mg/kg)	Ano-urethral distance (mm)	
		males	females
Vehicle	-	4.2 ± 0.04	1.5 ± 0.03
DEAS	1	4.3 ± 0.05	1.5 ± 0.03
	25	4.2 ± 0.03	1.6 ± 0.03

Table 4. Data on 21-day old rats

Treat-ment	Dose (mg/kg)	Males				Females			
		total number	body weight (g)	adrenals mg/100 g	testes mg/100 g	total number	body weight (g)	adrenals mg/100 g	ovaries mg/100 g
Vehicle	-	40	30.6 ± 0.5	39.1 ± 0.88	486.1 ± 6.11	39	30.2 ± 0.6	40.6 ± 0.88	48.8 ± 1.31
DEAS	1	33	33.0 ± 0.9	39.9 ± 0.76	479.2 ± 8.06	47	33.0 ± 0.6	40.4 ± 0.92	50.1 ± 1.15
	25	22	32.0 ± 1.1	36.2 ± 1.14	474.7 ± 10.1	29	32.0 ± 1.1	35.8 ± 0.79	38.3 ± 1.16

References

1. LAURITZEN, C.: Acta Endocr. Suppl. 119, 188 (1967).
2. LAURITZEN, C.: In: "Verhandlungen, 13. Symposion der Deutschen Gesellschaft für Endokrinologie" (Köln, 1967). Berlin: Springer 1967, p. 313.
3. LAURITZEN, C.: Hormone Metab. Res. 1, 96 (1969).
4. CRABBEN H., et al.: Geburtsh. Frauenheilk. 30, 71 (1970).
5. HAUSKNECHT, R. U., MANDELMAN, N.: Amer. J. Obstet. Gynec. 104, 433 (1969).
6. VULLIEMOZ, P., et al.: Med. Hyg. 917, 774 (1970).
7. KELLER, P. J., et al.: Lancet 2, 729 (1971).
8. CRABBEN, H., et al.: Geburtsh. Frauenheilk. 31, 844 (1971).
9. LAURITZEN, C.: Arch. Gynäk. 211, 247 (1971).
10. LAURITZEN, C.: In: "Proceedings 3rd International Congress on Hormonal Steroids", (Hamburg 1970). Editors: V. H. T. JAMES and L. MARTINI. Amsterdam: Excerpta Medica 1971, p. 37.
11. GOLDMAN, A. S.: Endocrinology 87, 432 (1970).

Variation in Maternal Urinary Excretion of Total Oestrogens Following Intra-Amniotic Administration of Dehydroepiandrosterone

S. Dell'Acqua, A. Lucisano, G. Plotti, E. Parlati, E. Arno,
U. Bellati, and A. Bompiani

At present, the determination of urinary oestriol in pregnant women is one of the most useful methods of evaluating the condition of the foetus, by assessing the steroid-metabolizing activity of the feto-placental unit.

In recent years several investigators have proposed for this evaluation the use of dynamic tests, which could complement and improve the diagnostic possibilities provided by the simple oestriol assay, in terms of long-term prognosis of fetal conditions.

The conversion of dehydroepiandrosterone sulphate (DHAS) into oestrogens takes place mainly in the placenta (DICZFALUSY, 1968). Such tests are based upon supplying a large amount of DHAS to the placenta, to test its steroid-metabolizing activity under load conditions. The LAURITZEN test (1967) consists of a rapid intra-venous administration of DHAS (20 to 200 mg according to different authors and at different stages of pregnancy) to the mother and then measuring the increase in the urinary excretion of oestriol or total oestrogens (KNAPSTEIN et al., 1970; VULLIEMOZ et al., 1970; CHEF & LAMBOTTE, 1972; STEMBERA & HERZMANN, 1972).

We describe a test, based on the intra-amniotic administration of DHAS.

200 mg of DHAS (Roche) is rapidly injected into the amniotic cavity and any increment in the urinary excretion of total oestrogens over the 24 hours following the injection is expressed as the percentage of the mean of the two 24-hours excretion values before DHAS administration.

The increase in urinary oestrogens occurs 6 - 8 hours after the injection of DHAS, as clearly shown by urinary assays performed on urine passed every 2 - 4 hours. For the above reason it is more convenient to measure any increment after 8 hours from the administration of DHAS. As urine collections in our Department start at 6 a. m., intra-amniotic injection is given at 10 p. m. of the previous day.

Fig. 1 shows 8 normal pregnancies, where the increment in the total urinary oestrogens during the first 24 hours always exceeded 100 %.

In Fig. 2 are illustrated 5 cases of pathological pregnancies, where the increase never reached 100 %. It is interesting to note that in such pathological pregnancies often the increase is slight in the first 24 hours, but it persists during the following days. This suggests that in placental insufficiency DHAS metabolism is delayed. In some cases a simple oestriol assay gave values within the normal range, while the test under load condition showed that there was a definite placental deficiency.

Fig. 3 shows two profiles of urinary oestrogen assays performed every 4 hours in 2 cases, one normal and one pathological. The two profiles show a different increment curve and it can be seen that in the first

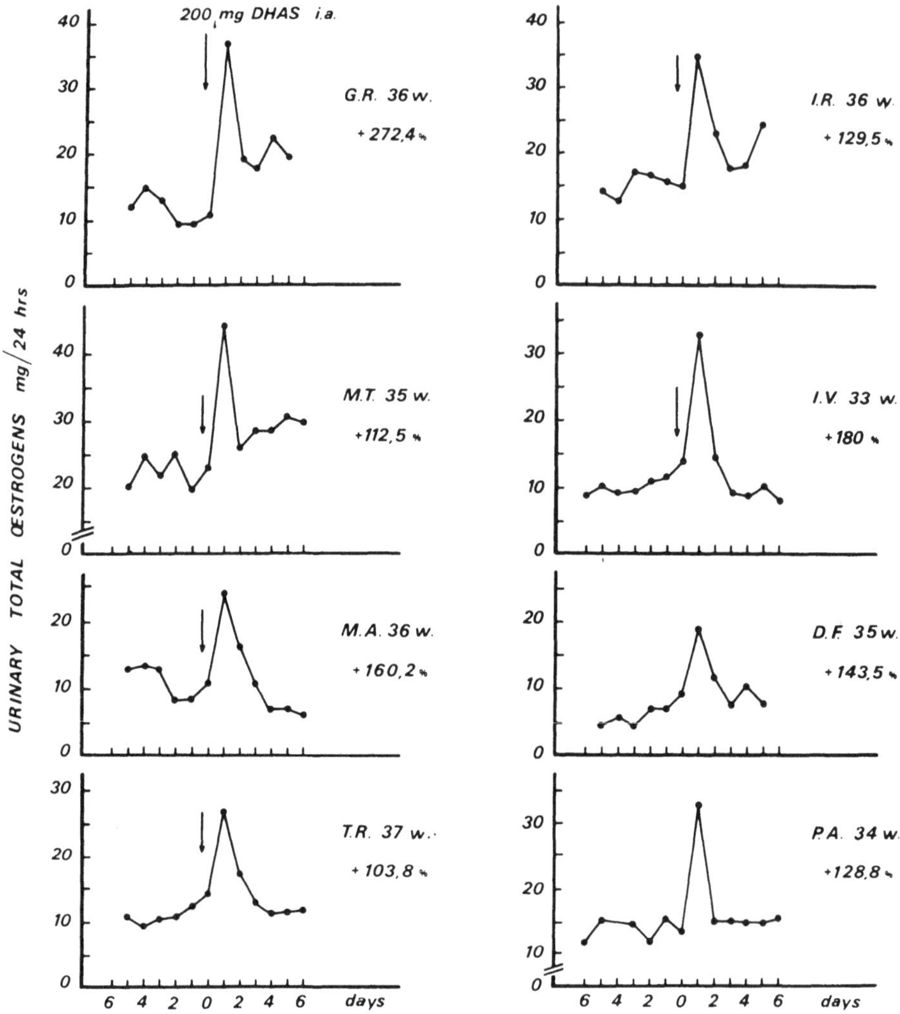

Fig. 1. Urinary excretion of total oestrogens in normal pregnant women before and after intra-amniotic administration of dehydroepiandrosterone sulphate

8 hours after administration, no significant increase in excretion is found.

Compared with the LAURITZEN test, where the DHAS administered is diluted in the maternal body compartments, the intra-amniotic test offers the advantage that the DHAS concentration in the amniotic fluid enables a much greater utilization of the steroid by placental enzymes. As a result there is a more marked increase in urinary excretion of oestrogens and thus a more precise evaluation of placental response.

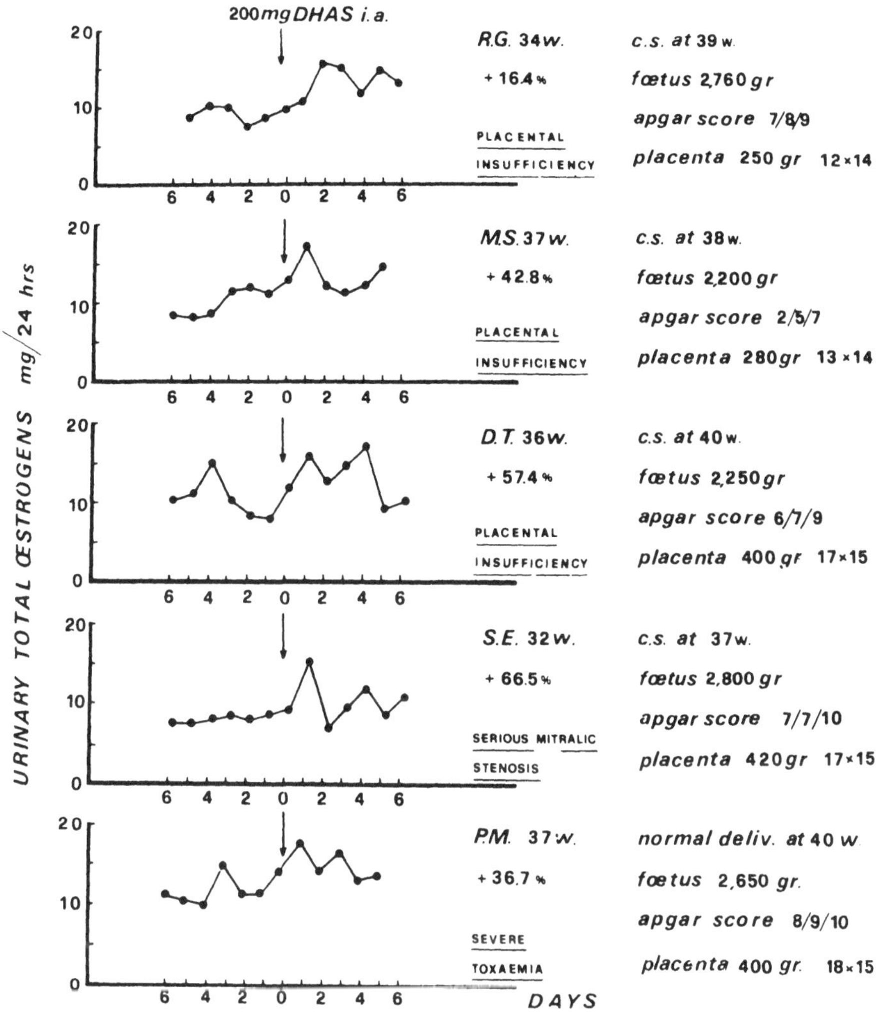

Fig. 2. Urinary excretion of total oestrogens in cases of pathological pregnancies, before and after intra-amniotic of dehydroepiandrosterone sulphate

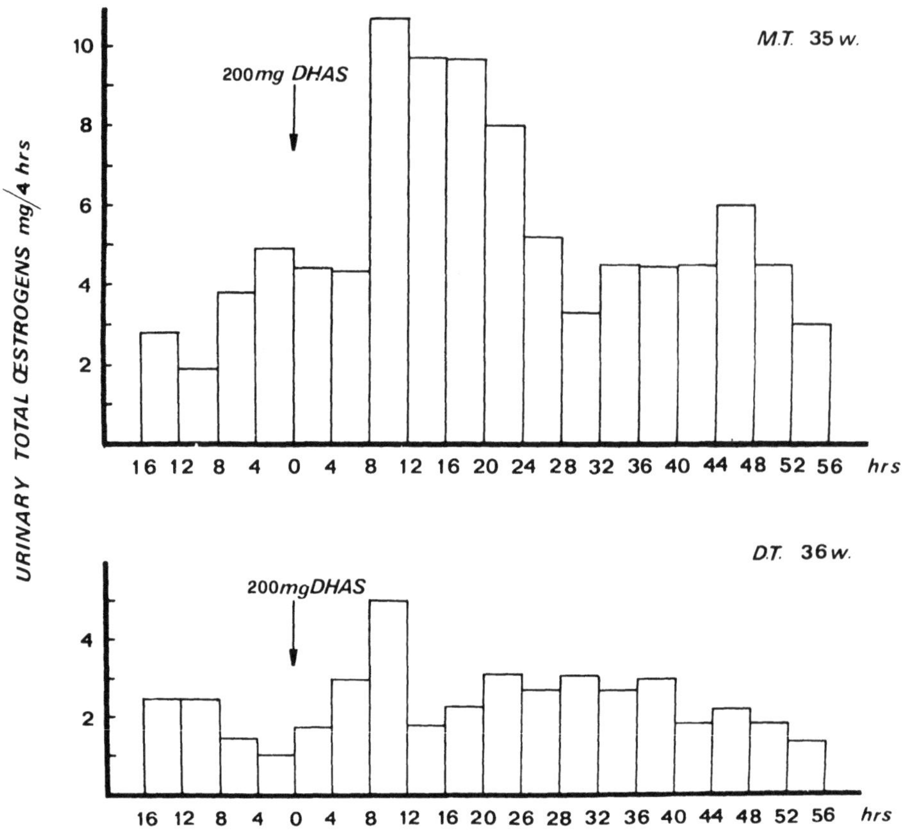

Fig. 3. Two profiles of urinary oestrogen excretion performed every four hours in a normal and in a pathological pregnancy, before and after, intra-amniotic administration of dehydroepiandrosterone sulphate

References

CHEF, R., LAMBOTTE, R.: In: BOSSART, H., et al., Ed., Perinatal Medicine 383, Bern: Hans Huber Publishers 1973.

DICZFALUSY, E.: Excerpta Medica Intern. Congress Series 183, 65 (1968).

KNAPSTEIN, P., MARTIN, K., HIERSCHE, H., HEIDENREICH, J., WORTMANN, W., OERTEL, G. W.: Arch. Ginäk. 211, 249 (1970).

LAURITZEN, C.: Acta Endocr. (Kbh), Suppl. 119, 188 (1967).

STEMBERA, Z., HERZMANN, J.: In: BOSSART, H., et al., Ed., Perinatal Medicine, Bern: Hans Huber Publishers 290, 1973.

VULLIEMOZ, P., OBOLENSKY, W., VARGA, L.: Méd. et Hyg. 917, 774 (1970).

Levels of Serum Unconjugated Oestrogens after DHEA-S Loading Tests in Human Pregnancy

U. Gaspard, J. Sulon, H. Thoumsin, and L. Demey-Ponsart

Different workers have investigated the variations in maternal urinary oestrogen excretion during pregnancy after an intravenous Dehydroepiandrosterone sulphate (DHEA-S) loading test (1, 2).

They have shown an inadequate conversion of DHEA to oestrogens during abnormal pregnancies. In this preliminary study we report the results of serum oestriol and oestradiol measurements measured after DHEA-S loading tests during the last trimester of pregnancy.

Assay Procedures: Prior to the assays the serum samples were extracted with di-ethylether so that only unconjugated oestriol and oestradiol were measured (3). The oestradiol radioimmunoassay was performed by using a new technique that we developed with a rabbit antiserum against oestriol-6-oxime-bovine serum albumin. This anti-serum was a generous gift from Prof. M. F. JAYLE (Paris). These radio-immunoassay procedures will be described in detail elsewhere.

Results and Discussion

a) 50 individual serum unconjugated oestriol measurements have been made from the 12th to the 38th week of normal pregnancies. The mean levels ± 1 standard deviation (S. D.) are illustrated in Fig. 1. A marked increase in serum-free oestriol is seen from the 20th week onwards; this increase is greater after the 32nd week and maximum levels are reached during the 37th and 38th weeks (8.1 ng/ml). These results are in complete agreement with other published figures (4, 5, 3, 6). The serial oestriol values obtained in 12 high risk pregnancies during the third trimester are in the same range as those obtained in normal pregnancy.

b) Fig. 2 shows the changes in serum oestriol levels determined at 2 hourly intervals for 12 hours after DHEA-S loading tests. The tests were performed in 12 patients with abnormal pregnancies and in 12 normals all in the third trimester.

The individual and mean serum oestriol levels showed no marked variation discernible from spontaneous fluctuations. Thus, there is an important discrepancy between serum-free oestriol and urinary oestriol variations after DHEA-S loading procedures. Urinary oestriol levels have repetitively shown statistically significant fluctuations in such circumstances.

c) Fig. 3 illustrates the simultaneous fluctuations of serum free oestradiol and oestriol levels after the injection of 50 mg DHEA-S (3 patients) and 100 mg (1 patient). The serum samples were obtained at 30-minute intervals for a period of 3 hours.

There is no variation of the oestriol serum levels but the oestradiol levels show a rapid increase within one hour after the DHEA-S injection. The existence of this discrepancy between serum unconjugated oestriol

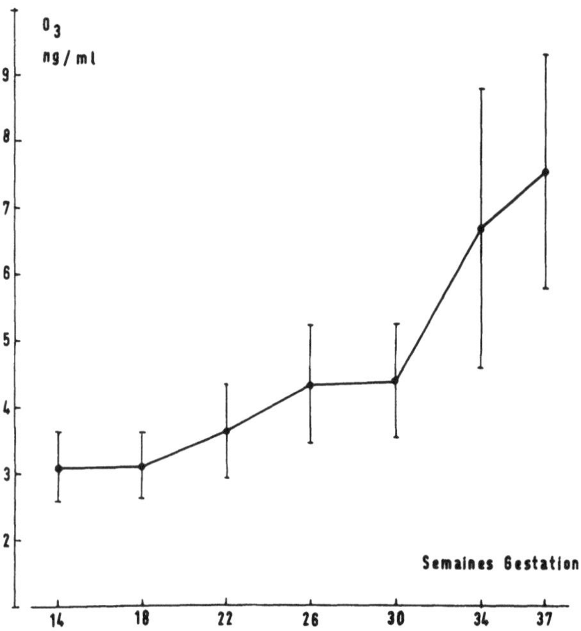

O_3
ng/ml
9
8
7
6
5
4
3
2
Semaines Gestation
14
18
22
26
30
34
37

Fig. 1

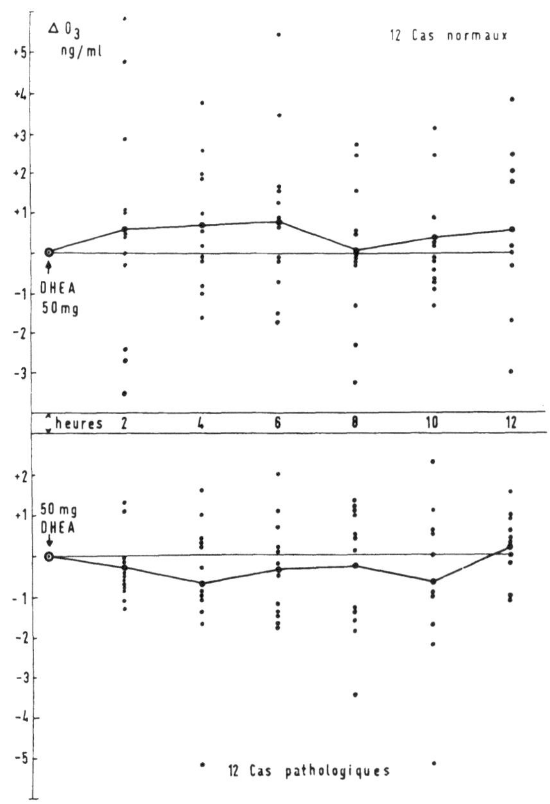

Δ O_3
ng/ml
12 Cas normaux
+5
+4
+3
+2
+1
-1
-2
-3
DHEA
50 mg
heures
2
4
6
8
10
12
+2
+1
50 mg
DHEA
-1
-2
-3
-4
-5
12 Cas pathologiques

Fig. 2

levels, urinary oestriol and serum-free oestradiol, seems to be due to metabolic differences.

Unconjugated plasma oestradiol represents 70 % of the total circulating oestradiol levels, and thus may be a valuable index of placental oestrogen production. Conversely, plasma-unconjugated oestriol accounts only for 5 % of total plasma oestriol (4). Moreover, this conjugated fraction is rapidly cleared and has an approximate biological half-life of 15 min. In that respect, free plasma oestriol cannot be expected to be an accurate index of steroid production by the feto-placental unit.

Thus we now plan to investigate the evolution of total serum oestriol and oestradiol during DHEA-S loading experiments.

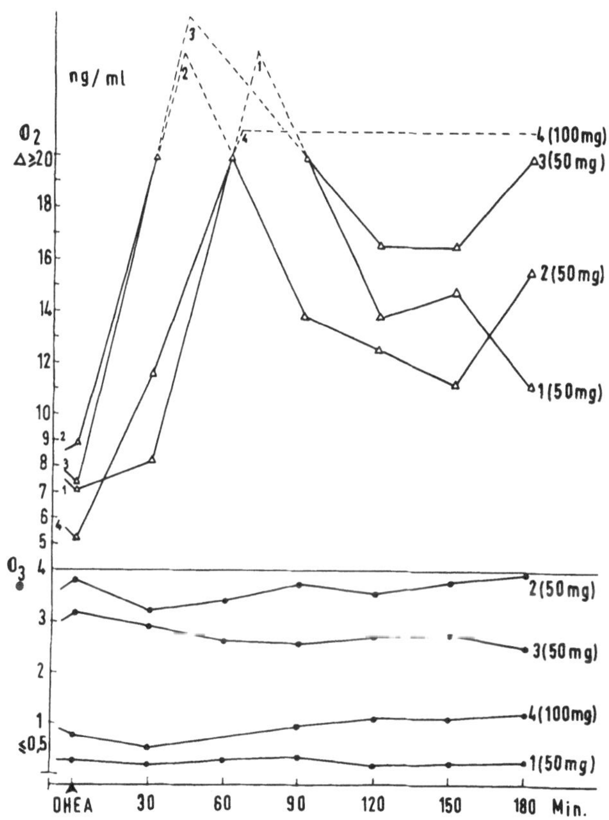

Fig. 3

References

1. LAURITZEN, CH.: Horm. Metab. Res. 1, 96 (1969).
2. THOUMSIN, H., GASPARD, U., DUVIVIER, J., LAMBOTTE, R.: C. R. XXème Congrès d'anesthésie et réanimation. Arnette Ed. (sous presse) 1973.
3. AHMED, J., KELLIE, A. E.: J. Ster. Bioche. 4, 1 (1973).
4. LORIAUX, D. L., RUDER, H. J., KNAB, D. R., LIPSETT, M. B.: J. Clin. Endoc. Metab. 35, 887 (1972).
5. TULCHINSKY, D., HOBEL, C. J., YEAGER, E., MARSHALL, J. R.: Am. J. Obst. Gynec. 112, 1095 (1972).
6. TULCHINSKY, D., HOBEL, C. J., KORENMAN, S. G.: Am. J. Obst. Gynec. 111, 311 (1971).

The Reliability of a Placental Function Test Using Dihydroepiandrosterone Sulphate (DHEA-S)

H. Thoumsin, U. Gaspard, R. Lambotte, and J. Duvivier

Assessing high-risk pregnancies by urinary oestriol excretion has limitations. In 1972 we reported our experience of LAURITZEN's in-vivo test which measures the ability of the feto-placental unit to metabolize a known amount of DHEA-S in oestriol. We now report similar work and comment in greater detail regarding the indications for, and the interpretation of, the test in clinical practice.

Of 75 pregnancies of 30 to 40 weeks, 24 were normal and 51 were classified as high-risk.

Urinary oestriol has been assayed by the BROWN-HEUSCHEM method. In-vivo tests have been performed by injecting 50 mg of DHEA-S into each patient, and measuring the quantity converted into oestriol during the next 24 hours. Results are expressed as percentage conversions. From our previous work a conversion rate higher than 6 % is defined as positive. In most patients, plasma human placental lactogen (HPL) has also been measured. Maternal diabetes mellitus led us to exclude the case as the interpretation of HPL concentrations is difficult in this condition. Only the last DHEA conversion before delivery has been considered.

Table 1 gives the criteria used in retrospective evaluation of the feto-placental function. This feto-placental score (IFP) has been used to group pathological pregnancies into a) Low scores (satisfactory) and b) high scores (unsatisfactory).

Table 1. Fetoplacental score (IFP); from 0 to 2: satisfactory; from 3 to 6: unsatisfactory

Fetal distress	No 0	APG 7 No dip 1	APG 7 Dip 2	APG 5 Dip 3
Dysmaturity	No 0	Moderate 1	Evident 2	
Placental sclerosis or degeneration	Missing 0	Present 1		
Total	0 to 6			

All normal pregnancies had a satisfactory IFP (24), but among the 51 high risk pregnancies 20 had a poor IFP (Table 2). It must be emphasized that among 25 high-risk pregnancies with oestriol rates in the normal range but below the mean value of gestational age, 18 had unsatisfactory IFP. In normal cases, urinary oestriol excretion corresponds to a satisfactory IFP, whereas the DHEA test shows 29 % false negative results (Table 3). In high-risk pregnancies, urinary oestriol is less trustworthy and has 35.3 % false positive results. Conversely, the DHEA test gives 34.3 % false negative results (Table 4) which are most frequent in cases of high basic oestriol values. Furthermore, HPL and DHEA tests, when combined, provide 100 % accuracy (Table 5).

Table 2

Pregnancy	Estrioluria (Vm = mean value for gestational age)	Number of cases	Mean value of DHEA conversion (M $\pm$ SD)
Normal (24)	03 $\geq$ Vm	17	10.9 % $\pm$ 1.9 %
Satisfactory	03 $<$ Vm	7	11.8 % $\pm$ 3.4 %
IFP	03 $<$ lower lim	0	-
High-risk (31)	03 $\geq$ Vm	24	6.0 % $\pm$ 1.4 %
Satisfactory	03 $<$ Vm	7	9.0 % $\pm$ 2.1 %
IFP	03 $<$ lower lim	0	-
High-risk (20)	03 $\geq$ Vm	2	1.1 % $\pm$ 1.1 %
Unsatisfactory	03 $<$ Vm	16	2.4 % $\pm$ 0.6 %
IFP	03 $<$ lower lim	2	1.8 % $\pm$ 1.8 %

Table 3. Normal pregnancies (24)

	Accurate results	False positive	False negative
Estriol	100.0 %	-	0.0 %
DHEA	70.8 %	-	29.2 %
HPL	90.0 %	-	10.0 %

Table 4. High-risk pregnancies (51)

	Accurate results	False positive	False negative
Estriol	64.7 %	35.3 %	0.0 %
DHEA	64.7 %	1.0 %	34.3 %
HPL	80.6 %	19.4 %	0.0 %

Table 5. High-risk pregnancies (excluding diabetes mellitus((37)

DHEA / HPL	Accurate	False
Accurate	48.7 %	29.7 %
False	21.6 %	0 %

For high-risk pregnancies in which oestriol excretion is below the mean for gestational age, the DHEA test becomes much more reliable than oestriol assay (84.0 % against 36.0 %).

The best method is to combine the results of urinary oestriol values with the DHEA test and to define accordingly 5 different clinical categories, each category indicating the clinical approach to be taken.

Table 6. High-risk pregnancies with low normal estrioluria (25)

	Accurate results	False positive	False negative
Estriol	36.0 %	64.0 %	-
DHEA	84.0 %	8.0 %	8.0 %

Table 7

Classe	Estrioluria compared to mean normal values	DHEA Conversion	IFP Sat. No. of patients	IFP Unsat. No. of patients	Feto-placental unit
I	$\geqq$	$\geqq$ 6 %	100 %	0 %	Good
II	$\geqq$	$<$ 6 %	90 %	10 %	Satisfactory
III	$<$	$\geqq$ 6 %	84 %	16 %	Sufficient
IV	$<$	$<$ 6 %	35 %	65 %	Unsufficient
V	$<$ Lower lim	$<$ 6 %	0 %	100 %	Bad

21- and 18-C Urinary Steroids after the Oral Administration of DHA-S in Pregnancy

E. Vadora, A. Merialdi, F. Coppola, L. Benassi, and B. Salvadori

13 patients with various obstetric complaints and a low basic value of urinary estrogen were given 75 mg of DHA-S daily for 10 days. In each case the values were taken for two days prior to starting and daily during the administration of DHA-S within the following hormonal parameters:

Total urinary estrogen (spectrophotometry, ROURKE, MARSHALL and SHELLEY method).
Urinary estriol (gas chromatography, SCOMMEGNA and CHATTORAJ method).
Urinary pregnenolone and pregnanediol (gas chromatography, SCOMMEGNA method).

Furthermore, the urinary creatinine was established for each urine sample using the modified Folin method. The values have been expressed as a ratio of the creatinine/steroid. In 10 cases we noticed an increase in the excretion of total estrogens and estriol higher than 25 % the basic value (in our method, the limit of individual daily variations). In 3 cases no increase or a reduction against the basic value was observed.

In 6 cases, 200 mg of progesterone were administered daily for one week prior to the oral trial with DHA-S, without any increase in total estrogens excreted being observed: and in two of these cases treatment with DHA-S did not improve the curve for the excretion of total estrogens. In patients with an estrogenic response higher than 25 % of the basic value we have studied the mean behaviour of the steroid excretions during the ten days of treatment.

There was a constant increase of total estrogens and of estriol up to the 6th and 7th day of treatment, with a tendency to diminish in the following days. An increase of more than 100 % was observed for total estrogens, while for estriol the percentage increase remained more limited: only on the 6th day did we observe a mean increase of more than 100 %. It is more difficult to interpret the behaviour of the 21-carbon steroids pregnenolone and pregnanediol. A mean percentage increase of pregnenolone was observed from the 6th day, coinciding with the peak for estrogen and estriol excretion with values which, in the following days, returned below the 20 % limit. A mean percentage increase of pregnanediol was already observed on the second day with a progressive increase up to the 7th day. In the first days however, the rate of increase was not distinguishable from the daily variations and only with the increases of the 7th and 9th days surpassing 60 % were we able to establish a real increase. Studying individually the curve behaviour of the various steroids using the correlation coefficients, we observed a positive correlation between estrogen and pregnenolone and between estriol and pregnenolone.

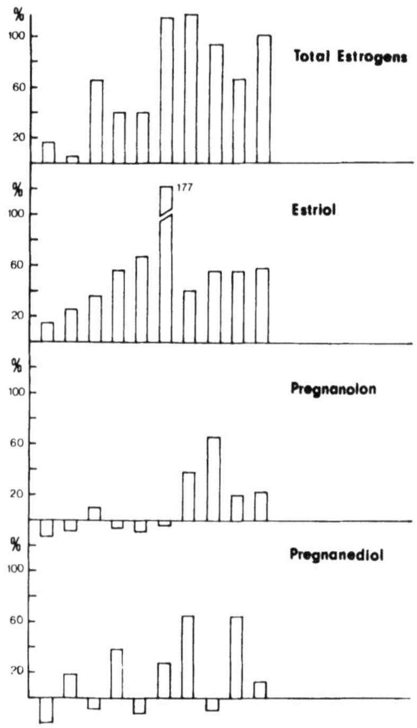

Fig. 1. Increase after oral DHA-S (75 mg daily) Mean values

	Correlation coefficient r
Total estrogens vs pregnenolone	0.504 $p < 0.005$
Estriol vs pregnenolone	0.629 $p < 0.005$
Total estrogens vs pregnanediol	0.403 $p < 0.005$
Estriol vs pregnanediol	0.435 $p < 0.005$
Pregnenolone vs pregnanediol	0.828 $p < 0.001$

In fact, between total estrogens and pregnenolone and between estriol and pregnenolone positive correlation coefficients were observed which were statistically significant and in no case was a negative correlation observed. Between estrogen and pregnanediol we observed correlation coefficients which were still positive but not statistically significant with only individual negative coefficients. These coefficient values indicate a correlation between estrogen and pregnenolone which is not evident from an analysis of the mean percentage increase since it does not give the ratio of excretion, but only the profile of individual curves. This last fact confirms the behaviour of steroid excretion after betamimetic therapy, where an analogous correlation was observed between the behaviour of estrogens and that of pregnenolone.

Mrs. D. BOLZONI and Mr. R. SPALLANZANI, Laboratory Technicians at the Obstetric and Gynaecological Clinic of the University of Parma collaborated actively in the hormonal analyses.

Subject-Index

MIX
Papier aus verantwortungsvollen Quellen
Paper from responsible sources
FSC® C105338
FSC
www.fsc.org

If you have any concerns about our products,
you can contact us on
ProductSafety@springernature.com

In case Publisher is established outside the EU,
the EU authorized representative is:
Springer Nature Customer Service Center GmbH
Europaplatz 3, 69115 Heidelberg, Germany

Printed by Libri Plureos GmbH
in Hamburg, Germany